Refuge and Resilien

The series publishes original scholarly books that advance our understanding of international migration and immigrant integration. Written by academic experts and policy specialists, each volume addresses a clearly defined research question or theme, employs critical analysis and develops evidence-based scholarship. The series includes single- or multi-authored monographs, volumes and edited collections.

The scope of the series is international migration and integration research. Topics include but are not limited to thematic and current issues and debates; comparative research of a regional, national or international nature; the changing character of urban areas in which migrants or refugees settle; the reciprocal influence of migrants/refugees and host communities; issues of integration and social inequality as well as policy analysis in migration research.

Series Editors:
Peter Li and Baha-Abu-Laban

For further volumes:
http://www.springer.com/series/8811

Laura Simich • Lisa Andermann
Editors

Refuge and Resilience

Promoting Resilience and Mental Health among Resettled Refugees and Forced Migrants

Volume 7

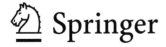

Editors
Laura Simich
Center on Immigration and Justice
Vera Institute of Justice
New York
New York
USA

Lisa Andermann
Department of Psychiatry Equity, Gender
 and Populations Division
University of Toronto and Mount Sinai
 Hospital
Toronto
Ontario
Canada

The findings, interpretations, and conclusions expressed herein are those of the author and do not necessarily reflect the views of the Vera Institute of Justice.

ISSN 2214-9805   ISSN 2214-9813 (electronic)
ISBN 978-94-017-7812-1   ISBN 978-94-007-7923-5 (eBook)
DOI 10.1007/978-94-007-7923-5
Springer Dordrecht Heidelberg New York London

© Springer Science+Business Media B.V. 2014
Softcover reprint of the hardcover 1st edition 2014
This work is subject to copyright. All rights are reserved by the Publisher, whether the whole or part of the material is concerned, specifically the rights of translation, reprinting, reuse of illustrations, recitation, broadcasting, reproduction on microfilms or in any other physical way, and transmission or information storage and retrieval, electronic adaptation, computer software, or by similar or dissimilar methodology now known or hereafter developed. Exempted from this legal reservation are brief excerpts in connection with reviews or scholarly analysis or material supplied specifically for the purpose of being entered and executed on a computer system, for exclusive use by the purchaser of the work. Duplication of this publication or parts thereof is permitted only under the provisions of the Copyright Law of the Publisher's location, in its current version, and permission for use must always be obtained from Springer. Permissions for use may be obtained through RightsLink at the Copyright Clearance Center. Violations are liable to prosecution under the respective Copyright Law.
The use of general descriptive names, registered names, trademarks, service marks, etc. in this publication does not imply, even in the absence of a specific statement, that such names are exempt from the relevant protective laws and regulations and therefore free for general use.
While the advice and information in this book are believed to be true and accurate at the date of publication, neither the authors nor the editors nor the publisher can accept any legal responsibility for any errors or omissions that may be made. The publisher makes no warranty, express or implied, with respect to the material contained herein.

Springer is part of Springer Science+Business Media (www.springer.com)

To my parents and grandparents, who were once refugees and New Canadians; To my wonderful husband and children; And to all the refugees who have shared their stories with me.

L.A.

To peace and sanity.

L.S.

Foreword

The refugee experience confronts us with humanity at its most challenged—forcibly uprooted and in flight from violence, caught between countries, facing an uncertain future—but it also provides some of the most striking examples of human resilience. This innovative and important book explores that resilience and its implications for resettlement and mental health services, policy and practice. The contributors have a wealth of research, clinical and community experience and have been at the forefront of interdisciplinary studies that advance our understanding of refugee mental health and adaptation. They approach the person seeking refuge and resettling in a new country not as a clinical, social or political problem but as the active agent of their own survival. In so doing, they encourage us to move from diagnosing and treating traumatic wounds and losses to fostering individual and collective adaptation and flourishing. They emphasize the importance of the larger community that receives those seeking asylum and call us to a more humane and effective response.

Migration has been a constant in human evolution and the ability to adapt to radically new environments is intrinsic to our psychology. The migrations of prehistory brought us into different ecological environments that gave rise to diverse cultures, with different ways of life that included changes in modes of subsistence, worldviews, systems of values and aspirations. The roots of human resilience are in self-regulating and self-righting adaptive systems that include our capacity to acquire new strategies for survival and to reorganize our ways of life to fit new contexts. Resilience then is part of 'human nature' built into our multiple systems of learning, grounded in neuroplasticity, psychological inventiveness, and cultural creativity, which allow us to embrace and adopt new, hybrid identities. At the same time, continuity of identity, relationships and community are central to many individuals' strength, sense of coherence, and self-efficacy.

Much of the scientific research on resilience has focused on individual characteristics, but resilience is not only the outcome of psychological processes but also of social process that reside in relationships among people, systems and institutions at the level of families, neighborhoods, communities, and organizations, governments and transnational networks. Recognizing the social dimensions of refugee resilience means we must look beyond the individual to understand the larger contexts in which they are embedded. Resettlement policies can support the refugee's efforts to build a new life or undermine them, leaving individuals or whole groups stranded without connection.

International conventions on refugees and asylum emerged in the wake of the Second World War during which countless numbers of people seeking safety were turned away by Canada and other countries that could have easily received them. Earlier generations of migrants from Europe and other war torn areas did not have the formal category of refugee to frame their identity but faced many of the same challenges in escaping danger, bringing their families and loved ones to safety, and building a new life in a new land. The categories of asylum-seeker, refugee and immigrant imply a clear distinction between those who migrate voluntarily for economic or other personal advancement and those who are forced to by threat of political violence. In fact, this distinction is often hard to make and does not fit the complex realities of individual struggles.

After achieving their escape from harm's way, refugees seek not just bare survival but a better life for themselves and their families. Those who are able to focus on a hopeful future, find meaningful work and relationships, and invest in the next generation, are likely to fare well. Those caught in a consuming nostalgia for what they have lost, may find it difficult to invest in the future or find the energy and flexibility needed to face all the many demands of their new environment.

For most refugees, the long-term outcome of migration will be positive. But this outcome depends on many factors involving the individual's history, the kinds of violence and losses they have endured, their migration trajectory, and especially, their reception in the country where they find a new home. A major lesson from the research on long-term adaptation collected in this volume is that the quality of the host country reception of newcomers is a major determinant of their health, well-being and social integration. This is good news because this reception is something that can be improved through public policy. The dilemma is that in the current environment of international insecurity, there is a risk of forgetting our recent history, reneging on our commitments, and closing the doors to those seeking asylum and making it harder for those accepted to build their new lives.

Our experience with refugees and asylum seekers at the Cultural Consultation Service in Montreal underscores their resilience as well as the major challenges they face. Many of these challenges stem not from having to navigate a new cultural environment, but from difficulties negotiating bureaucratic institutions that are divorced from the human realities of forced migration. For example, we know that detention can be extraordinarily harmful, that long delays in deciding outcomes are corrosive to well-being and confidence, that taking meaningful work and choice away from people renders them helpless, and that ensuring the safety of loved ones left behind and reuniting with one's family are all powerful determinants of mental health. Yet politically motivated policies and institutional practices strew obstacles in the refugee's path.

The emphasis on strength and resilience is a welcome shift from the emphasis in mental health research on vulnerability and pathology. In focusing on strengths and resilience, however, there is a risk that those who have a harder time will be further stigmatized as 'lacking resilience'. This is especially egregious when the barriers to adaptation clearly reflect social obstacles and adversity. It is important that resilience be understood not as the inevitable outcome of some inherent quality or capacity of the individual but as a dynamic process of interactions between individuals and the circumstances in which they find themselves. What is adaptive in one situation may be problematic in others and new strengths may emerge when the individual is afforded new opportunities. The resilience perspective is an invitation to clinicians, policy makers and others to think in terms of strengths and solutions rather than deficits and to ensure that our welcoming and hospitality to those most in need provides them with the basic structures and resources they need to rebuild their lives and, ultimately to contribute to the variegated tapestry of our communities.

The creation of refugee status and the moral and legal obligation to provide asylum reflect an emerging global ethic essential for our collective survival. Indeed, climate change and the resultant economic and politic instabilities are likely to dramatically increase the need for an international human rights regime in the years to come. In the wake of past failures, Canada became a model of progressive practices in the area of refugee resettlement. Unfortunately, recently enacted restrictive policies tightening the refugee determination process and reducing basic coverage of medical care for refugees (on the absurd argument that they are better treated than the average Canadian citizen) have undermined this commitment. These short-sighted policies have been widely denounced by many sectors of society including physicians and those most knowledgeable about the refugee experience. Hopefully, these regressive steps will soon give way to a more socially responsive view consonant with long-standing Canadian values so that we can once again contribute to advancing international human rights.

In addition to advocating for change at the level of policy, and health and social services professionals and researchers can contribute in many ways to the well-being and social integration of refugees. In the clinical encounter, we can work to understand refugees' stories, learning more about their unique predicaments and developing the skills needed to respond effectively. We can support others in the community in their efforts to provide a welcoming space and pathways toward integration and reunification for refugees and their families. As the contributors to this volume show, through research, advocacy and clinical engagement, we can contribute to building a civil society founded on the values of dignity and diversity.

Montreal, August 2013   Laurence J. Kirmayer

Contents

1. **Editor's Introduction** 1
   Laura Simich

2. **What Is Resilience and How Does It Relate to the Refugee Experience? Historical and Theoretical Perspectives** 7
   Wade E. Pickren

3. **Social Determinants of Refugee Mental Health** 27
   Farah N. Mawani

4. **The Debate About Trauma and Psychosocial Treatment for Refugees** .. 51
   Clare Pain, Pushpa Kanagaratnam and Donald Payne

5. **Reflections on Using a Cultural Psychiatry Approach to Assessing and Fortifying Refugee Resilience in Canada** 61
   Lisa Andermann

6. **Personal and Social Forms of Resilience: Research with Southeast Asian and Sri Lankan Tamil Refugees in Canada** 73
   Morton Beiser

7. **Social Support in Refugee Resettlement** 91
   Miriam J. Stewart

8. **Newcomer Youth Self-Esteem: A Community-Based Mixed Methods Study of Afghan, Columbian, Sudanese and Tamil Youth in Toronto, Canada** 109
   Nazilla Khanlou, Yogendra B. Shakya, Farah Islam and Emma Oudeh

9. **Newcomer Refugee Youth as 'Resettlement Champions' for their Families: Vulnerability, Resilience and Empowerment** 131
   Yogendra B. Shakya, Sepali Guruge, Michaela Hynie, Sheila Htoo, Arzo Akbari, Barinder (Binny) Jandu, Rabea Murtaza, Megan Spasevski, Nahom Berhane and Jessica Forster

10 **A Social Entrepreneurship Framework for Mental Health Equity: The Program Model of the Canadian Centre for Victims of Torture** 155
Sean A. Kidd, Kwame J. McKenzie and Mulugeta Abai

11 **The Role of Settlement Agencies in Promoting Refugee Resilience** ... 167
Biljana Vasilevska

12 **Mental Healthcare Policy for Refugees in Canada** 181
Kwame J. McKenzie, Andrew Tuck and Branka Agic

13 **Supporting Human Trafficking Survivor Resiliency through Comprehensive Case Management** 195
Lauren Pesso

14 **Migrant Mental Health, Law, and Detention: Impacts and Alternatives** 211
Chelsea Davis

Contributors

Mulugeta Abai Canadian Centre for Victims of Torture, Toronto, Canada

Branka Agic Health Equity Unit, Centre for Addiction and Mental Health, Toronto, Canada

Arzo Akbari Access Alliance Multicultural Health and Community Services, Toronto, Canada

Lisa Andermann Equity, Gender and Populations Division, Department of Psychiatry, University of Toronto and Mount Sinai Hospital, Toronto, Ontario, Canada

Morton Beiser Ryerson University, Toronto, Canada

Keenan Research Centre and Li Ka Shing Knowledge Institute, St. Michael's Hospital, Toronton, Canada

Cultural Pluralism and Health, University of Toronto, Toronto, Canada

Nahom Berhane Access Alliance Multicultural Health and Community Services, Toronto, Canada

Chelsea Davis Mailman School of Public Health (MPH), Columbia University, New York, USA

Jessica Forster Access Alliance Multicultural Health and Community Services, Toronto, Canada

Sepali Guruge Access Alliance Multicultural Health and Community Services, Toronto, Canada

Sheila Htoo Access Alliance Multicultural Health and Community Services, Toronto, Canada

Michaela Hynie Access Alliance Multicultural Health and Community Services, Toronto, Canada

Farah Islam Access Alliance Multicultural Health and Community Services, Toronto, Canada

Barinder (Binny) Jandu Access Alliance Multicultural Health and Community Services, Toronto, Canada

Pushpa Kanagaratnam Department of Psychiatry, Faculty of Medicine, University of Toronto, ON, Canada

Centre for Addiction & Mental Health, Toronto, ON, Canada

Nazilla Khanlou Echo Chair, Women's Mental Health Research, Faculty of Health, Lillian Wright Maternal Child Health Scholars Program, School of Nursing, York University, Toronto, ON, Canada

Sean A. Kidd Department of Psychiatry and Centre for Addiction and Mental Health, University of Toronto, Toronto, Canada

Farah N. Mawani Dalla Lana School of Public Health, University of Toronto, Toronto, Canada

Kwame J. McKenzie Department of Psychiatry and Centre for Addiction and Mental Health, University of Toronto, Toronto, Canada

Rabea Murtaza Access Alliance Multicultural Health and Community Services, Toronto, Canada

Emma Oudeh Access Alliance Multicultural Health and Community Services, Toronto, Canada

Clare Pain Department of Psychiatry, University of Toronto, and Mount Sinai Hospital, Toronto, ON, Canada

Donald Payne Health Network, Amnesty International (English Speaking) Canada, Toronto, Canada

Lauren Pesso My Sisters' Place, New York, USA

Wade E. Pickren Center for Faculty Excellence, Ithaca College, Ithaca, NY, USA

Yogendra B. Shakya Access Alliance Multicultural Health and Community Services, Toronto, Canada

Laura Simich Vera Institute of Justice, New York, NY, USA

Megan Spasevski Access Alliance Multicultural Health and Community Services, Toronto, Canada

Miriam J. Stewart Faculty of Nursing, University of Alberta, Edmonton, Canada

Andrew Tuck Department of Psychiatry and Centre for Addiction and Mental Health, University of Toronto, Toronto, Canada

Biljana Vasilevska Department of Health, Aging and Society, McMaster University, Hamilton, Canada

About the Authors

Mulugeta Abai is Executive Director of the Canadian Centre for Victims of Torture (CCVT). He has over 20 years of community involvement in the areas of community development, advocacy and anti-racism, and has written numerous articles and guides for community members that work with refugees who are survivors of torture and war.

Lisa Andermann M.Phil., M.D., FRCPC is an Assistant Professor in the Department of Psychiatry at the University of Toronto and psychiatrist at Mount Sinai Hospital, where she works in the Psychological Trauma Clinic and the Ethnocultural Assertive Community Treatment Team. Dr. Andermann is a consultant psychiatrist and former Board Member for the Canadian Centre for Victims of Torture, and continues to be active on their Health Committee. Her main areas of interest in research and teaching focus on cultural psychiatry. For the past few years, she has been very involved in an educational initiative to enhance the cultural competence of the postgraduate psychiatry residency curriculum and has led a faculty development initiative on culturally competent supervision and teaching which won the 2008 Ivan L. Silver Award for Excellence in Continuing Mental Health Education. She has been part of the Toronto-Addis Ababa Psychiatry Program since its inception in 2003, assisting in the development of the first psychiatry residency training program in Ethiopia. She has an undergraduate degree in Anthropology from McGill University, where she completed her medical studies, and a graduate degree in Social Anthropology from Cambridge University.

Dr. Morton Beiser CM, MD, FRCP is Professor of Distinction and Program Director Culture, Immigration and Mental Health, Dept of Psychology, Ryerson University; Crombie Professor Emeritus of Cultural Pluralism and Health, University of Toronto; and Founding Director and Senior Scientist, Ontario Metropolis Centre of Excellence for Research on Immigration and Settlement (CERIS). He has been Principal Investigator for studies including the *Refugee Resettlement Project*, a ten year study of refugees from Southeast Asia; *Flower of Two Soils*, a study of mental health and academic achievement among American Indian and First Nations reserves; *Immigrants and Tuberculosis; Community in Distress*, an investigation of the mental health of Sri Lankan Tamils in Toronto; *The New Canadian Children and*

Youth Study, a national, longitudinal investigation of the health and development of approximately 4,000 immigrant and refugee children in six Canadian cities; *Leavers and Stayers*, a comparison between Ethiopian children growing up in Toronto and in Addis Ababa; and *Promised Land, Land of Promise*, a study of Ethiopian youth in Israel and Canada. Dr. Beiser has authored more than 180 scientific papers, and a book entitled *Strangers at the Gate*, (University of Toronto Press 1999). Recognitions include National Health Scholar and Scientist Awards from Canada's National Health Research and Development Program; the University of Toronto Beverley Distinguished Professor Award; the Rockefeller Foundation Resident Scholar Award; the Canadian Psychiatric Association's Alexander Leighton Award for Research in Psychiatric Epidemiology, and the Order of Canada, the country's highest distinction for lifetime achievement.

Chelsea Davis is the Coordinator of the Mass Incarceration and Public Health Initiative at Columbia University, Mailman School of Public Health. She received her MPH in History and Ethics of Public Health and Medicine from Columbia University MSPH after getting her BA from Vanderbilt University. Her areas of expertise are research and policy at the intersection of public health and criminal justice.

Dr. Sepali Guruge is an Associate Professor in the Daphne Cockwell School of Nursing at Ryerson University.

Michaela Hynie is a social and cultural psychologist in the Department of Psychology, York University, and the Associate Director of the York Institute for Health Research.

Farah Islam is a Ph.D. candidate in the Kinesiology and Health Science Program at York University. Her dissertation focuses on mental health and mental healthcare utilization patterns of Canada's immigrant and ethnocultural populations.

Pushpa Kanagaratnam Ph.D. is a clinical psychologist and Assistant Professor at the Department of Psychiatry, University of Toronto and has affiliate status as a Research Scientist at the Center for Addiction and Mental Health. As an immigrant herself, her personal experience enlightens her clinical practice and writing.

Nazilla Khanlou, RN, Ph.D. ECHO's inaugural Chair in Women's Mental Health Research in the Faculty of Health at York University and an Associate Professor in its School of Nursing, conducts interdisciplinary research in community-based mental health promotion with youth and women.

Sean Kidd, Ph.D. is an internationally recognized authority in the area of youth homelessness research and has extensively examined stigma and marginality among persons with severe mental illness. Dr. Kidd is an Assistant Professor with the Department of Psychiatry, University of Toronto, and is head of Psychological Services for the Centre for Addiction and Mental Health (CAMH) Schizophrenia Division.

Farah N. Mawani is Visiting Scholar, Massey College, University of Toronto. She has global research, policy, teaching, and writing experience in social determinants of mental health inequalities. She focuses on the negative impact of workplace environments, human rights abuses, and on mental health inequalities. She also focuses on the transformative capacity of peer support to reduce mental health inequalities. She has national experience as Senior Policy and Research Analyst, Mental Health Strategy, Mental Health Commission of Canada, and as a Multicultural Mental Health Resource Centre Steering Committee member. She is a founding member of the Centre for Social Innovation—Regent Park, Toronto.

Kwame McKenzie, M.D., FRCPC Senior Scientist and Medical Director, Centre for Addiction and Mental Health and Professor, Department of Psychiatry, University of Toronto. Psychiatrist, academic, social commentator and advocate—Dr. McKenzie is committed to using scientific investigation to help to build inclusive, humane and effective models of mental health care for everyone. He is a sought after speaker in academic and community circles, including invited media appearances. Dr. McKenzie's research focuses on the science of improving mental health services. Key areas of interest include social determinants of health, society and mental health, social capital and mental health, redesigning mental health services for visible minority groups, efficacy of treatment in schizophrenia, psychiatric diagnosis, community engagement, racism, pathways to care, and suicide. **Branka Agic** is Manager, Clinical Health Equity, CAMH, and **Andrew Tuck** is Research Coordinator, Clinical Health Equity, CAMH.

Emma Oudeh, RN earned her BA at Carleton University and BScN at York University. She is completing her MScN and primary health care nurse practitioner certificate at York University.

Clare Pain M.D., FRCPC is Associate Professor at the Department of Psychiatry, University of Toronto. As a psychiatrist, she works as Director of the Psychological Trauma Program at Mount Sinai Hospital, Toronto, and in association with the Canadian Centre for Victims of Torture.

Donald Payne is a psychiatrist who has 34 years of experience in working with refugees through CCVT. He has provided expert testimony at refugee hearings, in the Ontario Superior Court and in the Federal Court of Canada.

Lauren Pesso, LMSW MPA is the Director of the Human Trafficking Program at My Sisters' Place (MSP) in Westchester County, New York. Prior to joining MSP, Lauren worked as a counselor for victims and witnesses of crime at Sanctuary for Families and the Crime Victims Treatment Center at St. Luke's-Roosevelt Hospital; managed gender-based violence research teams in Eastern Europe and East Africa; and coordinated various maternal and reproductive healthcare programs at Engender Health, an international women's health organization.

Dr. Wade Pickren is the director of the Center for Faculty Excellence at Ithaca College. He is also the President of the Society for General Psychology and Past-President of the Society for the History of Psychology. Wade's current scholarly interest is the transformation of knowledge and practice across time and place.

Yogendra B. Shakya, Ph.D. is the Senior Research Scientist at Access Alliance Multicultural Health and Community Services. **Sheila Htoo** and **Arzo Akbari** worked as Lead Peer Researchers at Access Alliance for the Refugee Youth Health study. **Barinder (Binny) Jandu**, a recent MPH graduate in Health Promotion and Community Development, has worked on many health promotion initiatives and assisted with data analysis for the study. **Rabea Murtaza** worked as Research Coordinator for the Refugee Youth Health study at Access Alliance and currently is a community facilitator and teaches in the departments of Social Service Work and Community Work at Sheridan College. **Megan Spasevski** is a Research Coordinator at Access Alliance. **Nahom Berhane** is the Hub Community Development Coordinator at Access Alliance and has been working with vulnerable populations for the past 10 years. **Jessica Forster**, Youth Worker at Access Alliance, holds an LLM in International Law with International Relations and has worked with communities with refugee experience for the past five years.

Laura Simich, Ph.D. joined the Center on Immigration and Justice, Vera Institute of Justice, New York, as Research Director in 2011. For the previous ten years, she was a Research Scientist at Canada's largest research and teaching hospital, the Centre for Addiction and Mental Health in Toronto, where she conducted mixed-methods research with immigrant and refugee communities. She has held appointments as Associate Professor, Department of Psychiatry, and Assistant Professor, Department of Anthropology, at the University of Toronto. From 2000 to 2010, Laura conducted studies on immigration and social determinants of mental health, specializing in community-based, policy-oriented research. Her prior research focused on social support, refugee resettlement, resilience and immigrant child wellbeing. She is currently the Principal Investigator on a study funded by the National Institute of Justice, U.S. Department of Justice, *Improving Trafficking Victim Identification: Evaluation and Dissemination of a Screening Tool*. She received her doctorate in cultural anthropology from Columbia University.

Miriam Stewart, PhD, FRSC, FCAHS conducts research on social determinants of health of vulnerable populations and salient interventions. Dr. Stewart has received three career awards in Canada and has served as Director, Atlantic Health Promotion Research Centre, Co-PI of Maritime Centre of Excellence on Women's Health, Director and Chair of Center for Health Promotion Studies (University of Alberta) and Scientific Director of the Canadian Institutes for Health Research Institute of Gender and Health. She has received the University of Alberta Kaplan Award for Excellence in Research.

Biljana Vasilevska, M.Ed. is a researcher in Hamilton, Canada, where she works on various projects related to health and vulnerable members of society. She was the Research Coordinator of the Refugee Resiliency study and the multi-site Refugee Mental Health Practices, both of which were conducted at the Centre for Addiction and Mental Health in Toronto.

Chapter 1
Editor's Introduction

Laura Simich

> *"God, I thought, did I really have to choose between peace and sanity". ("K'naan: An immigrant song," The Globe and Mail, May 10, 2010.)*

Abstract Every year, a relatively small number of refugees are given opportunities through official channels to resettle in host countries that have agreed to provide a safe haven under international law. Though challenging to survive under these circumstances, many refugees do survive in their adopted lands, and many even thrive. What makes such resilience possible? This book is about solutions, not just problems. It is about what it takes for refugees to overcome loss and adversity and to stay psychologically healthy while they recreate their lives in new places. The editors of this book have assembled recent research on this topic to demonstrate the importance of those factors that restore refugee health, and to suggest how resilience can be promoted by health and social service providers and by communities in refugee-receiving societies.

Keywords Asylum seekers · Mental health · Migration · Refugees · Resilience · Research · Social determinants of health

The acclaimed Somali-born rap artist, K'naan posed this problem in a personal essay published in 2010, voicing earlier unease, perhaps even fear of impending insanity. As a young man living in Toronto, he confessed that he felt conflicted and confused over having the good fortune to escape war in his homeland at the age of 13, only to be beset by depression and anxiety once he was presumably safe in Canada.

It is never easy being a newcomer in an alien society, especially when forced out of one's homeland by violence or persecution. A refugee may feel torn, thinking of loved ones left behind while facing new uncertainties and challenges in an unfamiliar place. But this is what happens every year to millions of refugees around the world whose lives have been disrupted by war and conflict. A relatively small number of refugees are given opportunities through official channels to resettle in host countries that have agreed to provide a safe haven under international law, but more people fleeing violence are "displaced" to neighboring countries where continuing hardships and little public support for their welfare undermine their existence. Though challenging

---

L. Simich (✉)
Vera Institute of Justice, New York, NY, USA
e-mail: lsimich@vera.org

to survive under these circumstances, many refugees do survive in their adopted lands, and many even thrive. What makes such resilience possible?

This book is about solutions, not just problems. It is about what it takes for refugees (or "asylees," as they are known in some countries) to overcome loss and adversity and to stay psychologically healthy while they recreate their lives in new places. Researchers are learning that the traumatic effects of war and conflict do not necessarily doom people to life-long suffering. Rather, the negative impacts of violence and forced migration can be significantly alleviated. The editors of this book have assembled recent research on this topic to demonstrate the importance of those factors that restore refugee health, and to suggest how resilience can be promoted by health and social service providers and by communities in refugee-receiving societies.

While the research highlighted in this book points to many things a society can do to enhance resilience, a migrant's personal strengths and cultural roots are clearly important components of the process. K'naan, for example, found some resolution through his art, which is imbued equally with evocative memories of his homeland and with strains experienced by a young African man coming of age in North America. As reported in his essay, his talent as a poet and musician and crucial support from family and community members helped him in his struggle. Personal qualms can be soothed by shared experiences. No doubt K'naan's songs have provided solace and enlightenment to others whose experiences of forced migration and social adaptation resonate with his own. He is not the first to express and overcome these stresses, nor will he be the last.

1.1 Refugees

The label "refugee" encompasses diverse worlds of experience, yet it is not widely understood. Individual nations and the international community have legal obligations to assist refugees under certain conditions, but refugees nevertheless often face discrimination. Refugees and other forced migrants are not always trusted as individuals deserving of help from society. Fulfilling humanitarian obligations to refugees may be viewed as a drain on a host country's resources, especially when that country is unprepared for forced migrants or if it perceives some refugees as threats to its security. People in general also may be discomfited by thoughts of the world's persecuted and displaced. While mass media are regularly consumed by vivid reports of ongoing violence around the world, the harsh existence of those who have fled the violence less often reaches public awareness. In-depth knowledge of refugee affairs is largely confined to specific government and non-profit agencies, much as refugees themselves are virtually hidden from view. But rather than push away knowledge of who refugees are, we might usefully seek to learn more.

Imagining refugees' lives as confined and concealed ignores the reality of their abilities and hopes. Whether they are detained in refugee camps, massing on borderlands, subsisting in cities of neighboring countries, or creating new lives in resettlement countries, they are survivors from whom valuable lessons about overcoming adversity can be learned. They are women, men, children and teenagers, parents and caregivers; they are professionals, teachers, farmers, artists and business people. They may be highly educated or they may have little formal education. They commonly suffer terrible losses, but they often retain reservoirs of strength. Many resettle permanently outside their homelands and patiently integrate into host societies, while others are in transient situations for long periods and hold dear plans of returning home. In either case, they live and strive among us with their sights set on mental horizons we may not readily comprehend. Understanding what helps them to move on and regain stability and productivity may benefit us all.

Millions of people currently live in refugee camps or have been displaced within the boundaries of their own countries. In 2011, more than 800,000 people were displaced as refugees across international borders, the highest number in over a decade.[1] In the last half of the twentieth century, an international system developed to formally resettle a portion of the world's forced migrants. Since then, Canada, the United States and several other countries have successfully managed government and non-governmental programs that provide limited assistance to small groups of refugees from selected countries. The numbers of refugees who are formally resettled and their countries of origin change over time according to fluctuations in world conflicts and in receiving societies' national and international priorities. Permanent or temporary resettlement in host countries is considered by the international community to be one solution for people who cannot return to their home countries. Other desirable options, such as return to the home country and repatriation, are seldom feasible in situations of prolonged conflict.

Wars are not likely to end, so the phenomenon of forced migration is not likely to abate. What might have to change is how we think about refugees and forced migration. In the near future, we will have to confront the human and social costs of other types of violence and environmental degradation that lead to forced population movements, even though these are not currently considered legal grounds for asylum. Here is just one example: beginning in the 1980s, tens of thousands of unaccompanied children from Central America and Mexico have embarked each year on dangerous journeys to the north, where they try to cross into the United States in search of safety. In 2011, the number of these children who were caught and detained in the U.S. (counting only those who were not turned back or never detected) has *more than doubled* over previous years to nearly 20,000. Advocates who have interviewed these children report that increasing numbers are being driven to escape gang violence and severe environmental problems such as drought.[2] A humanitarian crisis in the making, the situation cannot currently be addressed by existing asylum laws and research is needed immediately to help fashion solutions to these children's predicament. As our understanding of forced migration changes in the future, research on risk and resilience among other populations will necessarily follow.

---

[1] Migration Policy Institute 2012.
[2] Women's Refugee Commission 2011.

1.2 Why This Book, Why Now?

Concern about migrant and, in particular refugee, mental wellbeing and social adaptation in resettlement countries has given rise to public debates that challenge scientists and policy makers to assemble facts and solutions to perceived problems. This social context of refugee resettlement and the challenges and opportunities it presents have prompted the interdisciplinary research from which this book draws. Unified by the concept of resilience, this book presents selected refugee mental health research from the last quarter century. Taking an interdisciplinary approach and focusing on what works, it book reviews theory and evidence about what keeps refugees healthy. It presents up-to-date qualitative and quantitative research findings, including empirical evidence from psychiatric epidemiology, community-based studies and refugee and service provider narratives, and some emerging areas of concern.

Refugee mental health research has been productive, as a large number of studies on trauma and other mental disorders published since the 1980s demonstrate; but in general, the field has been more focused on identifying medical problems rather than on what helps to overcome these problems. A relatively smaller proportion of studies historically have emphasized the social context and role of resilience factors during resettlement.[3] As epidemiological research now demonstrates, social and cultural determinants of health and conditions of reception and resettlement play a larger role in refugee health and adaptation outcomes than do biological factors or traumatic pre-migration experiences.[4] We hope to expand upon this body of scholarship as well as to suggest new directions.

This book's goal is therefore to help shift the prevailing narrow perspective on refugee mental health to a broader view informed by social and cultural research. As a foundation for a more integrative perspective, the book outlines important approaches in diverse fields, including cultural psychiatry, psychology, epidemiology, social work, community development, education and nursing. To provide specific examples of how these approaches are applied, it presents recent quantitative and qualitative evidence from studies conducted with refugees and forced migrant populations, particularly in Canada, a leading resettlement country. In contrast to the conventional focus on mental disorders and risk factors in refugee mental health research, the studies in this book identify resiliency factors that contribute to positive mental health, which can provide leverage for health promotion and immigration policy. The book is intended for three audiences: students and scholars in social and health sciences for whom it can serve as course reading; service providers in immigrant and refugee settlement, social and health services who wish to have a strong scientific background for professional practice; and immigration and health policymakers who can benefit from a synthesis of theory and evidence about refugee mental.

---

[3] Excellent examples of these works include Beiser (1999), Ingleby (2005), and Miller and Rasco (2004).

[4] Porter and Haslam 2005.

Most contributors to this volume have been drawn together by their mutual interests in understanding and improving migrant health, and by their intersecting professional pathways in Canada and in the U.S. Within their respective fields, the editors and the authors have spent decades studying, teaching other professionals, mentoring and caring for refugee and ethnic minority community members and using what they have learned through the many years of applied research and practice. What became clear to everyone in the process is that where there are risks to refugee's mental health, from trauma, family separation, challenges to identity and discrimination, there are also personal and social sources of resilience that protect and propel refugees forward. These insights, many from collaborative research and synergy from a network of like-minded scientists, health professionals and refugee community leaders and students, formed the impetus for this book. For example, studying patterns of secondary migration among refugees from many countries of origin who had been resettled in Canada a decade ago, we found that recreating social ties and seeking social support from refugees who preceded them was key to their resettlement success and wellbeing.[5] This research led to and complemented other applied research with refugees that focused on the role of informal and formal supports in community wellbeing; it also led to applying what was learned about refugee resilience in post-disaster relief health promotion, and to additional studies that defined concepts of mental health and resilience among refugees from many diverse countries in Africa, Asia and the Americas.[6] Many of these studies were joint efforts by contributors to this book, and the cross-pollination of ideas and methods has been valuable.

The book does not present the complex topic of refugee resiliency in a linear fashion. The first part of the book introduces comprehensive approaches to individual and population mental health that provide foundations for refugee resilience research, while the second part spotlights research on factors that have been found to promote resilience among refugees and other forced migrants. Some chapters emphasize theory and others, research findings; however, most do both and the reader should in the end comprehend both principles and evidence. In the first part of the book, Pickren and Mawani were each asked to describe major theoretical approaches in psychology and in social epidemiology that underlie resiliency research. Not to neglect the essential practice of psychiatry in the given context of refugee resettlement, the chapters about psychosocial approaches to trauma by Pain and about cultural psychiatric approaches by Andermann demonstrate in theory and in practice how sensitive medical treatment can enhance refugee resilience. The chapters that follow exemplify rigorously designed studies led by Beiser and by Stewart using stress process and social support paradigms, respectively, in refugee mental health research. These two chapters in particular present findings that have inspired and set the stage for other integrative research approaches in the field. Recent community-based participatory research by Khanlou, Shakya and colleagues similarly demonstrate how positive resiliency factors such as identity, self-esteem, interdependencies and social

---

[5] Simich 2003.

[6] Simich et al. 2005, 2006, 2007, 2009, 2011.

supports can buffer the stresses of discrimination, loss and adversity during resettlement, and furthermore show how refugees can and should play a leadership role in the process of research and recovery. Studies in this book described by Kidd and by Vasilevska enlarge our understanding of the important role that social service providers and community-based organizations play in enhancing refugee resiliency. The chapter by McKenzie and Tuck shows a way to connect what we know about refugee resiliency to health and social policy. Finally, the book includes two chapters by Pesso and by Davis about important emerging issues in studies of forced migration and mental health in the U.S.—promoting resilience among victims of human trafficking and among immigrant detainees—which necessarily push the boundaries of resiliency research into more controversial areas where sound evidence will be needed to address present and future challenges.

References

Beiser, M. (1999). *Strangers at the gate: The 'Boat People's' first ten years in Canada*. Toronto: University of Toronto Press.

Ingleby, D. (Ed.). (2005). *Forced migration and mental health: Rethinking the care of refugees and displaced persons*. New York: Springer.

Migration Policy Institute. (2012, 22 Dec). The top ten migration issues of 2012, migration information source, Migration Policy Institute, December 2012. http://www.migrationinformation.org/.

Miller, K. E., & Rasco, L. M. (Eds.). (2004). *The mental health of refugees: Ecological approaches to healing and adaptation*. Mahwah: Erlbaum.

Porter, M., & Haslam, N. (2005). Predisplacement and postdisplacement factors associated with mental health of refugees and internally displaced persons: A meta-analysis. *Journal of the American Medical Association, 294*, 602–612.

Simich, L. (2003). Negotiating boundaries of refugee resettlement: A study of settlement patterns and social support. *The Canadian Review of Sociology and Anthropology, 40*(5):575–591.

Simich, L., Beiser, M., Stewart, M., & Mwakarimba, E. (2005). Providing social support for immigrants and refugees in Canada: Challenges and directions. *Journal of Immigrant Health and Minority Health, 7*, 259–268.

Simich, L., Rummens A., Andermann, L., & Lo, T. (2006). *Mental health in public health policy and practice: Providing culturally appropriate services in acute and post-emergency situations* (Working Paper #43, p. 24). Toronto: Centre of Excellence on Immigration and Settlement.

Simich, L., Wu, F., & Nerad, S. (2007). Status and health security: An exploratory study among irregular immigrants in Toronto. *Canadian Journal of Public Health, 98*(5), 369.

Simich, L., Maiter, S., & Ochocka, J. (2009). From social liminality to cultural negotiation: Transformative processes in immigrant mental wellbeing. *Anthropology & Medicine, 16*, 253–266.

Simich, L., Pickren, W., Vasilevska, B., & Rouse, J. (2011). Resilience, acculturation and integration of adult migrants: Understanding cultural strengths of recent refugees. A final report to Human Resources and Skills Development Canada, Ottawa.

Women's Refugee Commission. (2011). *Forced from home: Lost boys and girls of Central America*. New York: Women's Refugee Commission.

Chapter 2
What Is Resilience and How Does It Relate to the Refugee Experience? Historical and Theoretical Perspectives

Wade E. Pickren

Abstract In this chapter, the historical and theoretical foundations of the construct of resilience in North American social sciences are examined. Although the contemporary use of the term did not emerge until the 1960s, there is a longer tradition of theorizing on topics that are conceptually related to resilience. In the 1980s, research that shaped our contemporary understanding of resilience was conducted. Developmental scientists from various disciplines now dominate the field, resulting in a major focus on children and youth while leaving a noticeable gap in understanding resilience in adulthood. Implications for understanding refugee resiliency are discussed.

Keywords History of resilience concept · Culture and resilience · Resilience over time · Resilience and societal norms

The United States and Canada have continued to be primary destinations for refugees in the twenty-first century. Many refugees that have arrived in North America have demonstrated resilience and great adaptive skills, often in the face of negative expectations from the citizens of both countries. The editors and authors of this volume explore the multifaceted experience of refugees with an eye toward understanding and improving the resilience of refugees.

In this chapter, the historical and theoretical foundations of the construct of resilience in North American social sciences are examined. The historical analysis of resilience is then situated within the context of our rapidly globalizing world, in which millions of people, including refugees, are continually on the move. Such mass movement across cultural, national, and political boundaries makes it imperative that we broaden our approach to take into account the importance of cultural

---

I would like to thank my former students for their assistance in gathering materials for use in this chapter. Chanda Pundir's insights on family resilience were especially helpful. Nima Abdirizak, Sofia Puente, and Story Day were also helpful. I greatly appreciate their assistance.

W. E. Pickren (✉)
Center for Faculty Excellence, Ithaca College, 953 Danby Rd. I,
Ithaca, NY 14850, USA
e-mail: wpickren@ithaca.edu

dynamics. Understanding that the concept of resilience in North America emerged from the particular cultural values here should help us understand and use a cultural framework for the study of resilience today.

Although the contemporary use of the term resilience did not emerge until the 1960s, there is a longer tradition of theorizing on topics that are conceptually related to resilience. We examine the antecedents of the current construct of resilience, beginning with the "mind-cure" movement of the late nineteenth century, especially its expression in the work of William James. We then trace the utilization of related constructs in American psychology until the 1960s. Beginning at the time of cultural change and social upheaval, we move to a closer examination of the introduction of the concept of resilience and its rapid deployment in support of the emergence of the interdisciplinary field of developmental psychopathology. Finally, we problematize the current use of resilience, especially in relation to the absence of cultural considerations in a globalizing world. In that light, we explore the usefulness of the resilience construct in studies of refugees.

For psychology we can locate the intellectual and practical origins of the current understanding of resilience. More than a century ago, William James, the leading public intellectual of his day, wrote about what he termed "strenuousness," by which he meant the virtues of activity as a way to resist sickliness and ill health. From that starting point, there is a thread of theorizing and research related to human strengths and potential. For many years, the thread ran mostly through the writing of personality theorists, including Erich Fromm ("productive orientation," 1947) Gordon Allport ("propriate striving," 1955), Carl Rogers ("fully-functioning person," 1951), Abraham Maslow ("self-actualization," 1954), and Harvard personality theorist, Robert W. White ("competence," 1959). In the 1980s, research that shaped our contemporary understanding of resilience was conducted by Norman Garmezy, Ann Masten, Dante Cichetti, and Emily Werner. Developmental scientists from various disciplines now dominate the field, resulting in a major focus on children and youth while leaving a noticeable gap in understanding resilience in adulthood.

2.1 William James and the Religion of Healthy-Mindedness[1]

In the late nineteenth and early twentieth centuries, a number of self-help approaches to health and wellness arose. Some of these approaches focused on diet, some on exercise, others on the mind, and yet others some combination of these and more. There were diverse sources for these approaches, including ancient alchemical beliefs, Native American traditions, and practices introduced by Africans brought in as slaves, among others (Albanese 2007; Harrington 2008).

The teaching and writing of the former clockmaker, P. P. Quimby, melded mesmerism, spiritualism, and mental therapeutics into what his followers came to call New Thought or mind cure. Quimby's method of empathic rapport with the patient allowed him, he claimed, to see the false belief (about disease) that was the true

---

[1] William James, Lectures IV and V, *Varieties of Religious Experience*, 1902.

cause of the illness. This insight allowed Quimby to correct the false belief so that the person experienced healing. The resultant movement was a mélange rather than a focused set of practices. By the 1890s, along with Christian Science, the diverse practices of New Thought or mind cure was part of an even larger set of self-help practices embraced by millions of Americans. The popularity of these approaches lasted well into the twentieth century (Loss 2002; Taves 1999; Taylor 1999). Such popularity led the American psychologist and philosopher, William James, to call this the "religion of healthy-mindedness." The enduring influence of this "religion" can be felt even in our own day, as the popular embrace of the importance of mind and body connections in health and disease laid the cultural foundation for later receptivity to the ideas that these connections could be studied scientifically (Harrington 2008).

Along with the philosophical/religious approach of New Thought, the nineteenth century was also a period when diet and exercise, along with other treatments designed to prevent or cure disease, flourished in the United States (Andrick 2012; Haley 1978; Whorton 1982). Health, its absence, its attainment, was the predominant concern of many nineteenth century Americans, with diet, exercise, sport, and fitness each thought to play a key role in a healthy life (Owens 1985; Park 1994). For example, this was the era of diet as a cure-all, with the prescriptions of John Harvey Kellogg (cereals) and Dr. Sylvester Graham's advocacy of the salutary benefits of his cracker as part of the Graham diet (Whorton 1982). Each of these health practices, whether diet, exercise, or right thinking were pathways to healthy mental and physical functioning. The healthy person was one who was so in body, mind, and spirit.

Millions of Americans accepted the importance of mental and physical practices in the service of disease prevention and the maintenance of health (Whorton 2002). In this sense, these nineteenth century developments helped made the later direct involvement of psychologists possible (Harrington 2008).

Cognate to the discourse on health was a significant public discourse about the strenuous life in late nineteenth and early twentieth century America. Theodore Roosevelt coined the phrase, "strenuous life," in 1899 and linked it to the superiority of American manliness and vital for American political and national life (Bederman 1995). In the age of Theodore Roosevelt, William James, like millions of other Americans, took to activity—hikes, camping, and other outdoor activities—as central to well-being (Bederman 1995). This, in James's case, was despite other health problems. In this, James was like many of his fellow Americans and his writing about the "energies of men" was part of the popular literary conversation about male resourcefulness in the face of crises and danger. Like Jack London and Stephen Crane, among other popular writers, James sought to understand and explicate what was possible for humans in a difficult world (Dooley 2001). How, or under what conditions, James wondered, can a person be roused to extend themselves to reach a higher plane of life, despite the challenges faced? As he wrote in 1907,

> The human individual lives usually far within his limits; he possesses powers of various sorts which he habitually fails to use. He energizes below his maximum, and he behaves below his optimum. In elementary faculty, in coordination, in power of inhibition and control, in every conceivable way, his life is contracted.... (James 1907a, pp. 17–18)

What then, is the route to strenuousness? James saw it in the reaction of individuals and groups to extraordinary difficulty. He used the San Francisco earthquake of 1906 as an example of human resourcefulness and strength:

> Such experiences show how profound is the alteration in the manner in which, under excitement, our organism will sometimes perform its physiological work. The metabolisms become different when the reserves have to be used, and for weeks and months the deeper use may go on. (James 1907, p. 9)

There is no doubt that James saw the mind-cure or New Thought movement as one route to rousing human capabilities and energies to live fully despite risk, danger, challenge, or stress.

As he wrote in 1902,

> The greatest discovery of my generation is that man can alter his life simply by altering his attitude of mind. The blind have been made to see, the halt to walk; lifelong invalids have had their health restored. The moral fruits have been no less remarkable. The deliberate adoption of a healthy-minded attitude has proved possible to many who never supposed they had it in them. (James 1902, p. 95)

Connected to this healthy-mindedness, James made clear, was the release of great, internal resources to meet the challenges of life. James's embrace of what he called the strenuous life reflected his desire to elevate the human experience in times of emergency, challenge, risk, and stress. Strenuousness had implications for health and recovery from disease, if needed.

> We are just now witnessing—but our scientific education has unfitted most of us for comprehending the phenomenon—a very copious unlocking of energies by ideas, in the persons of those converts to 'New Thought,' 'Christian Science,' 'Metaphysical Healing,' or other forms of spiritual philosophy, who are so numerous among us to-day. The ideas here are healthy-minded and optimistic.... (James 1907, pp. 16–17)

Beyond James, the impact of the "religion of healthy-mindedness" was felt in every facet of American life. Fitness and physical hygiene became especially prominent in public discourse in the early twentieth century. Physical training, whether in the YMCAs or in public schools, was especially important for health, at least in the minds of many middle-class Americans. Thus, physical education became a regular part of the public school curriculum and gyms, playing fields, and specialized equipment became display symbols of the new emphasis (Park 1994).

Thus, we can see that from the late nineteenth century on, there was a new or renewed emphasis on the interrelation of mind and body in health and disease. The notion that physical activity, diet, and spirituality might be important for staying healthy and resisting illness took hold in the American imagination. The idea of human resourcefulness, or strenuousness, in the early twentieth century not only reflected the self-help ideology of the American past, it also foreshadowed later developments in psychology about how Americans could live a fulfilled life in a challenging world.

2.2 Personality, Stress, Lifestyle, and Well-Being in Post-War America

We have seen how psychological ideas about human strengths were related to a larger social context in early twentieth century America. In the post World War Two era, America had become an even more psychologically oriented society. This was the golden age of American psychology, with a flowering of new approaches to theory and practice (Pickren and Rutherford 2010). There were two threads of theory, research, and intervention that were important for later developments of research on resilience and its cognates. One thread was the new research on stress and lifestyle and their links to health outcomes. The other critical thread was the rich body of personality theory developed in the postwar period. We will begin with the work on stress and lifestyle and the historical context of social problems that could not be ignored in the 1960s and 1970s.

2.2.1 The Emergence of Stress and Lifestyle as Health Factors

Beginning in the 1930s, the endocrinologist Hans Selye developed a large and influential body of research on stress. The model he eventually promulgated, the General Adaptation Syndrome (GAS), linked stress with health outcomes and suggested an important role for personal reactivity in the stress process (Mason 1975; Selye 1950, 1956). In the extensive body of research that Selye conducted, he went well beyond the earlier work on psychosomatic factors in health that was so prominent in American medical theory and research from the 1930s to the postwar era (e.g., Dunbar 1935; Mittelman and Wolff 1942; Sparer 1956). By contrast, Selye's stress model of how stress was linked to health and disease was grounded in years of laboratory research. In Selye's GAS model, various stimuli could function as stressors. The crucial step in the syndrome is the organism's effort to adapt to the stressor in order to return to normal functioning. Neuroendocrinological reactions were part of the mobilization of the organism's defenses. Selye proposed that if the organism is unable to return to normal functioning then it became more likely that there would be negative health outcomes. This was especially likely if the pattern of stress and response occurred frequently.

To say that Selye's model was extremely influential is an understatement. Health care providers, as well as the general public, found the concept of stress useful in explaining a range of health outcomes. Because of the role of personal reactivity in Selye's model, there was a role for exploring psychological factors. One of the first major psychological models linking stress and health was the coping research of Richard Lazarus (1966), in which he and his colleagues proposed that cognitive appraisal is crucial in determining whether an event is stressful. By the 1970s, stress and coping research had become an important domain for psychologists, with strong links to health and disease. The role of cognitive factors, such as appraisal, and social factors, such as social support, were important influences on the research of Suzanne Kobasa and Salvatore Maddi at the University of Chicago as they developed their work on hardiness. We examine their work below, after a brief discussion of lifestyle and health in historical context.

A new understanding of health emerged in American cultural life in the 1960s. For the first time on such a large scale, scientists and health care professionals began to link human behavior to health outcomes. A new term, lifestyle, appeared to indicate the multifaceted nature of how we live. The new President, John F. Kennedy, initiated a campaign in public schools to encourage children to exercise and become fit, as part of a broader initiative of Cold War preparedness. Americans were less fit than ever before, due in part to the differences in work that occurred across much of American life. Factory labor and farm work were increasingly mechanized. Even recreation had become more oriented to spectator sports, rather than active participation. In the Cold War era, when preparedness was at a premium, the lack of physical fitness was a cause for concern.

It was in this era, too, that researchers began to discover links between many diseases and behavior. Much of this research was funded by the government, who had a vested interest in reducing health care costs. In 1957, the U. S. Surgeon General's office claimed that there was a connection between smoking tobacco and lung cancer. The 1964 government report, *Smoking and Health: Report of the Advisory Committee to the Surgeon General*, provided evidence that cancer rates rose with every increase in amount of smoking. Furthermore, tobacco use was implicated in other diseases, including bronchitis and coronary heart disease. The advisory committee noted that smoking during pregnancy reduced the average birth weight of infants. For the first time, federal legislation was passed that forbade advertising for cigarettes and required a warning label on each package of cigarettes. In retrospect, these events signaled a policy change that now included the assumption that behavior was clearly important in health and disease. For medical and psychological researchers, it became necessary to rethink extant models of health and disease. Physician George Engel proposed a new model in the 1970s that has continued to find favor among many psychologists, as well. Engel proposed a "biopsychosocial" model that asserts the need to think about health in terms of biological, social, and psychological factors and their interrelations (Engel 1977). This model seemed to vindicate the role of psychologists in health research and health care, as well, since psychologists are the behavior experts.

More evidence linking mental and behavioral states to health and disease emerged in the 1960s, as it became clear that patterns for death and disability had changed from acute diseases—TB, polio, influenza—to chronic diseases—coronary heart disease, cancer, stroke, and accidents. In each of these chronic diseases, mind and behavior played important roles in both cause and treatment.

After President Kennedy's death, Lyndon Johnson continued the new emphasis on the nation's health. Under Johnson's leadership, the Federal government began to pour more money into medical research, with special focus on heart disease, stroke, and cancer. Johnson continued the initiative begun by Kennedy on the nation's mental health by establishing the national network of Community Mental Health Centers (Pickren and Schneider 2005).

By the end of the 1960s the contribution to health and disease of what was now termed "lifestyle" seemed to be well established. Despite this emphasis, most American psychologists and, certainly, the largest professional organization, the APA, appeared to be out of the loop, to use a Washington phrase. In an effort to catch up, APA asked a well-known clinical psychologist, William Schofield, to lead the effort to identify where and how psychologists could contribute to the new government initiatives on improving the nation's health (Schofield 1969). In his review, Schofield found that the only domain of health research and practice where psychologists had a notable presence was in schizophrenia research, psychotherapy, and mental retardation. Astoundingly, psychologists did not appear to have a place in any of the areas of chronic disease research or intervention that had been identified as critical for the nation's health: coronary heart disease, stroke, and cancer. As it turned out, it was schizophrenia research that led directly to our current research and understanding of resilience. Before exploring that further, we turn to an account of psychologists and social problems, for the two areas are linked.

2.2.2 Psychology, Society, and Social Problems: The Crucible for Resilience

The social unrest of the 1960s highlighted the differences among various APA factions on whether psychology and psychologists had any role to play in resolving social problems. Significant numbers of APA members wanted APA to stay out of such problems in the belief that scientists should stay neutral about them. Others felt just as vehemently that psychology as a science and a profession could make positive contributions to resolving social problems. The astonishing events of 1968—the assassinations of Martin Luther King, Jr. and Robert F. Kennedy, the police brutality toward demonstrators at the Democratic National Convention, as well as the dramatic confrontation of APA leaders at the San Francisco convention by the newly established ABPsi all served to make it impossible to pretend that psychology or any science was immune to social ills. This was so apparent that it was decided that the theme of the 1969 APA convention would be "psychology and the problems of society" (Korten et al. 1970).

Kenneth B. Clark, who with his wife, Mamie Phipps Clark, had conducted the "Doll Tests" that convincingly portrayed the damaging effects of racial segregation and which were so crucial in the 1954 U. S. Supreme Court decision, *Brown v. Board of Education* that made segregation by race unlawful in public schools, became a leader of APA during this time. He was called upon because of his use of social science for social justice (Phillips 2000). In his 1965 book, *Dark Ghetto*, Clark had explicated many of the factors that lay behind the destructive inner city riots then occurring. Clark conceptualized the riots as a form of resistance and protest of the structural inequalities of American life, the enduring racism toward Black citizens and the consequent lack of opportunities for progress. Clark was distressed by the bad results of the "good intentions" of well-meaning white folk:

> The dark ghetto's invisible walls have been erected by the white society, by those who have power, both to confine those who have no power and to perpetuate their powerlessness. (Clark 1965, p. 11)

Clark believed that psychologists could and should use their science and their profession for social justice. He and Mamie Phipps Clark initiated several programs that did improve life for inner city children of all races, the most notable of which is the Northside Center for Child Development (est. 1946) (Markowitz and Rosner 2000).

While the Clarks were able for a period to move closer to mainstream of American psychology, at the same time a separate and equally powerful voice for psychology and social justice emerged, the Association for Black Psychologists (ABPsi) (Williams 2008). As noted above, ABPsi leaders like Joseph White articulated the strengths of Black communities as important resources in the face of 300 years of racism. The rich theorizing and interventions developed by ABPsi members provided evidence of human resilience, given the long history of racism and oppression in the United States (Nobles 1972; White 1972). The ultimate source of the strength of Black communities lay in the communalism of the West African tribal societies that were the origin societies for most of the human beings captured and sold into slavery in the U. S. Despite the oppression, the communalist ethos served as a survival resource for generations of African Americans and continued to do so in contemporary life.

An emphasis on strengths characterized Black psychology as it emerged in this period. To be certain, Black families and Black communities were typically mischaracterized in the white press and misunderstood by even well-meaning whites. Many whites considered Black children culturally deprived and Black families were characterized as a "tangle of pathology" (Moynihan 1965). ABPsi founder Joseph White, coined the term, Black Psychology, in a comment on such mischaracterizations written for *Ebony* magazine. White stressed the strengths of Black children and Black families:

> Most psychologists take the liberal point of view which in essence states that black people are culturally deprived and psychologically maladjusted because the environment in which they were reared as children lacks the necessary early experiences to prepare them for excellence in school, appropriate sex-role behavior, and, generally speaking, achievement within an Anglo middle-class frame of reference..... Possibly, if social scientists, psychologists, and educators would stop trying to compensate for the so-called weaknesses of the black child and try to develop a theory that capitalizes on his strengths, programs could be designed which from the get-go might be more productive and successful. The black family represents another arena in which the use of traditional white psychological models leads us to an essentially inappropriate and unsound analysis. Maybe people who want to make the Black a case for national action should stop talking about making the black family into a white family and instead devote their energies into removing the obvious oppression of the black community which is responsible for us catchin' so much hell. (White 1972, pp. 43–45)

As articulated by the leaders of ABPsi, Black Psychology was about the strengths and resilience of Black folks and Black communities. Black Psychology was an articulate vision substantiated by solid scholarship and a commitment to community involvement.

It was in this atmosphere of highly visible social problems and the need to address the role of mind and behavior in health that the research on resilience emerged.

2.2.3 Theories of Human Potential and Fulfillment in the Post-War Era

Theories and interventions from humanistic and existential psychologists suggested a large capacity or reservoir of potential in humans. Such approaches have been called "fulfillment" theories of personality (Maddl 1980). In fulfillment models, there is one basic motivating force and that force moves the person to seek the full unfolding or maximal expression of innate potentialities. Not surprisingly, each of these theories focused on the individual, thus reflecting the intense individualism of American culture (McLaughlin 1998). However, for our purposes, they are worth noting, as they posited human personality as a potential source of strength for dealing with adversity.

The neo-Freudian Erich Fromm contrasted what he called a "productive orientation" with a non-productive one. A productive orientation, according to Fromm, was a "mode of relatedness in all realms" (Fromm 1947, p. 85) and being in this mode made it possible for the person to fulfill his potential. Crucial to the productive orientation was the capacity to love on every level, including a healthy love of self (Fromm 1947) that could serve as a resource in difficult times. American personality psychologist Gordon Allport wrote about propriate striving, by which he meant the capacity to fulfill one's potential (1955).

Carl Rogers and Abraham Maslow were the best-known theorists of humanistic psychology in the United States in the post-war era. Carl Rogers formulated a new approach to counseling that he called client-centered psychotherapy, which was not predicated on the medical model of psychiatry and psychoanalysis (Rogers 1951; Sarason 1981). Abraham Maslow, after earning his doctorate studying sexual aggression in primates at Wisconsin, became interested in studying what humans could do and become rather than focusing on human deficits (Maslow 1954). His early attempts to develop such a psychology suggested a hierarchy of needs that moved from the biological upward to full self-expression as the highest level of human development. To describe the motivating force, he borrowed the term self-actualization from the neurologist, Kurt Goldstein, and the depth psychologist, Carl Jung (Pickren 2003). In many ways, the work of Rogers and Maslow adumbrated the development of positive psychology at the end of the twentieth century.

The rich theoretical formulations of Harvard personologist, Robert W. White, were a more immediate influence on the development of research related to personality and health, including resilience (Kobasa 1979; Ouellette 2012). Ironically, Robert White's work is now considered somewhat outside the mainstream of American personality research. It is ironic given that White and his first mentor, Henry Murray, were the most important pioneers of a distinctively American approach to personality conceptualizations (Murray 1938). White's orientation in his mature theorizing focused on the whole person. He argued that we must understand each life in the context of the full life, thus, for each person a personality description was always incomplete, as the person was still in the process of becoming. In the 1950s, Robert White began writing about what he called competence, by which he meant, "an organism's capacity to interact effectively with its environment" (White 1959, p. 297). The child learned competence through interaction with a stimulating and varied environment, one that presented appropriate challenges and risks. White believed that it was crucial that the child had opportunities to actively effect change in a constantly dynamic environment through the child's own actions. In doing so, the foundation for competence was established.

Salvatore Maddi and his student, Suzanne Kobasa (now Ouellette), expanded Robert White's notions to articulate the viability of what Maddi called authentic living. Kobasa coined the term hardiness in her studies of the relationships between personality and health (Kobasa 1979; Maddi 2002). She suggested that hardiness stemmed from personality dispositions and experiential learning. Kobasa (Ouellette) built on this early research to conduct nuanced studies of critical life stances, such as religious belief, in response to stress and disease and became a major contributor to narrative approaches to understanding life choices (e.g., Ouellete et al. 1995; Rodriguez and Ouellette 2000). Maddi, who supervised Ouellette's doctoral dissertation work on hardiness, has continued the empirical research and application of hardiness (2002).

It was popular misconceptions about stress that led Kobasa and Maddi to begin the studies that eventuated in the construct of hardiness. The proximate stimulus for it was the restructuring of Illinois Bell Telephone (IBT) in the wake of its parent company, AT&T, being required to divest itself of many of its subsidiaries. Kobasa initiated a retrospective survey of IBT managers' responses to the restructuring, which included significant layoffs. She found that the stress of the events had widely differing effects that varied by personality. For many of the managers there was little connection to illness or other negative effects. Kobasa suggested that certain attitudes or personality traits may have moderated the effects of stress (1979). She and Maddi and their research team followed up these earlier studies and found that these attitudes, along with social support and physical exercise, seemed to provide protection against stress-related health problems. Hardiness was the word they coined to describe these traits or attitudes, thus echoing William James in his use of strenuousness. Hardiness, Kobasa and Maddi posited, consisted of three attitudes: commitment, control, and challenge. Commitment referred to an orientation of involvement with others and with the events of life, and was contrasted with detachment or isolation. Kobasa suggested that control meant seeking to influence and shape one's life, rather than being passive, while challenge indicated that the person wanted to learn from life experiences, even when these were not positive. With this conceptualization, Kobasa, and later, Maddi, drew upon Robert White's concept of competence.

The other major theoretical orientation from this period that cannot be overlooked comes from the research and writing of a new generation of African American psychologists. As we noted above, beginning in the late 1960s, Joseph White and his colleagues emphasized the strengths of the Black community in the face of centuries of oppression, coining the term Black Psychology to describe their approach (Nobles 1972; White 1972). Black Psychology, as it developed, was a psychology of resiliency and strength situated in a sense of community.

2.3 An Overview of Resilience Research

Resilience can only be defined in context. That is, it is a process rather than a static phenomenon. While many definitions have been offered, it became generally agreed by researchers that resilience refers to "patterns of desirable behavior in situations where adaptive functioning or development have been significantly threatened by adverse experiences" (Masten et al. 1995, p. 283). Resiliency is most often understood differently, as a personality trait that helps in psychological adaptation in risky or adverse life situations. It has not always been clear which term was being used in various research reports.

Retrospectively, one can find early research that is clearly related to later resilience research. For example, in the 1950s Emory Cowen at the University of Rochester began studying what he called psychological wellness. This body of research morphed over the years, especially after Dante Cicchetti became involved, into one of the main streams of resilience research (e.g., Cicchetti and Rogosch 1997). In Hawaii, Emily Werner and her colleagues began a major investigation of resilience that continued for a number of years (Werner and Smith 1982, 1992).

The late Norman Garmezy had a long and illustrious career distinguished by insights in several dimensions of psychological functioning. By the late 1960s, Garmezy was deeply involved in efforts to understand schizophrenia. In this work, he began to notice that many children whose parent or parents were suffering from schizophrenia and who as a result were at much greater risk of developing the disorder were themselves free of the disorder and living reasonably happy lives and seemed remarkably well adjusted (Garmezy 1971, 1973). What, Garmezy wondered, made this possible? How did these children escape what appeared to be their inevitable future? Why do many of these children at risk go on to flourish in life? These were questions that Garmezy began pursuing in the late 1960s when he was quite aware of the vast social problems that put many children at risk. In doing so, Garmezy pioneered the modern study of resilience.

By this time, Garmezy was Professor of Psychology at the University of Minnesota and held an appointment, as well, in the Institute of Child Development at the University. Along with junior colleagues and graduate students, Garmezy wanted to know if the impact of racism, poverty, urban blight, divorce, neglect, war and other risk factors for children could be ameliorated. Perhaps the study of children whose developmental arc seemed normal despite these problems would hold clues that could lead to interventions that would help others. The influence of Robert White's concept of competence can be seen in Garmezy's work, in that he named the research program on resilience, Project Competence (Garmezy and Devine 1984).

Garmezy and his colleagues hoped that their research would help behavioral scientists understand risk factors and how they unfolded, as well as help identify any factors or conditions that might be protective against risks. While this approach might seem utterly reasonable today, it appeared to many in that time as foolish and unnecessary, as the greater good would be served by directly investigating deficits and finding interventions to address those deficits.

Initially, the pioneering group of researchers focused on individual factors. For example, a child who had good interpersonal skills may have been able to avoid interpersonal conflict. Over the next 20-plus years, resilience research blossomed and played an especially important role in the emerging field of developmental psychopathology. Various terms were tried out as descriptors, including stress-resistance, invulnerability, and finally, resilience.

As investigations at the University of Minnesota, in Rochester, and many other sites began to yield results, it became clear that resilience was multifaceted. Protective factors were elucidated, as well as events that were likely to prove overwhelming for most children. Over time, longitudinal studies began to reveal how resilience might change over the course of a person's life. By and large, however, the research has remained focused on children and adolescents.

In recent years, the focus on individual resilience has led psychologists to suggest evolutionary factors, potential neurobiological pathways, and genetic predispositions as causative factors in childhood resilience. Ann Masten has called resilience "ordinary magic." By this, she means that the factors that lead to resilience are all facets of what human beings have evolved to do in order to adapt to a sometimes hostile and threatening environment. In other words, resilience is part of what has helped humans survive (Masten 2001).

Psychologists have also contributed a number of cognate concepts to resilience. The list is too long to include here, but a few will be mentioned. Antonovsky wrote about a sense of coherence as important to mental health in adverse conditions (e.g., Antonovsky and Sourani 1988). Scheier and Carver have suggested dispositional optimism and attendant mastery as an important developmental aspect of successful coping (e.g. 1996). There is now a large literature on thriving and post-traumatic growth. Both constructs can be understood as cognate to the resilience literature (e.g., Joseph 2004; O'Leary and Ickovics 1995). And there are a number of other constructs that bear a family resemblance to resilience. What has not been so well-developed until recent years has been the role of cultural factors and their place in the lives of immigrants and refugees. Thus, resilience in migration is under-theorized (Simich et al. 2011).

2.4 Migration, Culture, and Resilience

It would not be fair to characterize American psychological research and theorizing on resilience as only focused on the individual. It is true that schools, social networks, and peers have all been suggested as important in facilitating individual resilience. In recent years, a body of work on familial resilience has also emerged (Defrain 1999; Haan et al. 2002). However, over the last 15–20 years, researchers from outside psychology and from a range of cultural backgrounds have begun complicating and enriching our understanding of resilience and its cognates. Such research is of vital importance in a world of people on the move. In recent years, the phenomena of migration around the globe have been studied as scholars have sought to understand the problems and positive possibilities of immigrant and refugee experiences.[2]

The modern nation-state that emerged in the sixteenth and seventeenth centuries was typically characterized by relatively homogeneous populations. In the twenty-first century, multicultural or global societies are becoming the norm (Pieterse 2009), with the trend especially visible in industrialized and post-industrial societies. Yet, host populations and governments still struggle to fully accommodate the new members of their societies and to recognize the strengths that immigrants bring with them, often patronizing migrants by thinking of them as disadvantaged or pathologizing them as different or even threatening. Often, migrants have a different understanding of social relations and obligations and an understanding of self and identity that is predicated upon different assumptions about being human. Many migrants bring approaches to health care, child-rearing, and close relationships, to name only three domains, that may be significantly different than the host country and that may create tension and stress between the migrant community and the host culture.

However, these cultural specific practices also serve as sources of strength and sustenance to migrants. This is a little understood and poorly appreciated facet of the migrant experience. Perhaps because migrants are different in their practices and beliefs, most research undertaken by social scientists in the host cultures have focused on migrants as problematic. That is, the intent of the research is meliorative. What has generally been lacking is an approach that focuses on the cultural strengths that immigrants bring with them. Every human being grows up in a culture that teaches them, explicitly and implicitly, how to be human, from dietary practices to relational practices to health care, and so on. These are resources with which to engage the world. Immigrants and refugees bring these resources with them, that is, they know how to relate, to self-care, to be human, reflexively. This is part of a person's sense of self or identity. In the migration context, of course, these reflexive ways of being may not always bring the same positive results as in the natal culture. The impact of difference may be felt in sense of self/identity and relationships, and may extend to health care and other practical activities. But, the core issue is that migrants bring with them resources that can help them adjust to the new society and that will also enrich the host society. All of these factors have important implications for understanding resilience among migrants, including refugees.

Migration to multicultural or pluralistic societies poses a potentially different case than migration to a relatively homogeneous society. The latter was often considered to be the norm until relatively recently (Handlin 1951; Smith 1939). In the U. S. and Canada since the 1960s, immigration has resulted in large influxes of immigrants and refugees who differ in many ways from the older European descended immigrants. Now, there is often no unitary "Us" to confront "Them." This poses challenges related to religion, health and dietary practices, and expected norms of children-parent relationships, and others. It also has important implications for identity and self understanding (Chryssochoou 2000). Pluralistic and multicultural societies are potentially rich contexts for examining these issues in relation to resilience (Beiser 1999, 2005).

---

[2] The material in this section is drawn primarily from Simich et al. 2011.

Rather than the individual focus of much North American psychological research on resilience among children and youth, it may be more informative to use the family as the unit of study for resilience among refugees and other migrants. For migrant families, the refugee or immigration experience is an extremely challenging transition. Some common stressors for families related to migration include loss of close relationships, uncertainty about decision to immigrate, uncertainty about being assigned refugee status, changes in financial status, loss of lifestyle, country and roots, change in cultural norms (Bennett and Colleen 1997), changes in the marital relationship (Scott 2001), employment (Aycan and Berry 1996), and ability to understand and communicate in a language other than one's own (Nwadiora and Mcadoo 1996), among many other potential stressors. Although these stressors can be overwhelming for immigrant and refugee families, still, there remains the potential to flexibly select appropriate coping behaviours that can keep the family in balance and assist in construing the world as ordered and predictable, and crises as manageable and meaningful (Antonovsky and Sourani 1988).

Modes of familial resilience will vary depending on the socio-cultural-historical contexts in which a family exists (Hawley 2000; Scott 2001). Nor is resilience a static construct based on a set of qualities found in some families and not in others. As Hawley (2000) states, it is a path which families often follow when dealing with challenges and stressors in life. It is therefore important to look for resilience not only in the face of challenges, but as a process, a potential strength a family may display over time (Hawley 2000).

Some adaptational systems that often help people in the face of stressors are emotional and social support among family and community members, open and honest communication, exploration of ethnicity, religion and spirituality, and family rituals and belief systems (Carranza 2007; Greeff and Holtzkamp 2007; Greeff and Human 2004). Perhaps, the greatest threat to migrant families and communities are adversities that undermine these basic protective processes. Family values and belief systems play a very important role in cushioning the effect of transitions and changing circumstances on the family unit (Silberberg 2001). An important challenge for migrants developing constructive family practices is the cultural differences they encounter in family practices within the host society. Particularly difficult for a migrant parent is the process of bridging the gap between the socialization and parenting he/she experienced as a child, and the practices and beliefs encountered in the dominant culture. As notable as these differences may be, recognizing many of them as significant sources of strengths for refugee families can help provide crucial systems of support during the challenging period of adaptation and resettlement.

Culture is used here to mean shared learned experience that is transmitted across generations. It includes internal representations of meaning, values, beliefs, world-views, etc and external representations such as clothing, food, technologies, etc. We further assume that culture is dynamic, fluid, and emergent, rather than a static and fixed entity (Dorazio-Migliore et al. 2005; Hermans and Kempen 1998). Given this dynamic conceptualization, that the role of culture is flexible and fluid, then, what are the cultural strengths, our proposed basis for resilience, which refugees bring with them? How can those strengths, given their dynamic and fluid nature, then facilitate the transition and resettlement process? What is the relationship of strengths/resilience to migrants' sense of identity and ability to negotiate the adaptation and integration process?

Maintenance of cultural identity is one widely used strategy by migrants that can serve as a source of resilience. Yet, the impact of migration on identity is still not well understood. We know it is complex and does not reduce to simple categories, as is sometimes portrayed in acculturation research (e.g., Cuellar et al. 1995; Sadat 2008). For example, Sadat has shown how Afghan refugees and immigrants use memories and stories from their natal culture to maintain a sense of "Afghanness" even while living in countries with markedly different cultural norms (Sadat 2008). Immigrants and refugees from many cultural groups have been reared in societies that foster a markedly different sense of self or identity than the mainstream of the host culture and that also differ from each other. In a much cited article, Markus and Kitayama (1991) found that, at the least, native Japanese and native Americans held fundamentally different ontological and epistemological assumptions about selfhood. In many ways, their work only scratches the surface of these fundamental differences (Misra 1994; Roland 1988, 2011; Sinha 1990). Migration may also pose a threat to identity, as assumptions about self and appropriate social relations are challenged by the host society (Timotijevic and Breakwell 2000). On the other hand, a strong sense of cultural identity may be an important resource for resilience (Schwartz et al. 2006).

As Phinney pointed out (2003), little attention has been paid to the potential multidimensionality of identity, identity change, and the refugee resettlement process. Too often, researchers have made an assumption that acculturation/resettlement is a linear process, with adjustment to the host culture being a matter of degree. Recently, however, a body of research has emerged that has begun to address these lacunae. Benet-Martinez and her colleagues have addressed the question of bicultural identity among immigrants and, especially, the children of immigrants (Hong et al. 2000). They have found that the cultural code-switching necessary for such an identity has an overall positive effect, especially on girls. Yet, their work does not shed light on the formation of a bicultural identity. Phinney, in a number of publications (Berry et al. 2006; Phinney 1990, 2003; Phinney et al. 2001; Phinney and Devich-Navarro 1997), has articulated the correlates of ethnic identity, including factors related to cultural maintenance, such as language and food. With the increase in migration, forced or otherwise, psychological researchers have begun to explore the question of multiple group identities. Roccas and Brewer (2002) proposed a theory of social identity complexity to represent how such group identities could overlap and the strategies that individuals use to move among them. In a thoughtful review of literature on collective identity, Ashmore et al. (2004) articulated a multidimensional approach that synthesized extant literature on such traditional social psychological identity concepts as self-categorization, evaluation, interdependence, and social embeddedness, to name only a few, and suggested potentially viable assessment strategies, including narratives, to tap the richness of collective identities. Ashmore and colleagues concluded that much remains to do in order to understand the development of collective identity, including a need to focus on the historical context and its interplay with the developmental process, while considering both the individual and the society.

Maintenance of natal cultural identity is typically a challenge for migrants. Host cultures are, as pointed out above, often based on a different assumption about identity, self, child-parent relationships, and health care, to name only a few. Social, legal, and economic structures are often in place to maintain the norms of the host culture and are largely taken for granted by natives of that culture. Researchers have found that migrants typically experience these extant norms as barriers to the maintenance of their natal culture, yet continue to prize their own culture and seek to maintain it (e.g., Inman et al. 2007). Language is often a primary maintenance tool, as parents encourage their children to learn their natal language and speak it at home (Inman et al. 2007; Phinney 2003). Maintaining natal culture religious practices, including festivals and religious observances, such as fasting, is also a common strategy (Inman et al. 2007). Most families appear to adopt pragmatic strategies to maintain their cultural practices through such activities as dress and diet that are appropriate for their home culture within their homes, but embracing some modifications when in public, such as the workplace (Inman et al. 2007).

2.5 Conclusion

Michael Ungar has reminded us of the importance of culture in understanding resilience (Ungar 2008). In his seminal article examining resilience across cultures, he pointed out that communities or cultural groups must be the final arbiter on what counts for resilience. Thus, a task before those of us who seek to understand resilience is to make sure that we seek our understanding in a mode that allows us to respect multiple cultures and contexts.

We may indeed find that when we ask the culture question about resilience that we may be surprised to discover practices that differ dramatically from what we in North America would define as necessary or typical of resilient behaviour. While we can expect that there will be many similarities across cultures, there will also be important variations. Even when we consider resilience as the ordinary magic of human adaptive processes, we must remember that adaptation is always about survival and thriving in a particular time, place, and context.

As Ungar and others have pointed out, we still find that typical definitions of resilience fail to capture both individual aspects and the social/cultural context or ecology that the individual exists within. Yet, both must be accounted for if we are to make progress in understanding and facilitating resilience.

On that note, we close with the definition of resilience offered by Ungar (2008):

> In the context of exposure to significant adversity, whether psychological, environmental, or both, resilience is both the capacity of individuals to navigate their way to health-sustaining resources, including opportunities to experience feelings of well-being, and a condition of the individual's family, community and culture to provide these health resources and experiences in culturally meaningful ways. (p. 225)

References

Albanese, C. L. (2007). *A republic of mind and spirit: A cultural history of American metaphysical religion*. New Haven: Yale University Press.
Allport, G. W. (1955). *Becoming*. New Haven: Yale University Press.
Andrick, J. (2012). Delsartean hypnosis for girls' bodies and minds: Annie Payson Call and the Lasell Seminary nerve training controversy. *History of Psychology, 15*(2), 124–144.
Antonovsky A., & Sourani T. (1988). Family sense of coherence and family adaptation. *Journal of Marriage and the Family, 50*(1), 79–92.
Ashmore, R. D., Deaux, K., & McLaughlin-Volpe, T. (2004). An organizing framework for collective identity: Articulation and significance of multidimensionality. *Psychological Bulletin, 130*, 80–114.
Aycan, Z., & Berry, J. W. (1996). Impact of employment-related experiences on immigrants' psychological well-being and adaptation to Canada. *Canadian Journal of Behavioural Science, 28*, 240–251.
Bederman, G. (1995). *Manliness & civilization*. Chicago: University of Chicago Press.
Beiser, M. (1999) Strangers at the gate: The 'Boat People's' first ten years in Canada. Toronto: University of Toronto Press.
Beiser, M. (2005) The health of immigrants and refugees in Canada. *Canadian Journal of Public Health, 96*, S30–45.
Bennett, H., & Colleen, R. (1997). The relationship between tenure, stress, and coping strategies of South African immigrants to New Zealand. *South African Journal of Psychology, 27*, 160–166.
Berry, J. W., Phinney, J. S., Sam, D., & Vedder, P. (2006). *Immigrant youth in cultural transition: Acculturation, identity, and adaptation across national contexts*. Mahwah: Erlbaum.
Bhatia, S., & Ram, A. (2001). Rethinking 'acculturation' in relation to diasporic cultures and postcolonial identities. *Human Development, 44*, 1–18.
Carranza, M. E. (2007). Building resilience and resistance against racism and discrimination among Salvadorian female youth in Canada. *Child and Family Social Work, 12*, 390–398.
Chryssochoou, X. (2000). Multicultural societies: Making sense of new environments and identities. *Journal of Community and Applied Social Psychology, 10*, 343–354.
Cicchetti, D., & Rogosch, F. A. (1997). The role of self-organization in the promotion of resilience in maltreated children. *Development and Psychopathology, 9*, 797–815.
Clark, K. B. (1965). *Dark ghetto*. New York: Harper & Row.
Cuellar, I., Arnold, B., & Maldonado, R. (1995). Acculturation rating scale for Mexican Americans-II: A revision of the original ARMSA scale. *Hispanic Journal of Behavioral Sciences, 2*, 199–217.
DeFrain J. (1999). Strong families. *Family Matters, 53*, 6–13.
Dooley, P. K. (2001). The strenuous mood: William James' 'Energies in Men' and Jack London's "The Sea-Wolf." *American Literary Realism, 34*, 18–28.
Dorazio-Migliore, M., Migliore, S., & Anderson, J. (2005). Crafting a praxis-oriented culture concept in the health disciplines: Conundrums and possibilities. *Health: An Interdisciplinary Journal for the Social Study of Health, Illness and Medicine, 9*, 339–360.
Dunbar, H. F. (1935). *Emotions and bodily changes: A survey of literature on psychosomatic relationships, 1910–1933*. New York: Columbia University Press.
Engel, G. L. (1977). The need for a new medical model: A challenge for biomedicine. *Science, 196*, 129–136.
Fromm, E. (1947). *Man for himself*. New York: Rinehart.
Garmezy, N. (1971). Vulnerability research and the issue of primary prevention. *American Journal of Orthopsychiatry, 41*, 101–116.
Garmezy, N. (1973). Competence and adaptation in adult schizophrenic patients and children at risk. In S. R. Dean (Ed.), *Schizophrenia: The first en Dean Award lectures* (pp. 163–204). New York: MSS Information.

Garmezy, N. & Devine, V. (1984). Project Competence: The Minnesota studies of children vulnerable to psychopathology. In N. F. Watt, E. J. Anthony, L. C. Wynne, & J. E. Rolf (Eds.), *Children at risk for schizophrenia: A longitudinal perspective* (pp. 289–303). New York: Cambridge University Press.

Greeff, A. P., & Human, B. (2004). Resilience in families in which a parent had died. *American Journal of Family Therapy, 32*, 27–42.

Greeff, A. P., & Holtzkamp, J. (2007). The prevalence of resilience in migrant families. *Family Community Health, 30*, 189–200.

Haan L. D., Hawley D. R., & Deal J. E. (2002). Operationalizing family resilience: A methodological strategy. *American Journal of Family Therapy, 30*, 275–291.

Haley, B. (1978). *The healthy body and Victorian culture*. Cambridge: The Belknap.

Handlin, O. (1951). *The uprooted: The epic story of the great migrations that made the American people*. Boston: Grosset & Dunlap.

Harrington, A. (2008). *The cure within: A history of mind-body medicine*. New York: Norton.

Hawley, D.R. (2000). Clinical implications of family resilience. *American Journal of Family Therapy, 28*, 101–116.

Hermans, H. J. M., & Kempen, H. J. G. (1998). Moving cultures: The perilous problems of cultural dichotomies in a globalizing society. *American Psychologist, 53*, 1111–1120.

Hong, Y., Morris, M. W., Chiu, C., & Benet-Martinez, V. (2000). Multicultural minds: A dynamic constructivist approach to culture and cognition. *American Psychologist, 55*, 709–720.

Inman, A. G., Howard, E. E., Beaumont, R. L., & Walker, J. L. (2007). Cultural transmission: Influence of contextual factors in Asian Indian immigrant parents' experiences. *Journal of Counseling Psychology, 54*, 93–100.

James, W. (1902). *The varieties of religious experience*. New York: Longman, Greens.

James, W. (1907a). The energies of men. *Philosophical Review, 16*, 1–20.

James, W. (1907b). The Absolute and the strenuous Life. *The Journal of Philosophy, Psychology and Scientific Methods, 4*, 546–548.

Joseph, S. (2004). Client-centered therapy, post-traumatic stress disorder and post-traumatic growth: Theoretical perspectives and practical implications. *Psychology and Psychotherapy: Theory, Research and Practice, 77*, 101–119.

Kobasa, S. C. (1979). Stressful life events, personality and health: An inquiry into hardiness. *Journal of Personality and Social Psychology, 37*, 1–11.

Korten, F. F., Cook, S. W., & Lacey, J. I. (1970). *Psychology and the problems of society*. Washington, DC: American Psychological Association.

Lazarus, R. (1966). *Psychological stress and the coping process*. New York: McGraw-Hill.

Loss, C. P. (2002). Religion and the therapeutic ethos in twentieth century American history. *American Studies International, 40*, 61–76.

Maddi, S. R. (1980). *Personality theories: A comparative analysis*. Homewood: Dorsey.

Maddi, S. R. (2002). The story of hardiness: Twenty years of theorizing, research, and practice. *Consulting Psychology Journal: Practice and Research, 54*, 175–185.

Markowitz, G., & Rosner, D. (2000). *Children, race, and power: Kenneth and Mamie Clark's Northside Center*. New York: Routledge.

Markus, H. R., & Kitayama, S. (1991). Culture and the self: Implications for cognition, emotion, and motivation. *Psychological Review, 98*, 224–253.

Maslow, A. (1954). *Motivation and personality*. New York: Harper.

Mason, J. W. (1975). A historical view of the stress field. *Journal of Human Stress, 1*, 6–12.

Masten, A. (2001). Ordinary magic: Resilience processes in development. *American Psychology, 56*, 227–238.

Masten, A. S., Coatsworth, J. D., Neemann, J., Gest, S. D., Tellegen, A., & Garmezy, N. (1995). The structure and coherence of competence from childhood through adolescence. *Child Development, 66*, 1635–1659.

McLaughlin, N. (1998). Why do schools of thought fail? Neo-Freudianism as a case study in the sociology of knowledge. *Journal of the History of the Behavioral Sciences, 34*, 113–134.

Misra, G. (1994). Psychology of control: Cross-cultural considerations. *Journal of Indian Psychology, 12,* 8–45.
Mittelman, B., & Wolff, H. G. (1942). Emotions and gastroduodenal function. *Psychosomatic Medicine, 4,* 5–61.
Moynihan, D. (1965). *The Negro family: A case for national action.* Washington, DC: U.S. Department of Labor.
Murray, H. (1938). *Explorations in personality.* New York: Oxford University Press
Nobles, W. W. (1972). African philosophy: Foundations for a Black psychology. In R. L. Jones (Ed.), *Black psychology* (pp. 18–32). New York: Harper & Row.
Nwadiora, E., & Mcadoo, H. (1996). Acculturative stress among Amerasian refugees: Gender and racial differences. *Adolescence, 31,* 477–487.
O'Leary, V. E., & Ickovics, J. R. (1995). Resilience and thriving in response to challenge: An opportunity for a paradigm shift in women's health. *Women's Health: Research on Gender, Behavior and Policy, 1,* 121–142.
Ouellette, S. C. (2012). Robert W. White: A life in the study of lives. In W. E. Pickren, D. A. Dewsbury, & M. Wertheimer (Eds.), *Portraits of pioneers in developmental psychology* (pp. 171–184). New York: Psychology.
Ouellete, S. C., Cassel, J. B., Maslanka, H., & Wong, L. M. (1995). GMHC volunteers and the challenges and hopes for the second decade of AIDS. *AIDS Education and Prevention, 7*(Suppl 5), 64–79.
Park, R. J. (1994). A decade of the body: Researching and writing about the history of health, fitness, exercise, and sport, 1983–1993. *Journal of Sport History, 21,* 51–82.
Phillips, L. (2000). Recontextualizing Kenneth B. Clark: An Afrocentric perspective on the paradoxical legacy of a model psychologist-activist. *History of Psychology, 3,* 142–167.
Phinney, J. S. (1990). Ethnic identity in adolescents and adults: A review of research. *Psychological Bulletin, 108,* 499–514.
Phinney, J. S. (2003). Ethnic identity and acculturation. In K. M. Chun, P. B. Organista, & G. Marin (Eds.), *Acculturation: Advances in theory, measurement, and applied research* (pp. 63–81). Washington, DC: American Psychological Association.
Phinney, J. S., & Devich-Navarro, M. (1997). Variations in bicultural identification among African American and Mexican American adolescents. *Journal of Research on Adolescence, 7,* 3–32.
Phinney, J. S., Horenczyk, G., Liebkind, K., & Vedder, P. (2001). Ethnic identity, immigration, and well-being: An interactional perspective. *Journal of Social Issues, 57,* 493–510.
Pickren, W. E. (2003). Kurt Goldstein: Neurologist and philosopher of the organism. In G. Kimble & M. Wertheimer (Eds.), *Portraits of pioneers in psychology,* (Vol. 5, pp. 127–139). Washington, DC: American Psychological Association & Erlbaum.
Pickren, W. E., & Rutherford, A. (2010). *A history of modern psychology in context.* New York: Wiley.
Pickren, W. E., & Schneider, S. F. (Eds.). (2005). *Psychology and the National Institute of Mental Health: A historical analysis of science, practice, and policy.* Washington, DC: APA Books.
Pieterse, J. (2009). *Globalization and culture: Global mélange* (2nd ed.). Lanham: Rowman & Littlefield.
Roccas, S., & Brewer, M. B. (2002). Social identity complexity. *Personality and Social Psychology Review, 6,* 88–106.
Rodriguez, E. M., & Ouellette, S. C. (2000). Gay and lesbian Christians: Homosexual and religious identity integration in the members and participants of a gay-positive church. *Journal for the Scientific Study of Religion, 39,* 333–347.
Rogers, C. R. (1951). *Client-centered therapy.* Boston: Houghton-Mifflin.
Roland, A. (1988). *In search of the self in India and Japan: Toward a cross-cultural psychology.* Princeton: Princeton University Press.
Roland, A. (2011). *Journeys to Foreign Selves: Asians and Asian Americans in a Global Era.* New York: Oxford University Press.

Sadat, M. H. (2008). Hyphenating Afghaniyat in the Afghan diaspora. *Journal of Muslim Minority Affairs, 2,* 329–342.

Sarason, S. B. (1981). An asocial psychology and a misdirected clinical psychology. *American Psychologist, 36,* 827–836.

Scheier, M. F., & Carver, C. S. (1996). Psychological resources matter, no matter how you say it or frame it. *The Counseling Psychologist, 24,* 736–742.

Schofield, W. (1969). The role of psychology in the delivery of health services. *American Psychologist, 24,* 565–584.

Schwartz, S. J., Montgomery, M. J., & Briones, E. (2006). The role of identity in acculturation among immigrant people: Theoretical propositions, empirical questions, and applied recommendations. *Human Development, 49,* 1–30.

Scott, D. (2001). Building communities that strengthen families. *Family Matters, 58,* 76–79.

Selye, H. (1950). *The physiology and pathology of exposure to stress.* Montreal: Acta.

Selye, H. (1956). *The stress of life.* New York: McGraw-Hill.

Silberberg, S. (2001). Searching for family resilience. *Family Matters, 58,* 52–57.

Simich, L., Pickren, W. E., & Beiser, M. (2011). Resilience, acculturation and integration of adult migrants: Understanding cultural strengths of recent refugees. Final Report to Human Resources Skills Development, Canada.

Sinha, J. B. P. (1990). The salient Indian values and their socio-ecological roots. *Indian Journal of Social Science, 3,* 477–488.

Smith, W. C. (1939). *Americans in the making: The natural history of the assimilation of immigrants.* New York: Appleton.

Sparer, P. J. (1956). *Personality, stress, and tuberculosis.* New York: International Universities Press.

Taves, A. (1999). *Fits, trances, and visions: Experiencing religion and explaining experience from Wesley to James.* Princeton, NJ: Princeton University Press.

Taylor, E. (1999). *Shadow culture: Psychology and spirituality in America.* Washington, DC: Counterpoint.

Timotijevic, L., & Breakwell, G. M. (2000). Migration and threat to identity. *Journal of Community and Applied Psychology, 10,* 355–372.

Ungar, M. (2008). Resilience across cultures. *British Journal of Social Work, 38,* 218–235.

Werner, E. E., & Smith, R. S. (1982). *Vulnerable but invincible: A study of resilient children.* New York: McGraw-Hill.

Werner, E. E., & Smith, R. S. (1992). *Overcoming the odds: High Risk children from birth to adulthood.* Ithaca: Cornell University Press.

White, R. W. (1959). Motivation reconsidered: The concept of competence. *Psychological Review, 66,* 297–333.

White, J. L. (1972). Toward a Black psychology. In R. L. Jones (Ed.), *Black psychology* (pp. 43–50). New York: Harper & Row.

Whorton, J. C. (1982). *Crusaders for fitness: The history of American health reformers.* Princeton: Princeton University Press.

Whorton, J. C. (2002). *Nature cures: The history of alternative medicine in America.* New York: Oxford University Press.

Williams, R. L. (2008). A 40-year history of the Association of Black Psychologists (ABPsi). *Journal of Black Psychology, 34,* 249–260.

Chapter 3
Social Determinants of Refugee Mental Health

Farah N. Mawani

Abstract Disparities in social determinants and in mental health outcomes between refugees, immigrants, and domestic-born individuals, and between sub-groups of refugees, are largely attributable to inequalities in social determinants, including socioeconomic factors, social support, and systemic racism and discrimination. This chapter outlines a multi-level framework of determinants of mental health inequities, including macro-, community-, family-, and individual levels of determinants, across a continuum from pre-migration to resettlement.

Keywords Social determinants · Mental health · Health equity · Health inequities · Refugees · Refugee health · Health disparities · Intersectionality

3.1 Introduction

Canada's population is one of the most diverse in the world, and is growing in diversity across multiple dimensions: migration status, ethno-cultural background, racialized status, religious and spiritual beliefs, languages spoken, sex and gender, sexual orientation, and disability status. There is growing recognition, in Canada and globally, of the importance of examining and responding to intersections of diversity rather than individual dimensions of diversity. In order to adequately understand the disparities in mental health determinants and resulting inequities in mental health for refugees, it is necessary to delve into the complex intersecting dimensions of diversity shaping their lives.

There are inequalities in mental health determinants and resulting disparities in mental health outcomes experienced by diverse groups. Such inequalities in mental health determinants exist between refugees and Canadian-born individuals, refugees and immigrants, and sub-groups of refugees (e.g. men and women, refugees with disabilities and those without). Disparities in mental health outcomes between refugees, immigrants and Canadian-born individuals, and between sub-groups of

---

F. N. Mawani (✉)
Dalla Lana School of Public Health, University of Toronto, Toronto, Canada
e-mail: farah.mawani@utoronto.ca

refugees, are largely attributable to inequalities in social determinants, including socioeconomic factors, social support, and systemic racism and discrimination.

This chapter will outline a multi-level framework of determinants of mental health inequities, including macro-, community-, family-, and individual levels of determinants across a continuum from pre-migration to resettlement. Canadian evidence of social determinants of mental health, dynamically interacting at these levels, will be reviewed and critically analyzed within a global context. Gaps in evidence will be highlighted and recommendations made for filling those gaps in order to improve the potential for policy and programs to improve refugee mental health.

3.2 Framework of Determinants

A multi-level framework of determinants of mental health includes macro, community, family and individual levels of determinants of health. Individuals are nested within their families and/or households, which are nested within multiple communities, which are in turn nested in a broader societal context. Some factors are repeated in multiple categories of the causal framework because they may operate at societal and/or community levels and filter down to influence family and individual experiences or vice versa. The dynamic interaction of these factors operating at multiple levels affects mental health outcomes (Collins and Guruge 2008; Bierman et al. 2009).

Such a model is increasingly being applied to refugee mental health, including specific sub-populations of refugees. For example, as outlined by Lustig et al. (2004), such a multi-level transactional model has been applied to refugee children's trauma and well-being.

In consultations for the development of the Mental Health Commission of Canada's Mental Health Strategy Framework document, participants urged the Commission to adopt a plural form of the term community to reflect the fact that individuals belong to multiple communities, including communities of interest, geographic communities, and social movements (Ascentum 2009). Refugees may belong to a greater range of diverse communities, including for example, their ethnic and religious communities in addition to their neighbourhood and work/school communities. Their communities are also likely to be spread across national borders.

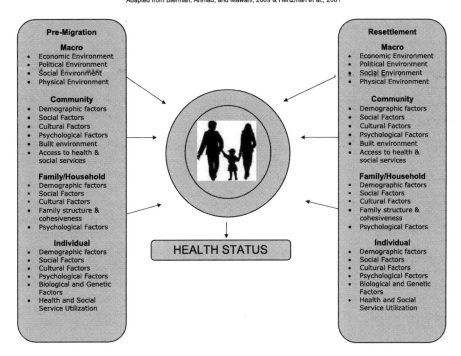

Determinants of Immigrant Health - A Conceptual Framework
Adapted from Bierman, Ahmad, and Mawani, 2009 & Hertzman et al., 2001

It is important to stress that although refugees may be more likely to experience certain determinants and are therefore more *at risk* of certain mental health outcomes, they may not actually experience those outcomes, due to a combination of individual, family and community strengths (e.g. resilience, social support). To date the public health field has largely approached research from a deficit perspective that emphasizes risk factors for illness. Such a focus has a role to play in identifying the need for intervention, but there is a growing recognition of the importance of an asset perspective that focuses on protective factors that prevent negative health outcomes and/or promote health (Morgan and Ziglio 2007).

Morgan and Ziglio (2007) emphasize the opportunity an asset-based approach provides "to create a more robust evidence base that demonstrates why investing in the assets of individuals, communities and organisations can help to reduce the health gap between those most disadvantaged in society and those who achieve best health (Morgan and Ziglio 2007)." Despite the importance of such an approach to diversity, shifting the focus and approach of research, policy and practice is taking time.

3.3 Macro-level Factors

Refugees' mental health is influenced by macro-level factors including the economic, political, social and physical environments in their countries of origin as well as their countries of resettlement. The economic, political, social and physical contexts refugees have experienced pre-migration affect their perceptions, understandings and expectations of the economic, political, social and physical environments they experience in Canada. Therefore, the environments refugees experience need to be considered on a continuum from pre-migration to resettlement in order to understand the contextual effects on their health (Beiser 2005; Bierman et al. 2009).

The economic, political, social and physical environments in their countries of origin, can continue to affect them and their families even after they have settled in Canada. The emergence and development of crises in those environments (e.g. natural disasters, political violence), the associated repercussions on their families and communities, and the potential re-traumatization they experience, can have particularly detrimental effects on their mental health.

3.3.1 Economic Environment

Economic environments influence mental health in multiple ways, including societal-level income distribution impacting mental health; economic factors influencing migration; and economic inequalities impacting post-migration mental health.

A considerable body of research demonstrates the impact of societal-level distribution of income on health, and mortality (Marmot and Wilkinson 1999; Raphael 2004; Auger and Raynault 2006; Gronqvist et al. 2012). People who live in areas with higher income inequality have poorer health and higher mortality rates (Gronqvist et al. 2012). The gap between people's income levels within a society is a stronger predictor of health status than absolute income (Marmot and Wilkinson 1999; Raphael 2004; Auger and Raynault 2006; Gronqvist et al. 2012). In analyses of prevalences of mental illness for 12 countries, Wilkinson and Pickett (Wilkinson and Pickett 2009) found an association between higher national levels of income inequality and higher prevalence of mental illness. They highlight, "in contrast with studies of physical morbidity and mortality, as countries get richer, rates of mental illness increase (Pickett et al. 2006)."

Economies of the countries of origin of immigrants and refugees influence who migrates, and shape migration experience (Bierman et al. 2009). Refugees often have to leave their countries of origin without money due to the threat to their lives from natural disaster, war, political context, etc. Economic refugees are forced to leave their countries of origin to escape oppressive poverty (Project Economic Refugee 2012).

Socioeconomic inequalities in refugees' countries of origin and settlement are important determinants of their post-migration mental health (Beiser 2005; Bierman et al. 2009). First, taking a lifecourse approach to mental health, early life experiences impact on later life mental health outcomes. Second, refugees are very likely to experience a change in exposure to inequalities in country-level income distribution in their migration process.

3.3.2 Political Environment

Multiple dimensions of the political environment in refugees' countries of origin and resettlement may impact on mental health including: the political system and ideology; the role of government in the economy; political instability; the country's international political relationships; civic engagement (public involvement in the political process); and government policies at multiple levels (i.e. national, regional, local).

The historical and current political environment in refugees' country of origin may impact on individual-level immigrant mental health by causing trauma and re-traumatization; affecting personal power; and shaping their perceptions, understandings and expectations of the political environment in Canada. The extent to which refugees perceive personal agency in the political process, including in informing policy change, may depend partly on the political context they have experienced in their countries of origin. For example, refugees, who come from countries where opportunities for civic participation[1] are limited or even violently suppressed, may not understand or feel safe with their opportunities for civic participation in Canada. They may also experience multiple barriers to civic participation, including lack of information, limited social networks and lack of commitment on the part of governments to engaging them. The combination of their expectations and barriers to participation may influence their sense of control over their life circumstances and thereby their health (Taylor and Seeman 1999). Government policies at different levels (federal, provincial, municipal) and in different sectors (health, settlement, social, etc.) also affect refugee mental health.

3.3.3 Social Environment

The key dimensions of the macro-level social environment of immigrants' countries of origin and resettlement that impact on mental health are **social inclusion**/exclusion and formal **social support**. Refugees' experiences with social exclusion/inclusion and social support in Canada are affected by their contexts of social exclusion/inclusion in their countries of origin, but very limited research considers this.

Social exclusion refers to the exclusion of groups and individuals from society, based on dimensions of diversity, including age, gender, race, ethnicity, social class, migration status, sexual orientation, etc. Immigrants are at risk of being excluded on the basis of all these factors, at an individual or systemic (institutional) level. Social exclusion can affect mental health by limiting opportunities for education, employment, housing, etc.

---

[1] 'Civic participation' refers to "the citizen's (or resident's) active role in shaping, defining and changing policies and procedures that impact his or her life (Jones 2008)," and includes the dimensions volunteering, political activism, voting, and acquisition of citizenship (Boyd 2009).

Social exclusion can also reduce individuals' self-esteem and mastery (perceived control over their life circumstances), thereby creating stress that affects physical and mental health.

Particularly concerning, in the context of the impact of social exclusion, are examples of increasing national government level discrimination against Muslims. France, Canada and Australia have banned Muslim face coverings to varying degrees (Cherfils 2010; Baldauf 2011; McGuirk 2012), and Switzerland has banned minarets (Cumming-Bruce and Erlanger 2009). In December 2011, Canadian Immigration Minister, Jason Kenney, issued a policy prohibiting Muslim women from wearing face veils during citizenship ceremonies. Minister Kenney stated that women who did not want to take off their face veils could choose not to come to Canada, or not to become Canadian citizens (Mawani 2012). Refugees do not choose to migrate to Canada. Rather, they are forced out of their countries of origin by threats to their safety and lives. While most refugees do not choose their country of resettlement, issues of gender inequality within many refugee families mean that women, in particular, often have no say on where they will migrate (Mawani 2012).

The veil policy also demonstrates a lack of understanding and inclusion of the diversity of Muslims. In Canada, Muslims from many different sects and countries, have varying belief systems with regard to women's dress. Some Muslim women choose their dress based on their belief systems. Others are forced to cover themselves to varying degrees by men in their families and communities (Mawani 2012). For the latter, Kenney's policy creates a no-win situation: Men in their families/communities force them to wear the veils, but, according to Kenney's policy, if they do, they are prevented from becoming Canadian citizens. This makes it even more difficult for them to overcome their oppression because, if they cannot become Canadian citizens, they are denied the complete set of rights, legal protections, access to services, and social support provided by such status. This marginalizes them even further, prevents them from being able to live freely in our country, and potentially threatens their safety (Mawani 2012).

Evidence from around the globe indicates that immigrants and refugees who experience racial, ethnic, and religious discrimination are at increased risk of developing mental-health issues and illness (Williams et al. 2008; Dunn and Dyck 2000; Omidvar and Richmond 2003; Krieger 2000). This risk is magnified for those who have been persecuted by governments in their countries of origin, as they may be re-traumatized by the experience of discrimination by the government in what they expect to be their safe new home. Within the context of such pre-migration experiences, and the distinct risks faced by Muslims amidst the increasing Islamophobia around the globe since 9/11 (Sheridan 2006; Laird et al. 2007; Rousseau et al. 2011), being forced to remove a veil could be very traumatic for a Muslim woman.

Using an asset-based approach, the focus can be shifted from social exclusion to social *inclusion*, made up of the dimensions, identified by the Laidlaw Foundation, of valued recognition, human development, involvement and engagement, proximity, and material well-being (Hanvey 2003). Such an approach could dramatically shift policy making processes.

Social support at the macro-level refers to formal support available at the federal or provincial level, via policies or programs (e.g. health insurance, income support, unemployment insurance; Canadian Interim Federal Health Program; Canadian Prenatal Nutrition Program, Canadian Action Program for Children).

3.3.4 Physical Environment

The physical environment is an important determinant of mental health. Inequalities in exposure to environmental contaminants, chemical warfare, natural disasters, and climate change have severe and long-term impacts on the physical and mental health of refugees. In many cases those exposures have inter-generational effects.

At certain levels of exposure, contaminants in our air, water, food and soil can cause a variety of adverse health effects. There are inequalities in exposure to environmental contaminants by country/region of origin, as well as within country inequalities. Refugees may also be exposed to contaminants due to war (e.g. chemical warfare) (Dworkin et al. 2008; Hashemian et al. 2006). Chemical warfare has been linked to current and lifetime post-traumatic stress symptoms, and poor general functioning (Dworkin et al. 2008); and post-traumatic stress disorder, major anxiety, and severe depression (Hashemian et al. 2006).

The physical and mental health consequences of chemical warfare are long-term (Dworkin et al. 2008; Hashemian et al. 2006), and can extend to the next generation (e.g. Kurdish refugees with children born in Canada with numerous physical and developmental disabilities) (Mawani 2001). The impact on children also has a great impact on the mental health of their parents, families, and communities (Mawani 2001). The injustices inherent in inequalities in exposure can be especially detrimental to mental health.

Natural disasters impact mental health via primary and secondary stressors (Lock et al. 2012). Primary stressors include injuries sustained, and witnessing deaths. The mental health impact of secondary stressors is often underestimated. They include economic stressors; loss of possessions and resources; health stressors; education stressors; media stressors; family and social stressors; loss of leisure and recreation; and changing world views (Lock et al. 2012).

Children and adolescents, and mothers with young children, are especially psychologically vulnerable to disasters (Beaton et al. 2009). Children and adolescents may experience long-term emotional distress, mental illness, functional impairment, and/or developmental challenges resulting from experiencing a natural disaster (Beaton et al. 2009). These in turn can affect their school performance and social behavior (Beaton et al. 2009).

There is growing recognition of climate change as a determinant of forced migration. The International Organization for Migration (IOM), United Nations High Commissioner for Refugees (UNHCR), and the United Nations University (UNU) (IOM et al. 2009) state,

While there are no scientifically verified estimates of climate change-related displacement or of overall population flows triggered by the effects of climate change, it is evident that gradual and sudden environmental changes are already resulting in substantial human migration and displacement.

The United Nations has projected between 50 and 200 million people displaced as a result of climate change by 2050 (IOM et al. 2009).

3.4 Community-level Factors

Refugees are part of many different, and sometimes overlapping communities, including their neighbourhood, ethnic communities, religious communities, work communities, and social/peer communities. There is increasing recognition that neighbourhood factors, including the built environment, access to services, and amenities affect mental health. This has important implications for refugee mental health as refugees tend to concentrate in particular neighbourhoods. It is important to recognize, however, that refugees' mental health is also affected by the demographic, social, cultural and psychological make up of communities they are part of beyond their neighbourhoods. These other communities have not received as much attention as neighbourhoods in mental health research in general nor in refugee mental health research in particular (Ray and Bergeron 2007), although some research has been conducted focusing on faith-based neighbourhoods in the Greater Toronto Area (Agrawal and Qadeer 2008).

3.4.1 Social Factors

Social support is a well-recognized determinant of health that is conceptualized and measured in numerous ways in the literature. The two main aspects of social support that affect health are structural and functional support. Structural support refers to the existence and quantity of social relationships (e.g. marital status, group membership, number of friends) and interconnectedness of a person's social network, while functional support refers to the degree to which support (formal and informal) serves particular functions (e.g., emotional support, instrumental support, informational support, affirmational support[2]) (Sherbourne and Stewart 1991).

Social support is usually considered a protective factor that buffers the negative impact of stressors on health. In the context of migration, however, there is a substantial loss of social support. Sometimes loss or separation from immediate family members, including partners and/or children, occurs during the process of migration.

---

[2] Affirmational or appraisal support refers to the "provision of information that is useful for self-evaluation purposes, that is, constructive feedback, affirmation, and social comparison" (Heaney and Israel 1997).

The loss of immediate family, extended family and community, combined with the value placed on independence over interdependence in Canada, leads to a feeling of great isolation in many immigrants (Mawani 2001). This is especially challenging during resettlement, when the need for emotional and affirmational support is acute. It can be even more challenging for refugee women who are often significant providers of support to their families and communities. The social support literature recognizes that men and women give and receive different levels of social support, need different types of support and seek support in different ways (Heaney and Israel 1997). Therefore, social support has a differential impact on their health and it is important to include a gender analysis in research on this topic (Mulvihill et al. 2001), especially with the added layers of issues for refugee women.

Research indicates that receiving social support contributes to more stable and positive self-esteem (Turner et al. 1999). Suffering a loss of support or experiencing a lack of needed support can thereby contribute to lowered self-esteem. Refugees have described feeling downtrodden and helpless with a sense of desperation, disappointment and despair when they did not receive support they needed (Simich et al. 2004). Although they do not see themselves as helpless given the extent of resourcefulness and work required for them to settle and integrate, when a lack of formal social support limits their access to the housing, education and employment that they feel entitled to, based on their merits or skills and/or basic rights, it lowers their self-esteem and perceived control (Simich et al. 2004). They describe an intensified and longer-term impact on their mental health when they feel that this limitation of their access to basic needs is due to discrimination (Mawani et al. 2005). Social support is also a key factor in recovery from mental health issues and illnesses (Topor et al. 2011).

Pregnancy and the postpartum period are points in the life course when immigrant and refugee women are in particular need of social support. Lack of support may be especially isolating and disempowering for women who would have received considerable social support from family and community members in their country of origin during these times (Zelkowitz et al. 2004). Single parent refugees are at high risk of isolation and its mental health consequences, especially if they are not proficient in the official language(s) of their settlement countries (Lenette et al. 2012). They are also at high risk of poverty and homelessness. In Canada, most immigrant and refugee families that have experienced homelessness are single mother headed households (Paradis et al. 2008). Children can also act as "a resource and opportunity for resilience (Brodsky et al. 2012)" by providing women with strong motivation to connect to family and community.

Immigrants and refugees may turn to numerous groups for support: immediate and extended family, like-ethnic community, religious community, neighbourhood and mainstream society. Expectations of the support that may be received from these groups are influenced by the support those communities provided in refugees' countries of origin.

The presence of a significant, established like-ethnic community in the city where an immigrant resides has been found to have a positive effect on immigrant mental health (Fenta et al. 2004; Beiser 1999). The like-ethnic community is said to provide some material advantages (e.g., help in finding jobs) and a sense of belonging, cultural identity and historical continuity, which have particular relevance for mental health (Fenta et al. 2004). Also, the more established a particular ethnic community is, the more likely that ethnospecific services (including first-language services) are available.

The literature is particularly limited in its analysis of gender differences in the effect of like-ethnic community support. If women are expected to give more support than they receive, having an established like-ethnic community in the community they resettle in may be draining rather than protective for women.

Research focusing on the social support experiences of immigrants and refugees in Canada has identified the following key issues: lack of informal support, lack of awareness of available formal support, barriers to access to formal support, and discomfort seeking formal support (Mawani 2001). Affirmational support from others who have successfully adapted and emotional support from family, friends and other members of their communities are critical to immigrants' settlement processes during a time when they are separated from family and friends in their countries of origin (Simich et al. 2003).

Quantitative research on social support among refugees has been limited both in quantity and ability to capture the complexity of the issues. In a recent analysis of the Canadian Community Health Survey, 65 % of Whites, 74 % of South Asians, 50 % of Koreans, 52 % of Chinese, 52 % of Southeast Asians and 54 % of Latin Americans (54 %) reported a strong sense of 'community' belonging (Shields 2008), although the 'community' referred to in the question was not explicit[3]. Sense of community belonging was strongly related to self-perceived general and mental health, even when other potentially confounding factors[4] were taken into account (Shields 2008).

Although there has been little research on the health impact of informal or formal social support provided by **religious communities**, there is increasing evidence of an association between religion and **spirituality** and positive health outcomes (Collins and Guruge 2008). Suggested pathways include increased self-esteem, sense of well-being, meaning and purpose in life, increased social support, and sense of community. These benefits take on heightened importance in the context of migration. Many newcomers feel more comfort staying within their own social/ethnic groups for support and a particular discomfort seeking formal mainstream support for what they consider private issues (Mawani 2001; Simich et al. 2004). Some religious communities (e.g. Ismaili Muslim community) provide particularly accessible support in health promotion and chronic disease management that can complement mainstream services, including information sessions and support groups for community members. Such support plays a critical role for immigrants who face informational, language and cultural barriers to seeking formal mainstream support, however, it is important

---

[3] Respondents may have been referring to neighbourhood or ethnic community, and data was not collected on the proportion of like-ethnic community in their neighbourhoods.

[4] Sex, age, marital status, presence of children in household, education, household income, home ownership, language spoken most often at home, cultural or racial group, percent urban composition in health region of residence, province or territory, employment status, smoking status, number of physical chronic conditions, and mood or anxiety disorder in past year.

to note that many communities do not have the resources to provide such services without government support.

Given that there is considerable social and cross-cultural interaction in workplaces (Ray and Bergeron 2007), the impact of workplace social environments on health warrants additional attention in research. More research is also required to focus specifically on the impact of work environments on refugee health. To date, most research has focused on the impact of refugee employment and earnings on health. It is also important to consider how their working conditions impact on their physical and mental health.

Immigrants to Canada face greater occupational health and safety risks to their short- and long-term health than Canadian-born individuals (Smith and Mustard 2009). Immigrants and refugees in Canada for 5 years or less are more likely to have higher qualifications than their jobs require, to have physically demanding jobs and work fewer hours than they want to. Those who are from racialized groups, whose mother tongue is not English or whose advanced degrees are from outside Canada do worse in these situations. Immigrants and refugees in Canada 5 years or less are also less likely to have supervisory responsibilities, be unionized or have non-wage employment benefits (Institute for Work and Health 2008). Recent immigrant and refugee men are twice as likely to sustain workplace injuries than their Canadian-born counterparts (Smith and Mustard 2009). Refugee women are often de-skilled and forced to take on jobs in manufacturing or service industries, characterized by long hours, hard physical labour, instability, and poor earnings and benefits (Mulvihill et al. 2001; Berman et al. 2006; Attanayake 2010).

A number of qualitative studies have captured the impact of such working conditions on their mental health. One narrative study of refugee women in Canada described isolation, with those arriving several decades ago more likely to be isolated in their homes. Many of the study participants described a sense of resignation and experiences of depression (Berman et al. 2006). In another study of unsponsored refugee women in Vancouver, women described lowered self worth, loss of social status, disempowerment and shame associated with their downward spiral of social and economic mobility, and frustration and depression associated with their inability to get out of that spiral (Attanayake 2010).

Despite workplace accommodation laws and policies, many workplaces do poorly at accommodating employees with mental health issues. Accommodation needs of refugees dealing with trauma may be especially misunderstood, and the risks to their mental health of such misunderstanding and resulting unmet accommodation needs are great.

3.4.2 Cultural Factors

Cultural aspects (shared beliefs, values, traditions and behaviors) of communities that refugees are part of affect health. Culture affects health and illness by shaping perceptions of and beliefs about health and illness. Perceptions of illness refers to the identification of symptoms of illness along with their categorization according to levels of severity (Kleinman 1980). Beliefs about illness refers to beliefs about health maintenance, illness causation, and effectiveness of treatment (Ware et al. 1992).

In addition to recognizing the diversity within cultural groups, it is important to recognize that all cultures are dynamic, with their inherent beliefs, values and practices constantly changing and developing (Kirmayer et al. 2000; Mawani 2001). Changes may accelerate in a new country when people are exposed to many new and different ideas. Immigrants may start to question rather than merely accept traditions (Mawani 2001), when those traditions are challenged by the new context they are living in. On the other hand, they may feel more pressure to hold onto beliefs, values, and practices held by their families and cultures of origin when faced with the risk of losing them. This pressure may be magnified in the context of limited opportunity to contribute their values to transforming their new home.

It is challenging to capture the complexity of the many dimensions of culture in health research. As a result, much research reduces the concept to discrete variables such as ethnicity, and overlooks the importance of examining cross-cultural validity of health outcome measures. This has important implications for the interpretation of findings. For example, differences in self-reported health status between racialized and non-racialized groups (Prus and Lin 2005), and immigrants and the Canadian-born (Newbold 2005a, b), may represent artefacts of measurement (reflecting differences in perceptions of health) rather than real health differences. Racialized individuals and refugees may also use different reference groups than non-racialized and/or Canadian-born individuals when asked to rate their health.

A richer understanding of cultural determinants of health is important for informing an understanding of designing and assessing culturally competent health services.

3.4.3 Psychological Factors

Most research focused on psychological determinants of refugee health examines psychological factors at the individual level. The psychological context of the communities that refugees are a part of can affect their health. For example, if a large proportion of a community has experienced trauma it may be difficult for individuals within the community to give or receive support. A Somali participant in a national study describes her experience in Canada: "*Here, there is no one to help you. Everyone is in 'survival mode'* (Simich et al. 2004)." Communities can also demonstrate inspiring resilience in the face of immense challenges. For example, in response to the Asian tsunami, the Toronto Tamil community mobilized, identified needs and accomplished a great deal for communities and families in Sri Lanka as well as those here who needed support (Simich et al. 2006). The Somali community in Canada legally challenging the federal government policy delaying their landed immigrant status (Simich et al. 2004) is another example of such resilience in the face of insurmountable-seeming barriers.

3.4.4 Built Environment

Research on the built environment and health has focused primarily on physical health, namely obesity and diabetes (Lovasi et al. 2009; Glazier and Booth 2007), but has often overlooked the important impact of physical environment on mental health. Physical environments are determinants of mental health issues and illness, and of recovery and well-being. Housing, indoor air quality, and the design of communities and transportation systems can significantly influence physical *and* psychological well-being. Neighbourhood design affects health via factors such as safety, location and quality of playgrounds, access to food and services, and traffic-related pollution (CIHI 2006). Good housing quality and neighbourhood green space promote mental health (CRICH 2012; Guite et al. 2006).

Refugees are often unable to choose their cities, towns, or neighbourhoods, due to national dispersal policies (Andersson 2003; Stewart 2012; Simich et al. 2002; Netto 2011), severe financial limitations that relegate them to high-density low-income neighbourhoods and social housing developments, and/or discrimination (Netto 2011). Close to half of the world's refugees live in urban areas (UNHCR 2009; Netto 2011), while in many cities, refugees are increasingly settling in peri-urban areas due to government dispersion and/or lower cost housing. Whether they settle in urban, peri-urban, or small towns, refugees face unique challenges to their mental health, and show remarkable resilience.

The lack of choice of neighbourhood, specific characteristics of their physical environment, and limited agency to change those characteristics, can negatively impact their mental health. Whether in the heart of cities, or on their perimeters, they are likely to live in neighbourhoods with limited access to healthy food, health and social services, high levels of traffic-related pollution, limited green space, and poor safety, etc. Those in peri- or semi-urban areas have especially limited access to health and social services, and poorer public transportation infrastructure to get to services at a distance from their neighbourhoods. Refugees are also likely to live in neighbourhoods where they feel unsafe, due to a high incidence of crime, violent crime, and/or threats of racial harassment and violence. Physical characteristics, such as segregated and isolated housing, dead-end streets, and poor lighting, may increase both the incidence of crime, and perceptions of neighbourhood safety. Mental health can be detrimentally affected by witnessing of violent acts, or knowledge of violence in their neighbourhoods, in addition to direct experience of violence (Self-Brown et al. 2012).

The built environment has heightened importance for refugees recovering from trauma. It can be re-traumatizing if it presents reminders of trauma associated with imprisonment, torture, violence, etc., or healing if it provides a contrast to environments where traumatic experiences took place. Research on the effect of the built environment on recovery from trauma is limited, but some innovative organizations are incorporating what they have learned from practice.

The Center for Victims of Torture in Minnesota designed the St. Paul Healing Centre, "to meet the needs of torture survivors, with domestic furnishings, large windows and rooms with rounded or angled corners to create an environment much different from the stark square rooms with glaring lights that most torture survivors experienced (Center for Victims of Torture 2012)." Freedom from Torture, based in London, England developed their "Natural Growth Project," to combine horticulture with psychotherapy and facilitate the recovery of their clients (Freedom from Torture 2012). They highlight its instrumental role by explaining,

> Many torture survivors have difficulties talking about their past experiences—or the uncertainty and difficulties of their present. For some of the most physically and mentally damaged clients, being in the open and in touch with the elements can bring instant relief and can open the path to extraordinary change. (Freedom from Torture 2012)

3.5 Family-level factors

There are numerous aspects of the family and household environments that are relevant to mental health. It is especially critical to focus on the family level within a lifecourse approach where the family takes on critical importance in determining health from gestation through to childhood and youth. For refugee communities where immediate and extended family plays a more integral role in individuals' lives, it is necessary to examine and understand family-level determinants in order to design family-level interventions.

Women without official migration status are especially vulnerable to homelessness. They often live in deep poverty with limited access to health care, social assistance and benefits. They are also often in precarious employment situations where they are prone to exploitation. According to Paradis et al. (2008), "for these women, pregnancy and childbirth represent a crisis, making employment impossible, incurring health care costs, and disrupting precarious housing arrangements. Most enter family shelters where they are required to try to regularize their status, although many will not qualify as refugees. Some are deported, while others wait years and spend substantial sums on fees and legal counsel before they and their families can enjoy a life of stability." Under such challenging circumstances, family shelters function as transitional and supportive housing rather than a crisis intervention (Paradis et al. 2008).

Refugees from many 'non-Western' regions of the world have a broad concept of family that includes extended family and often friends/community members, and an interdependent rather than individualistic perspective of life. As a result, family takes on more importance in the provision of support and in individuals' responsibility for providing support, including family remaining in their country of origin, or resettling in other countries. Increased access to transportation and cheaper communication technologies have enabled some groups of immigrants to retain close ties with family and friends in their countries of origin.

Family dynamics and the availability of family support change during the process of migration and these changes impact on health. Family loss or separation, gender role changes, intergenerational tensions and post-migration lifestyle changes often result in increased stress coupled with a loss of post-migration support from extended family and community members (Simich et al. 2004). Those who are unable to retain close ties with family and friends due to financial, geographic and/or political barriers are affected by the stress of separation and anxiety about the welfare of their loved ones (Mawani 2001; Simich et al. 2003).

Sometimes separation of immediate family members occurs during the process of migration. During the process of migration, families may lose members either as victims of war or political violence or may get separated from each other while fleeing. Some family members may come first while other family members follow a few months or years later. Such prolonged separation affects the quality of relationships upon reunification. Separation and reunification can be particularly painful for mothers and children. Parents may also separate from each other during the process of resettling for various reasons, including the stress of migration and resettlement on the family (Mawani 2001). The negative health outcomes of prolonged separation include emotional distress and post-reunification stress on the family (Canadian Council for Refugees 2004).

Even if all immediate family members come to Canada together and stay together, many refugees come from societies where relationships with extended family and community are valued greatly. As a result, they greatly feel the loss of those relationships in Canada, where emphasis is on relationships within the nuclear family (Mawani 2001). Single mothers in particular feel the lack of support and isolation for themselves and their children. The loss of extended family and community relationships due to migration can have a profound influence on children's development (Mawani 2001).

In addition to the impact of prolonged separations on relationship quality, the process of migration and resettlement can place great stress on family relationships. As previously mentioned, parents may separate from each other due to the stress of migration and resettlement. Children experience their own stress during the migration and resettlement process, while at the same time their parent(s) may be emotionally unavailable due to the stress of the process of migration and resettlement (Mawani 2001). Some studies have found that parental unemployment and poor emotional well-being are associated with increases in refugee children's symptoms of mental health issues (Davis et al. 2010).

3.6 Individual-level Factors

3.6.1 Migration Status and Context

Official migration status determines the particular policies that govern the settlement process of immigrants and refugees in Canada. Refugees face particular restrictions in accessing health care, education and employment; refugee claimants have even more limited access to services and resources; and non-status immigrants face the most serious barriers to accessing the services, rights and protections enjoyed by most people living in Canada (Khandor et al. 2004).

Official migration status may not adequately reflect context and reasons for migration. In a study of recent immigrants to Quebec, more than 50 percent of independent and sponsored immigrants cited the political situation in their country of origin as their primary reason for migration (Rousseau and Drapeau 2004). Women, in particular, may not have a choice about their migration due to the dominance of their spouse or male family member(s) in decision-making. It is therefore important to consider migration choice and exposure to premigration trauma as important factors regardless of official migration status.

In addition to reasons for migration, other factors—including country of origin, age at migration, fluency in an official language and length of time in Canada—influence the impact of migration on mental health. Although fluency in an official language has a significant impact on resettlement, there is a need to balance promotion of ESL/FSL with maintenance of mother tongues and recognition of speaking multiple languages as assets.

There is a paucity of research on determinants of mental health for non-heterosexual sexual orientations. Existing research does not focus on the intersection of sexual orientation with race or migration status (Doctor and Bazet 2008). Bisexual people are particularly poorly represented in studies (Doctor and Bazet 2008). For immigrants of diverse sexual orientation, age at migration and legal status have particularly strong implications for mental health. Depending on their age at migration, they may experience migration and coming out concurrently. A lack of permanent residency or citizenship status can reinforce existing feelings of alienation. Individuals with diverse sexual orientation may feel particularly threatened due to fears that disclosing their sexuality could influence their chances of gaining permanent residency or citizenship status (Doctor and Bazet 2008). For refugees in particular, sexual orientation may be one of the reasons for their persecution or torture in their countries of origin, with the nature of persecution potentially differing by gender (women experiencing violence in the home, men experiencing it from strangers outside the home) (Doctor and Bazet 2008).

3.6.2 Socioeconomic Status

Despite the extent to which immigrants and refugees select, or relocate to, the largest cities of Canada, in search of employment, in the 1990s, immigrants and refugees were not as successful in finding employment as their predecessors. This, despite the fact that their average level of education was higher than that of any previous cohort and even higher than that of Canadian born individuals (Omidvar and Richmond 2003; McIsaac 2003; Ruddick 2003).

The change has been dramatic. In the early 1980s, immigrants and refugees (including recent immigrants) had higher labour market participation rates than Canadian-born individuals. In 1991, however, participation rates for immigrants fell below the national average and the gap grew even wider for recent immigrants. The gap persisted and unlike previous cohorts, immigrants who arrived in Canada in the 1990s are not catching up to their Canadian-born counterparts (McIsaac 2003).

Canadian census data (2001) also indicates that higher education was positively associated with higher income for Canadian-born individuals. Individuals with a university degree made up 60 % of those in the top income category (McIsaac 2003). This association between education and income did not apply to immigrants, even including those with a university degree and knowledge of an official language (McIsaac 2003). There was an overrepresentation of university-educated immigrants and refugees in low-skill and low-income jobs, and in occupations of all skill levels, recent immigrants and refugees earned less than Canadian-born individuals (McIsaac 2003)

Recent immigrants and refugees to Canada report higher unemployment rates than non-immigrants (Kinnon 1999). Not surprisingly, unemployment has similarly negative effects on the health of immigrants and refugees as it does for the general Canadian population. Some evidence indicates, however, that unemployment may affect immigrants differently, with more considerable negative effects on mental health (Beiser et al. 1993; Kinnon 1999). The availability and accessibility of job opportunities is important, not only because of the potential income level, sense of purpose, identity and social contact that jobs themselves provide, but because of the important impact of physical and psychosocial environments of workplaces on health (Lynch and Kaplan 2000). Immigrants who are underemployed are likely not only dealing with the psychological impact of a lack of recognition of their skill level, but also with the unhealthier physical and psychosocial environments that often accompany low skill jobs.

Despite the high variability of income and its cumulative impact, most studies measure income at only one point in adulthood. As a result, they are unable to capture the impact of sustained exposure to low income or transitions into and out of low-income groups. Such transitions are important to measure as changes in income tend to be more frequent in low-income groups, who are more likely to experience unstable employment (Lynch and Kaplan 2000). A number of studies have demonstrated strong dose-response relationships between the number of periods of economic hardship and physical, psychological and cognitive functioning (Lynch and Kaplan 2000).

Immigrants are over-represented in low-income groups. Data from the 1994 National Population Health Survey (NPHS) shows that recent immigrants are twice as likely to be living in poverty as Canadian-born individuals (Beiser et al. 1997). Data from the 1994/95 National Longitudinal Study of Children and Youth (NLSCY) indicate a slightly higher proportion of poor immigrant families (Beiser et al. 2002). Beiser et al. (2002) found that 36.4 % of new immigrant children, aged 4–11, lived in poor families, compared with only 13.3 % of children in non-immigrant families. This is clearly an alarming difference and more research is required to examine the duration of and transitions into and out of low income in immigrant populations.

Immigrants in Canada 5 years or less are also less likely to have supervisory responsibilities, be unionized or have non-wage employment benefits (Institute for Work and Health 2008). Results of a study of Sudanese newcomers indicate that unmet employment expectations are associated with psychological distress (Simich et al. 2006).

It is difficult to analyze socioeconomic determinants of mental health by migration status due to limitations in sampling and data collection in Canada's Census and other national surveys. A 1998 Citizenship and Immigration Canada study utilizing the Longitudinal Immigration Database (IMDB) database revealed that Canadian refugees reported substantially lower employment earnings than economic applicants, but similar earnings patterns relative to three other immigrant entry categories (Ruddick 2003). The study also found that refugees who had been in Canada for twelve or more years reported average employment earnings at or near the Canadian-born average. Of more concern are its findings that refugees admitted prior to 1990 reported the highest rates of unemployment benefit usage when compared to any other immigrant category or the Canadian-born population. In addition, after 2 years in Canada, refugees reported the highest rates of social assistance usage (Ruddick 2003).

An analysis of the Longitudinal Survey of Immigrants to Canada (LSIC), found that skilled workers have the highest employment rates both at 6 months and 2 years since arrival, while refugees have the lowest employment rates (20 per cent and over 40 per cent respectively). Highlighting their resilience, refugees demonstrated the greatest improvement (over 20 %) between the two interviews (Yu et al. 2007).

3.7 Discrimination Experience

With the changing demographic profile of immigrants to Canada, and the incongruence between their increasing levels of education and decreasing economic returns, discrimination is a factor that is being increasingly discussed (Dunn and Dyck 2000; McIsaac 2003; Omidvar and Richmond 2003; Ruddick 2003). In the 1990s, 73 % of recent immigrants to Canada were racialized groups[5] (up from 68 % in 1980s and 52 % in 1970s) and by 2016, racialized groups are projected to account for one fifth of Canadian citizens (McIsaac 2003). Analysis of 2001 Census data also demonstrates a remarkable growth in Islam, Hinduism, Sikhism and Buddhism, consistent with changing immigration patterns toward increased immigration from Asia and the Middle East (Statistics Canada 2003a).

Discrimination can be defined as "a socially structured and sanctioned phenomenon, justified by ideology and expressed in interactions, among and between individuals and institutions, intended to maintain privileges for members of dominant groups at the cost of deprivation of others" (Krieger 2000). Refugees may experience diverse levels of discrimination, including: systemic, institutional, and interpersonal. *Systemic discrimination* is "the totality of ways in which societies foster discrimination" (Krieger 2000). *Institutional discrimination* is "discriminatory

---

[5] 'Racialized group' is a term increasingly used by researchers and organizations that recognizes race as a social construct. The Ontario Human Rights Commission clarifies their stance: "Recognizing that race is a social construct, the Commission describes people as "racialized person" or "racialized group" instead of the more outdated and inaccurate terms "racial minority", "visible minority", "person of colour" or "non-White" (Ontario Human Rights Commission 2013)".

policies or practices carried out by state or nonstate institutions" (Krieger 2000). *Interpersonal discrimination* is "directly perceived discriminatory interactions between individuals" (Krieger 2000).

Despite the growing diversity in Canada, the United States, and many countries in Europe, epidemiological research on discrimination as a determinant of mental health is in its infancy (Noh et al. 1999; Krieger 2000). Clearer definitions, and stronger conceptualization and operationalization of discrimination are needed.

Much of the research that has been done is American with simplistic racial divisions (Noh et al. 1999) and no differentiation between newcomers and racialized groups who may have been in the country for generations (Dunn and Dyck 2000). In addition, most of the research is focused on racial discrimination, with only a few including gender discrimination in their analyses (Krieger 2000), and fewer still including discrimination based on age, immigration status, religion or nationality. Combined analyses of the intersecting types of discrimination are important because individuals' health may face discrimination of multiple forms simultaneously (Krieger 2000). They may not be able to disentangle the types of discrimination they are experiencing, and facing more than one may have an additive or multiplicative impact on their mental health.

A systematic review of 138 studies of self-reported racism and health, found a relationship between self-reported racism and ill-health after adjusting for numerous confounders, ranging from demographic factors, to socioeconomic factors, to health risk factors (Paradies 2006). Paradies (2006) highlights a key finding "The strongest and most consistent association is between racism and poor mental health outcomes."

There is a gap in the literature, however, on the pathways by which discrimination influences mental health (Krieger 2000). Discrimination may affect mental health directly or indirectly by limiting access to intermediate determinants such as employment and educational opportunities (Krieger 2000), housing, health care, and social services. It can also do so by traumatizing, re-traumatizing, and disempowering people and groups. Refugees who have already been persecuted by governments in their countries of origin, may be re-traumatized by the experience of discrimination in the countries they settle in, especially when they reasonably assume that they have fled danger to settle in a safe new home.

Some cross-sectional studies have shown a link between discrimination and depression (Noh et al. 1999; Kaspar and Noh 2001) but they have used different and often simplistic measures of discrimination that do not differentiate between levels, sources and types of discrimination. According to Kaspar and Noh (2001), "*Development of comprehensive, multi-dimensional measures that assess the frequency, nature, source, and contexts of discrimination experiences are needed.*" Paradies (2006) advocates for psychometrically validated measures of racism, and a better understanding of the perception, attribution, and reporting of racism. Such measurement improvements can also be applied to measures of other types of discrimination.

Studies that have been conducted do not include explicit focus on the impact of individual perceptions of employment discrimination on depression. Yet this type of discrimination is clearly important to examine. Canada's Ethnic Diversity Survey reveal that of all the places and situations in which people identified experiencing discrimination, the most common was discrimination at work or when applying for a job or promotion (Statistics Canada 2003b). Of those who had sometimes or often experienced discrimination because of their ethno-cultural characteristics in the 5 years prior to the survey, 56 % experienced discrimination at work or when applying for work (Statistics Canada 2003b).

3.8 Conclusion

Applying a multi-level framework, including macro, community, family, and individual level determinants, highlights the complexity of factors affecting refugee mental health. Understanding the complex interplay of diverse factors at different levels, across the lifespan and through the migration process, along with the gaps in our understanding, enable the development of approaches to improve refugee mental health.

In order to address the broad range of determinants of refugee mental health, a "whole-of-government" approach is needed, that involves coordination and integration of efforts across multiple government departments. Australia has been a leader in applying such an approach to mental health, describing it as "public services agencies working across portfolio boundaries to achieve a shared goal and an integrated government response to particular issues. Approaches can be formal or informal. They can focus on policy development, program management, and service delivery" (Christensen and Lægreid 2007). Canada has been applying whole-of-government approaches in various sectors, and recently recommended one be applied to transforming the national mental health system (Mental Health Commission of Canada 2012).

In addition to a multi-portfolio approach, a multi-level government approach is required to address multi-level determinants of mental health. This involves integrated policy development and implementation at federal, provincial, and municipal levels. Workplaces, schools, health, and social service agencies can then develop and implement policies guided by multi-level integrated policy frameworks. Partnerships between diverse mainstream, settlement, and ethno-specific agencies build capacity to improve mental health among refugees. It is essential to take a systemic approach to improving refugee mental health, with determinants at all levels being addressed by a wide range of actors at macro, community, family and individual levels.

References

Agrawal, S., & Qadeer, M. (2008). Faith-based ethnic residential communities and neighbourliness. 63.

Andersson, R. (2003). Settlement dispersal of immigrants and refugees in Europe: Policy and outcomes. 03. Vancouver: Vancouver Centre of Excellence: Research on Immigration and Integration in the Metropolis.

Ascentum. (2009). *Public consultation report: Toward recovery and well-being -A framework for a mental health strategy for Canada*.

Attanayake, V. (2010). *Health issues and needs of unsponsored refugee women in Canada: A qualitative study*. Faculty of Health Sciences, Simon Fraser University.

Auger, N., & Raynault, M. (2006). Summarizing health inequalities in a balanced scorecard: Methodological considerations. *Canadian Journal of Public Health, 97*(5), 350–352.

Baldauf, S. (December 13, 2011). Burqa ban: Canada prohibits Muslim veil in citizenship ceremonies. The Christian Science Monitor.

Beaton, R. D., Murphy, S. A., Houston, J. B., Reyes, G., Bramwell, S., McDaniel, M., Reissman, D. B., & Pfefferbaum, B. (2009). The role of public health in mental and behavioral health in children and families following disasters. *Journal of Public Health Management and Practice, 15*(6), E1–E11.

Beiser, M. (1999). *Strangers at the gate: The 'boat people's first 10 years in Canada'*. Toronto: University of Toronto Press.

Beiser, M. (2005). The health of immigrants and refugees in Canada. *Canadian Journal of Public Health, 96*(Suppl 2), S30–S44.

Beiser, M., Johnson, P. J., & Turner, R. J. (1993). Unemployment, underemployment and depressive affect among Southeast Asian refugees. *Psychological Medicine, 23*(3), 731–743.

Beiser, M., Devins, G., Dion, R., Hyman, I., & Lin, E. (1997). *Immigration, acculturation and health: Report to National Health Research and Development Program. 6606-6414-NPHS*. Ottawa.

Beiser, M., Hou, F., Hyman, I., & Tousignant, M. (2002). Poverty, family process, and the mental health of immigrant children in Canada. *American Journal of Public Health, 92*(2), 220–227.

Berman, H., Giron, E. R., & Marroquin, A. P. (2006). A narrative study of refugee women who have experienced violence in the context of war. *The Canadian journal of nursing research/ Revue canadienne de recherche en sciences infirmieres, 38*(4), 32–53.

Bierman, A., Ahmad, F., & Mawani, F. N. (2009). Gender, migration and health. In V. Agnew (Ed.), Toronto: University of Toronto Press.

Boyd, M. (2009). Official Language Proficiency and the Civic Participation of Immigrants, paper presented at Metropolis Language Matters Symposium, Ottawa, October 22.

Brodsky, A. E., Talwar, G., Welsh, E. A., Scheibler, J. E., Backer, P., Portnoy, G. A., Carrillo, A., & Kline, E. (2012). The hope in her eyes: The role of children in Afghan women's resilience. *The American Journal of Orthopsychiatry, 82*(3), 358–366.

Canadian Council for Refugees. (2004). *More than a nightmare: Delays in refugee family reunification*. Montreal.

Center for Victims of Torture. (2012). Our story. www.cvt.org/who-we-are/history. Accessed June 2012.

Cherfils, M. (June 15, 2010). French Muslim girls flee to private school. Global post.

Christensen, T., & Lægreid, P. (2007). The whole-of-government approach to public sector reform. *Public Administration Review, 67*(6), 1059–1066.

Collins, E., & Guruge, S. (2008). Theoretical perspectives and conceptual frameworks. In S. Guruge & E. M. Collins (Eds.), Toronto: Centre for Addiction and Mental Health.

CRICH. (2012). Neighbourhoods & mental health: CRICH inner city health primer. http://www.stmichaelshospital.com/pdf/crich/neighbourhoodsmental-health.pdf. Accessed 5 Aug 2012.

Cumming-Bruce, N., & Erlanger, S. (2009). November 29, 2009. Swiss Ban Building of Minarets on Mosques. *New York Times*.

Davis, E., Sawyer, M. G., Lo, S. K., Priest, N., & Wake, M. (2010). Socioeconomic risk factors for mental health problems in 4–5-year-old children: Australian population study. *Academic Pediatrics, 10*(1), 41–47.

Doctor, F., & Bazet, S. (2008). Counselling lesbian and bisexual immigrant women of colour. In S. Guruge & E. Collins (Eds.), *Working with immigrant women: Issues and strategies for mental health professionals*. Toronto: Centre for Addiction and Mental Health.

Dunn, J. R., & Dyck, I. (2000). Social determinants of health in Canada's immigrant population: Results from the National Population Health Survey. *Social Science & Medicine (1982), 51*(11), 1573–1593.

Dworkin, J., Prescott, M., Jamal, R., Hardawan, S. A., Abdullah, A., & Galea, S. (2008). The long-term psychosocial impact of a surprise chemical weapons attack on civilians in Halabja, Iraqi Kurdistan. *The Journal of Nervous and Mental Disease, 196*(10), 772–775.

Fenta, H., Hyman, I., & Noh, S. (2004). Determinants of depression among Ethiopian immigrants and refugees in Toronto. *The Journal of Nervous and Mental Disease, 192*(5), 363–372.

Freedom from Torture. (2012). Natural Growth Project. http://www.freedomfromtorture.org/what-we-do/10/11/5109. Accessed June 2012.

Glazier, R., & Booth, G. (2007). *Neighbourhood environments and resources for healthy living—A focus on diabetes in Toronto*. Institute for Clinical Evaluative Sciences.

Gronqvist, H., Johansson, P., & Niknami, S. (2012). *Income inequality and health: Lessons from a refugee residential assignment program*. 11. Institute for Evaluation of Labour Market and Education Policy.

Guite, H. F., Clark, C., & Ackrill, G. (2006). The impact of the physical and urban environment on mental well-being. *Public Health, 120*(12), 1117–1126.

Hanvey, L. (2003). Social inclusion research in Canada: Children and youth: What do we know and where do we go? www.ccsd.ca. Accessed 31 Jan 2013.

Hashemian, F., Khoshnood, K., Desai, M. M., Falahati, F., Kasl, S., & Southwick, S. (2006). Anxiety, depression, and posttraumatic stress in Iranian survivors of chemical warfare. *JAMA: The Journal of the American Medical Association, 296*(5), 560–566.

Heaney, C. A., & Israel, B. A. (1997). Social support and social networks. In K. Glanz, B. Rimer, & F. Lewis (Eds.), *Health behavior and health education: Theory, research, and practice* (2nd ed., pp. 179–205). San Francisco: Jossey-Bass.

Institute for Work and Health. (2008). Immigrant workers experience different health and safety issues. At work.

IOM, UNHCR, & UNU. (2009). Climate change, migration, and displacement: impacts, vulnerability, and adaptation options.

Jones, A. R. (2008). The Maple Bamboo Initiative: Fostering Civic Participation of Canadian Immigrants in Public Processes. Unpublished master's thesis, University of British Columbia, Vancouver, British Columbia.

Kaspar, V., & Noh, S. (2001). Discrimination and identity. An overview of theoretical and empirical research. www.metropolis.net. Accessed 31 Jan 2013.

Khandor, E., Mcdonald, J., Nyers, P., & Wright, C. (2004). *The regularization of non-status immigrants in Canada 1960–2004*. Toronto.

Kinnon, D. (1999). *Canadian research on immigration and health: An overview*. Ottawa: Minister of Public Works and Goverment Services.

Kirmayer, L. J., Brass, G. M., Tait, C. L. (2000). The mental health of Aboriginal Peoples: Transformation of identity and community. *Canadian Journal of Psychiatry, 45*(7), 607–616.

Kleinman, A. (1980). Patients and healers in the context of culture: an exploration of the borderland between anthropology, medicine, and psychiatry. Berkeley: University of California Press.

Krieger, N. (2000). Discrimination and health. In L. F. Berkman & I. Kawachi (Eds.), *Social epidemiology* (pp. 36–75).

Laird, L. D., Amer, M. M., Barnett, E. D., & Barnes, L. L. (2007). Muslim patients and health disparities in the UK and the US. *Archives of Disease in Childhood, 92*(10), 922–926.

Lenette, C., Brough, M., & Cox, L. (2012). *Everyday resilience: Narratives of single refugee women with children*. Qualitative Social Work.

Lock, S., Rubin, G. J., Murray, V., Rogers, M. B., Amlot, R., & Williams, R. (2012). Secondary stressors and extreme events and disasters: A systematic review of primary research from 2010–2011. *PLoS Currents, 4,* 10. 1371/currents.dis.a9b76fed1b2dd5c5bfcfc13c87a2f24f.

Lovasi, G. S., Hutson, M. A., Guerra, M., & Neckerman, K. M. (2009). Built environments and obesity in disadvantaged populations. *Epidemiologic Reviews, 31*(1), 7–20.

Lustig, S. L., Kia-Keating, M., Knight, W. G., Geltman, P., Ellis, H., Kinzie, J. D., Keane, T., & Saxe, G. N. (2004). Review of child and adolescent refugee mental health. *Journal of the American Academy of Child & Adolescent Psychiatry, 43*(1), 24–36.

Lynch, J., & Kaplan, G. (2000). Socioeconomic position. In L. F. Berkman & I. Kawachi (Eds.), *Social epidemiology* (pp. 13–35).

Marmot, M., & Wilkinson, R. (Eds.). (1999). *Social determinants of health*. Oxford: Oxford University Press.

Mawani, F. N. (2001). Sharing attachment across cultures: Learning from immigrants and refugees. Health Canada.

Mawani, F. N. (January 17, 2012). Unveiling a discriminatory policy. *The Mark News*.

Mawani, F., Simich, L., Noor, A., & Wu, F. (2005). Discrimination, social support, and mental health among refugees. McGill Department of Psychiatry Division of Social & Transcultural Psychiatry Advanced Study Institute. April 28–29, 2005.

McGuirk, R. (March 4, 2012). Australian state toughens law for Muslim veils. Huffington Post.

McIsaac, E. (2003). Immigrants in Canadian cities: Census 2001—What do the data tell us? *Policy Options, 24*(5), 58–63.

Mental Health Commission of Canada. (2012). *Changing directions changing lives: The mental health strategy for Canada*. Calgary.

Morgan, A., & Ziglio, E. (2007). Revitalising the evidence base for public health: An assets model. *Promotion & Education, 14*(2), 17–22.

Mulvihill, M., Mailloux, L., & Atki, W. (2001). *Advancing policy and research responses to immigrant and refugee women's health in Canada*. Winnipeg: The Centres of Excellence in Women's Health.

Netto, G. (2011). Strangers in the city: Addressing challenges to the protection, housing and settlement of refugees. *International Journal of Housing Policy, 11*(3), 285–303.

Newbold, K. B. (2005a). Health status and health care of immigrants in Canada: A longitudinal analysis. *Journal of Health Services Research & Policy, 10*, 77–83A.

Newbold, K. B. (2005b). Self-rated health within the Canadian immigrant population: Risk and the healthy immigrant effect. *Social Science & Medicine, 60*, 1359–1370.

Noh, S., Beiser, M., Kaspar, V., Hou, F., & Rummens, J. (1999). Perceived racial discrimination, depression, and coping: A study of southeast Asian refugees in Canada. *Journal of Health and Social Behavior, 40*(3), 193–207.

Omidvar, R., & Richmond, T. (2003). *Immigrant settlement and social inclusion in Canada*. The Laidlaw Foundation.

Ontario Human Rights Commission. (2013). Racial discrimination, race, and racism (fact sheet). http://www.ohrc.on.ca/en/racial-discrimination-race-and-racism-fact-sheet. Accessed Jan 2013.

Paradies, Y. (2006). A systematic review of empirical research on self-reported racism and health. *International Journal of Epidemiology, 35*(4), 888–901.

Paradis, E., Novac, S., Sarty, M., & Hulchanski, J. D. (2008). *Better off in a shelter?: A year of homelessness & housing among status immigrant, non-status migrant, & Canadian-born families*. Centre for Urban and Community Studies, Cities Centre, University of Toronto.

Pickett, K. E., James, O. W., & Wilkinson, R. G. (2006). Income inequality and the prevalance of mental illness: A preliminary international analysis. *Journal of Epidemiology and Community Health (1979-), 60*(7), 646–647.

Project Economic Refugee. (2012). What does economic refugee mean? www.economicrefugee.net/what-does-economic-refugee-mean/ Accessed Nov 2012.

Prus, S., & Lin, Z. (2005). Ethnicity and health: an analysis of physical health differences across twenty-one ethnocultural groups in Canada (SEDAP Research Paper No. 143, McMaster University). Hamilton, ON: SEDAP, McMaster University.

Raphael, D. (Ed.). (2004). *Social determinants of health: Canadian perspectives*. Toronto: Canadian Scholars' Press.

Ray, B., & Bergeron, J. (2007). Geographies of ethnocultural diversity in a second-tier city. *Our Diverse Cities, 4*, 44–47.

Rousseau, C., & Drapeau, A. (2004). Premigration exposure to political violence among independent immigrants and its association with emotional distress. *The Journal of Nervous and Mental Disease, 192*(12), 852–856.

Rousseau, C., Hassan, G., Moreau, N., & Thombs, B. D. (2011). Perceived discrimination and its association with psychological distress among newly arrived immigrants before and after September 11, 2001. *American Journal of Public Health, 101*(5), 909–915.

Ruddick, E. (2003). *Immigrant economic performance—A new paradigm in a changing labour market*. Citizenship and Immigration Canada.

Self-Brown, S., Leblanc, M. M., David, K., Shepard, D., Ryan, K., Hodges, A., & Kelley, M. L. (2012). The impact of parental trauma exposure on community violence exposed adolescents. *Violence and Victims, 27*(4), 512–526.

Sherbourne, C. D., & Stewart, A. L. (1991). The MOS social support survey. *Social Science & Medicine (1982), 32*(6), 705–714.

Sheridan, L. P. (2006). Islamophobia pre- and post-september 11th, 2001. *Journal of Interpersonal Violence, 21*(3), 317–336.

Shields, M. (2008). Community belonging and self-perceived health. *Health Reports, 19*(2), 10.

Simich, L., Beiser, M., & Mawani, F. (2002). Paved with good intentions: Canada's refugee destining policy and paths of secondary migration. *Canadian Public Policy, 28*(4), 597–607.

Simich, L., Beiser, M., & Mawani, F. N. (2003). Social support and the significance of shared experience in refugee migration and resettlement. *Western Journal of Nursing Research, 25*(7), 872–891.

Simich, L., Mawani, F., Wu, F., & Noor, A. (2004). Meanings of social support, coping, and help-seeking strategies among immigrants and refugees in Toronto. CERIS Working Paper (67).

Simich, L., Hamilton, H., & Baya, B. K. (2006). Mental distress, economic hardship and expectations of life in Canada among Sudanese newcomers. *Transcultural Psychiatry, 43*(3), 418–444.

Smith, P. M., & Mustard, C. A. (2009). Comparing the risk of work-related injuries between immigrants to Canada and Canadian-born labour market participants. *Occupational and Environmental Medicine, 66*(6), 361–367.

Statistics Canada. (2003a). *2001 census: Analysis series—Religions in Canada*. Ottawa: Minister of Industry.

Statistics Canada. (2003b). Ethnic diversity survey: Portrait of a multicultural society.

Stewart, E. S. (2012). UK dispersal policy and onward migration: Mapping the current state of knowledge. *Journal of Refugee Studies, 25*(1), 25–49.

Taylor, S., & Seeman, T. (1999). Psychosocial resources and the SES-health relationship. *Annals of the New York Academy of Sciences, 896*, 210–225.

Topor, A., Borg, M., Di Girolama, S., & Davidson, L. (2011). Not just an individual journey: Social aspects of recovery. *International Journal of Social Psychiatry, 57*(1), 90–99.

Turner, R. J., Lloyd, D. A., & Roszell, P. (1999). Personal resources and the social distribution of depression. *American Journal of Community Psychology, 27*(5), 643–672.

UNHCR. (2009). *UNHCR policy on refugee protection and solutions in urban areas*. Geneva: UNHCR.

Ware, N., Christakis, N., & Kleinman, A. (1992). An Anthropological Approach to Social Science Research on the Health Transition. New York: Auburn House.

Wilkinson, R. G., & Pickett, K. E. (2009). Income inequality and social dysfunction. *Annual Review of Sociology, 35*, 493–511.

Williams, D. R., Neighbors, H. W., & Jackson, J. S. (2008). Racial/ethnic discrimination and health: Findings from community studies. *American Journal of Public Health, 98*(9 Suppl), S29–37.

Yu, S., Ouellet, E., & Warmington, A. (2007). Refugee integration in Canada: A survey of empirical evidence and existing services. *Refuge, 24*(2), 17–34.

Zelkowitz, P., Schinazi, J., Katofsky, L., Saucier, J. F., Valenzuela, M., Westreich, R., & Dayan, J. (2004). Factors associated with depression in pregnant immigrant women. *Transcultural Psychiatry, 41*(4), 445–464.

Chapter 4
The Debate About Trauma and Psychosocial Treatment for Refugees

Clare Pain, Pushpa Kanagaratnam and Donald Payne

Abstract Accepted Western guidelines for the treatment of trauma survivors who are diagnosed with Posttraumatic Stress Disorder (PTSD) demonstrate an emerging consensus with regard to treatment. All of the guidelines cite strong evidence for the inclusion of an exposure component to treatment. However, the accumulated evidence base for the treatment of patients with PTSD is drawn from trials that almost exclusively do not include refugees. The question this chapter explores is the advisability of using an exposure component to the treatment of refugees who have suffered traumatic experiences and who remain symptomatic. Do we have clear evidence that exposure techniques are necessary or even advisable to resolve the psychological difficulties that refugees experience? Based on a number of reasons, the authors suggest that in the first years of resettlement and adaptation, successful treatment should be focused on settlement issues.

Keywords Psychological trauma · Exposure therapy · Evidence based treatments

The accepted Western guidelines from the USA, UK and Australia (American Psychiatric Association 2004; Australian Centre for Posttraumatic Mental Health 2007; VA/DoD Clinical Practice Guideline Working Group 2004/2010; Foa, E. B. et al. 2008; National Institute for Health and Clinical Excellence 2005; Institute of Medicine 2007; Cohen, J. A. et al. 2010) for the treatment of trauma survivors who are diagnosed with Posttraumatic Stress Disorder (PTSD) demonstrate an emerging consensus with regard to treatment. All of the guidelines cite strong evidence

---

C. Pain (✉)
Department of Psychiatry, University of Toronto; Mount Sinai Hospital,
Room 934, 600 University Avenue, Toronto, ON M5G 1X5, Canada
e-mail: cpain@mtsinai.on.ca

P. Kanagaratnam
Department of Psychiatry, Faculty of Medicine, University of Toronto, ON, Canada

Centre for Addiction & Mental Health, Toronto, ON, Canada

D. Payne
Health Network, Amnesty International (English Speaking) Canada, 1992 Yonge Street,
3rd floor, Toronto M4S 1Z7, Canada

for the inclusion of an exposure component to treatment, most usually Trauma Focused Cognitive Behavioural Therapy (TF-CBT) and Prolonged Exposure. For TF-CBT, the patient is required to write a trauma narrative of their experience. For the treatment called Prolonged Exposure there are two components of exposure. One is imaginal exposure which involves a recounting of the traumatic experience to desensitize the individual to memories of their trauma, and the second is a behavioural desensitization to ambient reminders of trauma which function as triggers for fear and avoidance. Of importance, the accumulated evidence base for the treatment of patients with PTSD is drawn from trials that almost exclusively do not include refugees (Bisson and Andrew 2007; Stein et al. 2006).

The question this paper will explore is the advisability of using an exposure component to the treatment of refugees who have suffered traumatic experiences and who remain symptomatic. Do we have clear evidence that exposure techniques are necessary or even advisable to resolve the psychological difficulties that refugees experience? Based on a number of reasons that this chapter will identify, we lobby against requiring refugees with PTSD to have an exposure component in their treatment. We suggest that in the first long phase of resettlement, and re-adaptation (estimated in years not months) successful treatment is focused on settlement issues.

Refugees make up a special population not only because they are newcomers to Canada but because by definition they have "a well-founded fear of being persecuted for reasons of race, religion, nationality, membership of a particular social group or political opinion, is outside the country of his nationality and is unable or, owing to such fear, is unwilling to avail himself of the protection of that country; or who, not having a nationality and being outside the country of his former habitual residence as a result of such events, is unable or, owing to such fear, is unwilling to return to it" (UN General Assembly, 28th July, 1951).

Traumatic experiences such as politically organized collective violence against civilians, war and intimidation or targeted individual violence are almost an inevitably a part of the experience of refugees. Although immigrants are usually in good health upon arrival to Canada, vulnerable subgroups including refugees have been identified especially with respect to mental health issues. Forty primary care practitioners in Canada with experience of working with refugees identified torture and PTSD as major concerns (Swinkels et al. 2010). The priority issues associated with mental health identified within the refugee population were abuse, domestic violence, anxiety, adjustment disorders and depression, all of which could be directly or indirectly related to experiences of torture and organized violence, and subsequent resettlement difficulties.

That some or even many refugees may be distressed and have psychological symptoms and difficulties is not contested. Fazel et al. (2005) notes in a systemic review of research into the mental health of 7,000 refugees that they "could be about ten times more likely to have Posttraumatic Stress Disorder than age-matched general populations in those countries." However, do we know how best to treat PTSD in refugees? In a recent study in Afghanistan, the diagnosis of PTSD was found to be valid but noted to have limited clinical utility (Miller et al. 2009). How do we know if the distress and symptoms of PTSD arise as a result of previous traumatic experiences or whether they arise or are exacerbated by the struggles and complications of settlement: the refugee hearing; separation from family, friends and colleagues; financial stress; the almost inevitably lower job status and pay if the refugee does find work; and the problems of adapting to life in Canada? There is a lack of research concerning non-traumatic events including settlement that cause distress and mental illness in refugees (Basoglu et al. 1994; Silove et al. 1998) and as has been noted by Mollica (2004), distress in a refugee is usually assumed to be restricted to PTSD.

The appropriate treatment for psychologically distressed refugees will depend on the clinician's diagnosis or the attribution of the refugee's symptoms and suffering. However, deciding whether a refugee has a mental health disorder is difficult for several reasons, five of which we explore in this chapter: (1) differences between the explanatory models held by refugee and Western clinician that confound the clinical assessment; (2) lack of culturally valid assessment tools; (3) complications of using interpreters; (4) the issue of whether PTSD is the most appropriate illness construct for traumatized refugees with multiple symptoms, and (5) the dearth of studies concerning the psychiatric/psychological treatment of refugees.

1. *There are differences between the explanatory models held by refugees and western clinicians that confound the clinical assessment;*

In recognising the gap between the refugee's need and the provision of appropriate services it is important to take account of the conceptual and interactional differences between refugees and the health system that potentially provides primary and mental health services.

Kleinman (1980) suggests that the explanatory models or ideas about the cause and treatment of an episode of illness held by the medical profession are radically different from those held by people from different non Western cultures. The clinical interview of a distressed refugee by a primary health care practitioner or a mental health professional offers no easy access to understanding the refugee's distress. The clinician's observations, used as a basis for diagnosis are organized by the refugee's expression (or lack of expression) of distress. This in turn is structured by the refugee's culture of origin which shapes communication style (e.g. direct or indirect eye contact, and nonverbal communication), family roles, beliefs and ideas about the causes of distress, and ways of regulating aggression and other emotions. Because of these profound differences between the refugee and clinician, the risk of the clinician either under or overcalling psychiatric diagnoses is great (Andermann and Lo 2010; Fazel 2005). Crumish and O'Rourke (2010, p. 237) write "stigma, shame, numbing, therapist bias and culturally differing conceptualizations of trauma and illness may equally hinder communication."

Psychiatrists and other mental health professionals are trained to detect and treat mental illness. Taylor (2003) suggests that medical professionals belong to a culture just as surely as refugees, although to the medical professional concerned it is invisible and un-experienced. Taylor calls it "the culture of no culture." One of the expectations of this culture is that a health care professional looks for pathology (not resilience) in a refugee and makes a diagnosis which is often PTSD, as though this and possibly treatment with medications and therapy ends their encounter satisfactorily. The diagnosis of PTSD is frequently made whether or not the refugee has some symptoms but remains functional and optimistic. Within the invisible culture of health professionals, refugees are patients, largely because of their history of trauma and the fact they are meeting with a health care professional also designates them patients. Many health professionals do not usually recognise the refugee as highly resilient and probably having a difficult time getting settled in Canada. To complicate matters refugees themselves very often indicate the traumatic experiences that bring them to Canada assuming this is the appropriate history for the clinician; the clinician may also have their narrative account from Immigration Services available. Inevitably the refugee is distressed as a result of telling the story again, but the clinician assumes the trauma is the sole cause of the distress. With little else to inform the clinician, he or she is at great risk of projecting on to the refugee his or her own imagined response to the horror of the stories they hear, and fail to inquire further into what the refugee is finding difficult in their current life. Little or no attempt is made to explore the refugee's aspirations, dreams, ambitions and hopes. Too often, refugees are pathologised by attributing all distress to their past traumatic experiences and the causes of their current distress remain unexplored.

Two examples illustrate this problem: a 28 year old engineer and refugee who had been in Canada for 3 months was referred for a psychiatric assessment for distress. He was accompanied by an interpreter and the clinician heard how his father had been killed in front of him, how his leg was severely and permanently disabled by a bomb blast, and finally that his girlfriend has been killed by her family for dating him. His life was endangered by her family and he had fled to Canada. In the interview he had a lot to say, his speech was fluent and his distress congruent with the painful events he related. At the end of reporting his story he emphasised his suffering, the clinician responded to him with sympathy for his losses and congratulations that he had reached a safe country. The clinician also asked if there was a current issue frustrating and upsetting him. Exasperated, he said that he was the only son of his parents, and spoiled, and had never learned to cook. He now lived in an apartment with another young man and needed assistance. Cooking lessons proved to be the most beneficial therapy as well as encouragement to learn English.

The second example is of a middle aged African woman who came to the clinic for assessment of her anxiety. She was a very well groomed woman and reported that most of her family had been killed in a civil war in her country over 20 years ago and she worried about her remaining children there. The clinician did not understand the link between the clients immaculate appearance, the long standing problem of her family tragedy and her relatively new onset anxiety. After offering her condolences on the significant losses the client had suffered, the clinician raised her failure to understand what the problems were that caused the client's symptoms. The client explained she was in level 3 English as a Second Language (ESL) where she was learning to read and write for the first time. She had become anxious as she moved into the third level because everyone in her level were well educated professionals. She said, unlike her classmates, she had never been to school so had no idea how to do homework. She was very scared of no longer being able to keep up academically, but it mattered to her very much to do so. Taking pride in her appearance was linked to her pride in her literacy and English language training, an achievement now under threat.

At the Canadian Center for Victims of Torture where this client was assessed, the clinician was able to request two hours of tuition a week which was gratefully accepted by the client as the treatment of choice.

Ideally, future mental health training curricula will focus equally on the social determinants of health, which as Chokshi (2010) reports "reveal the mechanisms by which living conditions cause disease," as well as on a disease approach to mental illness where the focus is on molecular and organ system pathology. As a consequence, health and mental health professionals would have a more complex understanding of the proximal causes of mental distress which include social circumstances, environmental conditions, and behavioural choices which go beyond the deleterious effects of torture and war. As Kleinman and others wrote (Kleinman et al. 1997): "Social suffering... brings into a single space an assemblage of human problems that have their origins and consequences in the devastating injuries that social forces can inflict on human experience. Social suffering results from what political, economic, and institutional power does to people and, reciprocally, from how these forms of power themselves influence responses to social problems. Included under the category of social suffering are conditions that are usually divided among separate fields, conditions that simultaneously involve health, welfare, legal, moral, and religious issues. They destabilize established categories. For example, the trauma, pain, and disorders to which atrocity gives rise are health conditions; yet they are also political and cultural matters."

Refugees are less patients and more people caught in a system that is not sufficiently designed for their needs, but which if attended to can be expected to reduce their distress and the likelihood of mental illness.

2. *The lack of culturally valid assessment tools*

When questionnaires are used to assess or diagnose distress in refugees it has been frequently recognized that measurement is made with instruments developed in the west with little or no attention to cultural validity (Hollifield et al. 2002; Campbell 2007; Johnson and Thompson 2008; Crumlish and O'Rourke 2010; Kanagaratnam 2012). As a consequence of the differences in manifestations of distress and the lack of culturally valid assessment approaches to capture these issues, survivors of torture and politically organized violence are considered to present particularly complex challenges with regard to diagnosis and treatment (Nicholl and Thompson 2004).

3. *The complications of using interpreters*

The use of interpreters can also complicate the clinical interview by introducing another person who according to Miller et al. (2005) must be properly trained to deal sensitively with vulnerable scenarios. An inattentive or insensitive interpreter can make the client less able to disclose their concerns. Miller goes on to note that some interpreters interject their own opinion and views, or decide what questions they feel are appropriate to ask the client. Interpreters can understate or amplify the client's symptoms particularly when a family member is used as a substitute for an interpreter (Eytan et al. 2002). Confidentiality is also an issue as some clients feel more comfortable if the interpreter is not from their community (Kirmayer et al. 2011). Farooq and Fear (2003) suggest that the use of interpreters inevitably interferes with the quality of communication; Pugh and Vetere (2009) suggest this is particularly true for the communication of empathy. Importantly, Kanagaratnam (2012) suggests that some interpreters are biased toward preferring a Western based biomedical model of mental health and have a tendency to downplay their own indigenous understandings and practices as primitive or backward. This can impact their ability to interpret a client's issues from the client's perspective.

4. *Is PTSD the most appropriate illness construct for traumatized refugees?*

As Hollifield (2005) writes "culture, language and polytrauma complicate illness experience and diagnosis." A major controversy in refugee mental health has been the universality versus the cultural applicability of the diagnosis and framework of PTSD to capture the mental distress of refugees who have been exposed to traumatic events (Kienzler 2008). The argument in favour of the use of PTSD as valid across cultures is that the symptoms constitute a universal fear response to terrifying events, and in the last 25 years there have been countless studies of structural and functional brain changes in patients suffering from PTSD. However, Spitzer, the architect of the DSM-III and others (Rosen et al. 2008) note many problems with the diagnosis PTSD; that although the diagnosis requires the aetiological precursor to the symptoms as part of the criterion, there is plenty of evidence that PTSD can occur without a significant life threatening trauma (Cameron et al. 2010) and that even when PTSD does result from a life threatening event, the pre trauma variables and the availability of social support post trauma do more to influence the emergence of PTSD than the trauma itself (Ozer et al. 2003). The role of empathic and practical social support in the context of resettlement is helpful in reducing symptoms and optimizing function in newly arrived refugees.

PTSD has also been criticised as a diagnosis for non-Western cultural groups because the framework is derived mainly from the experience of American Vietnam veterans in the West, and has been reflexively extended to non-western populations (Almedom and Summerfield 2004; Bracken 2001; Summerfield 1999).

There is limited research concerning the psychiatric/psychological treatment of refugees. Kleinman (1977) coined the term "category fallacy" to describe the pitfall of projecting one cultural diagnosis into another culture, without considering its coherence and validity in the other culture. This appears to be a tendency in many studies that mostly look for PTSD and other depressive symptomatology following trauma; once found, they argue for its existence and validity in the other cultures. Hollifield et al. (2002) also addresses this issue, pointing to studies that fail to describe the connection between diagnosis and their relevance to clinically significant impairment. They indicate the need for a better theoretical framework to disentangle the glitches in assessment in the field of refugee trauma.

5. *The dearth of studies concerning the psychiatric/psychological treatment of refugees*

Although the problems of capturing emotional distress in refugees has been pointed out for more than two decades (e.g., Kleinman 1977; Zur 1996; Bracken 2001), this has not resulted in a consensus on best practices for refugees or an attempt to integrate alternative approaches into clinical work as recommended.

In a recent systematic review of treatments for refugees and asylum seekers diagnosed with PTSD, Crumlish & O'Rourke (2010) found only 10 randomized controlled trials for the psychotherapy of refugees with PTSD. They were small trials and sufficiently flawed that the authors concluded that no treatment was found to be firmly supported. Of note, they also wrote that there are no empirical studies designed or led by professionals who are or were refugees or who belong to the culture of the group they are studying. Thus, they write a local understanding of trauma and psychological distress among the refugee population is not reflected in the literature. They quote Summerfield (1999) "social healing and the remaking of worlds cannot be managed by outsiders." This important observation becomes more complicated for the refugee who is also trying to become an "insider" within the country of migration.

4.1 Conclusion

In spite of growing research in the field, there is not yet an evidence-based method of assessing and treating refugee survivors of torture, (Johnson and Thompson 2008; Crumlish and O'Rourke 2010) a deficit noted in the several Western guidelines for the treatment of PTSD which do not recognise refugees as a different group. Until now, there is no agreement on the appropriate mental health care for war traumatized individuals (Kienzler 2008), and the existing literature is not adequate to derive any conclusions regarding treatment efficacy and treatment of choice for torture survivors (Campbell 2007).

The few randomized controlled trials that exist in the area of refugee trauma treatment are limited to PTSD. Wampold et al. (2010) concluded there is a lack of evidence for exposure as the treatment of choice for refugees with PTSD. Related here is the recommendation by Bernardes et al. (2010) that the NICE guidelines' emphasis on a PTSD diagnosis and CBT as a treatment be re-considered when it comes to refugees. They argue that although many asylum seekers in the UK can be diagnosed with PTSD, they had other valid concerns regarding post-migration factors that need to be focused on more usefully in psychological treatment. It has also been pointed out that symptoms of PTSD may not always indicate past trauma or torture, but instead reflect current trauma in their country of resettlement through isolation, hostility, violence, and racism (Summerfield 1996). Beiser (1999) in an elegant study of the Vietnam boat people who resettled in Canada in the 1970s, noted that those who spent more time thinking of the past than the present and future had a worse outcome.

We would add that our clinical experience at the Canadian Centre of Victims of Torture, an agency specializing in the provision of various kinds of assistance to refugees, has provided a rich source of clinical learning about the needs of tortured refugees. The psychiatrists in the centre are an important component for the occasional refugee with, for instance, suicidal feelings, addictions and psychotic disorders. But working at this agency has taught us to look beyond the refugees' symptoms and explore and ameliorate the causes of distress in the 'here and now' of the complexity of resettlement in Canada. We find a refugee's symptoms improve once they have been accepted as a convention refugee, and seldom find medications and therapy popular or useful options for the clients. Most usually English lessons, the pairing of a befriender (volunteer) with the refugee, homework club for refugee children, music and art groups, cooking club and other similar group activities form the most popular and useful "treatments." The routine employment of exposure techniques to desensitize the refugee to their experiences of war, torture and other atrocities seems, in our experience and in reading the literature on the subject, to have no role in their successful treatment. However, follow-up studies of distressed refugees, and community-based research on the long term adjustment and mental well-being of accepted convention refugees are necessary, to evaluate current services. They would also identify the need for developing individual or collective approaches to further support the successful settlement and prosperity of convention refugees in their new home.

References

Almedom, A., & Summerfield, D. (2004). Mental well-being in settings of complex emergency: An overview. *Journal of Biosocial Science, 36,* 381–388.
American Psychiatric Association. (2004). *Practice guideline for the treatment of patients with acute stress disorder and posttraumatic stress disorder.* Arlington, VA.
Andermann, L., & Lo, H.-T. (2010). Cultural competence in psychiatric assessment. In D. Goldbloom (Ed.), *Psychiatric clinical skills* (Revised 1st ed.). Toronto: CAMH. (Originally published by Elsevier Canada 2006).
Australian Centre for Posttraumatic Mental Health. (2007). *Australian guidelines for the treatment of adults with acute stress disorder and posttraumatic stress disorder.* Melbourne, Australia.
Basoglu, M., Parker, M., Ozman, E., Tasdemir, O., & Sahin, D. (1994). Factors related to long-term traumatic stress responses in survivors of torture in Turkey. *The Journal of the American Medical Association, 272,* 357–363.
Beiser, M. (1999). *Strangers at the gate: The "Boat People's" first 10 years in Canada.* Toronto: University of Toronto Press.
Bernardes, D., Wright, J., Edwards, C., Tomkins, H., DIfoz, D., & Livingstone, A. G. (2010). Asylum seekers' perspectives on their mental health and views on health and social services: Contributions for service provision using a mixed-methods approach. *International Journal of Migration, Health and Social Care, 6*(4), 3–19.
Bisson, J., & Andrew, M. (2007). Psychological treatment of post-traumatic stress disorder (PTSD). Cochrane Database Syust Rev: CD003388.
Bracken, P. J. (2001). Post-modernity and post-traumatic stress disorder. *Social Science and Medicine, 53*(6), 733–743.

Cameron, A., Palm, K., & Follette, V. (2010). Reaction to stressful life events: What predicts symptom severity? *Journal of Anxiety Disorders, 24*(6), 645–649.

Campbell, T. A. (2007). Psychological assessment, diagnosis and treatment of torture survivors: A review. *Clinical Psychology Review, 27,* 628–641.

Chokshi, D. (2010). Teaching about health disparities using a social determinants framework. *Journal of General Internal Medicine, 25*(Suppl 2), 182–185.

Cohen, J. A., Bukstein, O., Walter, H., Benson, R. S., Christman, A., Farchione, T. R., et al. (2010). Practice parameter for the assessment and treatment of posttraumatic stress disorder in children and adolescents. *Journal of the American Academy of Child and Adolescent Psychiatry, 49,* 414–430.

Crumlish, N., & O'Rourke, K. (2010). A systematic review of treatments for post-traumatic stress disorder in refugees and asylum seekers. *The Journal of Nervous and Mental Disease, 198*(4), 237–251.

Eytan, A., Bischoff, A., Rrustemi, I., Durieux, S., Loutan, S., Gilbert, M., & Bovier, P. A. (2002). Screening of mental disorders in asylum seekers from Kosovo. *The Australian and New Zealand Journal of Psychiatry, 36,* 499–503.

Farooq, S., & Fear, F. (2003). Working through interpreters. *Advances in Psychiatric Treatment, 9,* 104–109.

Fazel, M., Wheeler, J., & Danesh, J. (2005). Prevalence of serious mental disorder in 7000 refugees resettled in western countries: A systemic review. *Lancet, 365,* 1309–1314.

Foa, E. B., Keane, T. M., Friedman, M. J., & Cohen, J. (Eds.). (2008). *Effective treatments for PTSD: Practice guidelines from the International Society for Traumatic Stress Studies* (2nd ed.). New York: Guilford Press.

Hollifield, M. (2005). Taking measure of war trauma. *Lancet, 365*(9467), 1283–1284.

Hollifield, M., Warner, T. D., Lian, N., Krakow, B., Jenkins, J. H., Kesler, J., Stevenson, J., & Westermeyer, J. (2002). Measuring trauma and health status in refugees. *Journal of the American Medical Association, 288,* 611–621.

Institute of Medicine. (2007). *Treatment of PTSD: Assessment of the evidence.* Washington, DC: National Academies Press.

Johnson, H., & Thompson, A. (2008). The development and maintenance of post-traumatic stress disorder (PTSD) in civilian adult survivors of war trauma and torture: A review. *Clinical Psychology Review, 28,* 36–47.

Kanagaratnam, P. (2012). Personal communications.

Kienzler, H. (2008). Debating war-trauma and post-traumatic stress disorder (PTSD) in an interdisciplinary arena. *Social Science and Medicine, 67,* 218–227.

Kirmayer, J., Narasiah, L., Munoz, M., Rashid, M., Ryder, A. G., Guzder, J., Hassan, G., Rousseau, C., & Pottie, K. (2011). Common mental health problems in immigrants and refugees: General approach in primary care: Canadian Guidelines for Immigrant Health. *Canadian Medical Association Journal, 183*(12), E959–E966.

Kleinman, A. (1977). Culture and illness: A question of models. *Culture, Medicine and Psychiatry, 1*(3), 229–231.

Kleinman, A. (1980). Major conceptual and research issues for cultural (anthropological) psychiatry. *Culture Medicine & Psychiatry, 4*(1), 3–13.

Kleinman, A., Das, V., & Lock, M. (Eds.). (1997). *Social suffering.* Berkeley: University of California Press.

Miller, K. E., Martell, Z. L., Pazdirek, L., Caruth, M., & Lopez, D. (2005). The role of interpreters in psychotherapy with refugees: An exploratory study. *The American Journal of Orthopsychiatry, 75,* 27–39.

Miller, K. E., Omidian, P., Kulkarni, M., Yaqubi, A., Daudzai, H., & Rasmussen, A. (2009). The validity and clinical utility of post-traumatic stress disorder in Afghanistan. *Transcultural Psychiatry, 46,* 219–237.

Mollica, R. F. (2004). Global health: Surviving torture. *The New England Journal of Medicine, 351*(1), 5–7.

National Institute for Health and Clinical Excellence. (2005). *Post-traumatic stress disorder*. London: Royal College of Psychiatrists and The British Psychological Society.

Nicholl, C., & Thompson, A. (2004). The psychological treatment of post traumatic stress disorder (PTSD) in adult refugees: A review of the current state of psychological therapies. *Journal Mental Health, 13,* 351–362.

Ozer, E. J., Best, S. R., Lipsey, T. L., & Weiss, D. S. (2003). Predictors of posttraumatic stress disorder and symptoms in adults: A meta-analysis. *Psychological Bulletin, 129,* 52–73.

Pugh, M. A., & Vetere, A. (2009). Lost in translation: An interpretive phenomenological analysis of mental health professionals' experience of empathy in clinical work with an interpreter. *Psychology and Psychotherapy, 82,* 305–321.

Rosen, G. M., Spitzer, R. L., & McHugh, P. R. (2008). Problems with the post-traumatic stress disorder diagnosis and its future in DSM-V. *The British Journal of Psychiatry, 192,* 3–4.

Silove, D., Steel, Z., McGorry, P., & Mohan, P. (1998). Trauma exposure, post-migration stressors, and symptoms of anxiety, depression and post-traumatic stress in Tamil asylum seekers: Comparison with refugees and immigrants. *Acta Psychiatrica Scandinavica, 97,* 175–181.

Stein, D. J., Ipser, J. C., & Seedat, S. (2006). Pharmacotherapy for post traumatic stress disorder (PTSD). Cochrane Database Syst Rev. CD 002795.

Summerfield, D. (1996). *The impact of war and atrocity on civilian populations: Basic principles of NGO interventions and a critique of psycho-social trauma projects*. London: Relief and Rehabilitation Network, Overseas Development Institute.

Summerfield, D. (1999). A critique of seven assumptions behind psychological trauma programmes in war-affected areas. *Social Science and Medicine, 48,* 1449–1462.

Swinkels, H., Pottie, K., Tugwell, P., Rashid, M., & Narasiya, L. (2010). Development of guidelines for recently arrived immigrants and refugees to Canada: Delphi consensus on selecting preventable and treatable conditions. *Canadian Medical Association Journal*, early release, published at www.cmaj.ca on June 28, 2010; Subject to revision.

Taylor, J. (2003). Confronting "culture" in medicine's "culture of no culture". *Academic Medicine, 78,* 555–559.

UN General Assembly. (28 July, 1951). Convention relating to the status of refugees (Electronic Version). United Nations, Treaty Series, vol. 189, p. 137. http://www.unhcr.org/refworld/docid/3be01b964.html. (Accessed 6 July 2012)

VA/DoD Clinical Practice Guideline Working Group. (2004/2010). *Management of post-traumatic stress*. Washington, DC: VA Office of Quality and Performance.

Wampold, B. E., Imel, Z. E., Laska, K. M., Benish, S., Miller, S. D., Fluckiger, C., Del Re, A. C., Baardseth, T. P., & Budge, S. (2010). Determining what works in the treatment of PTSD. *Clinical Psychology Review, 30,* 923–933.

Zur, J. (1996). From PTSD to voices in context: from an "experience-far" to an "experience-near" understanding of responses to war and atrocity across cultures. *International Journal of Social Psychiatry, 42*(4), 305–317.

Chapter 5
Reflections on Using a Cultural Psychiatry Approach to Assessing and Fortifying Refugee Resilience in Canada

Lisa Andermann

> *Yeah, believe it or not,*
> *What kept me alive is my dreams ...*
>
> K'naan, Dreamer, from the album Troubadour (2009)
>
> *Ever since my childhood, I have felt that memory is a living and effervescent reservoir that animates my being ...*
>
> *... Sometimes things I'd seen during the war would slip through from walled-in basements of memory, demanding the right to exist. But they did not have the power to bring down the pillars of oblivion and the will to live. And life itself said then: Forget! Be absorbed!*
>
> Aharon Appelfeld, The Story of a Life (2004)

Abstract Refugees in Canada, as in many countries around the world, face many difficulties in their journeys towards resettlement and stability. This chapter describes some of the clinical issues around using a cultural competence approach to working with refugees. Use of the cultural formulation is a helpful tool in gaining an appreciation of cultural identity, explanatory models, stressors and supports, as well as cultural factors in the relationship between client and clinician. This approach must also include an understanding of phase-oriented trauma treatment, which begins with safety, symptom reduction and stabilization. Fortifying refugee resilience with an emphasis on current functioning and settlement needs, and avoiding an overly medicalized approach to those who have experienced psychological trauma and torture is recommended. Several vignettes are presented. The importance of post-migration social support is highlighted as one of the most important factors in the promotion of refugee mental health.

Keywords Refugee mental health · Cultural psychiatry · Post-traumatic stress · Resilience · Acculturation

---

L. Andermann (✉)
Department of Psychiatry, University of Toronto, 9th Floor, Mount Sinai Hospital, 600 University Avenue, M5G 1X5 Toronto, Ontario, Canada
e-mail: landermann@mtsinai.on.ca

5.1 Introduction

Refugees in Canada, as in many countries around the world, have been facing unprecedented difficulties, and their resilience continues to be challenged. The past year has brought a number of harsh new legislative restrictions to Canada, including strict limits to access to health care for refugees in this country as well as limitations on countries from which refugees can be accepted (Beder et al. 2012; U of T Department of Psychiatry 2012). Canada has created an initial list of "designated countries of origin" (DCO's) from which refugees will not be accepted, including 25 countries in the European Union (Citizenship and Immigration Canada 2012). This has serious implications for particular groups such as the Roma who have been experiencing significant discrimination and persecution in European countries such as Hungary, as well as others (Chase 2013). As a result of these policies, advocacy organizations such as Canadian Doctors for Refugee Care (2013) and Health for All (2013) have been very active in working to challenge and reverse these changes with support from many other national and provincial medical and social organizations. As expressed by Beiser et al. (2011), "Wealthy countries like Canada that have chosen to resettle refugees assume an obligation that does not end with admitting them". For further discussion of Canada's refugee policies, please see the chapter by McKenzie and Tuck (this volume).

Not since the days of *'none is too many'* in the 1930's and early 40's, when Canada's immigration policy led to the refusal of thousands of Jewish refugees fleeing Nazi occupied Europe has the situation been as dire (Abella and Troper 1983). These policies reached their nadir in May 1939 when 907 German Jewish passengers aboard the M.S. St. Louis were not allowed to land in Halifax and sent back to Europe, where many were subsequently sent to concentration camps and died.

In addition to reducing the number of refugee claimants entering the country now, the current new legislation in Canada has been limiting refugees' access to basic health care in addition to all the challenges they are already facing as newcomers. For those persons fortunate to reach safety on Canadian shores after fleeing persecution, many also face time in detention centres, which have been shown to have significantly negative impacts on mental health for adults and children (Cleveland et al. 2012a, b).

Thirty years after the first publication of the book *None is too Many* (Abella and Troper 1983), Abella states that "it has become an ethical yardstick against which contemporaneous government policies are gauged ... Today's Canada is far different—generous, open, decent, humane. Multiculturalism is now an integral part of Canadian policy and diversity is encouraged. Yet at a moment when intolerance seems to be the global growth industry of the new century, the lessons of *None Is Too Many* should not be ignored. Immigration and refugee policies still divide Canadians. There remain significant pockets of discrimination and racism. Nazi war criminals and collaborators, thousands of whom were welcomed into this country immediately after the war, still live freely among us. Clearly, we still have much left to learn from our checkered past" (Abella 2013). Xenophobia continues to be a significant problem in Canada and many other immigrant-receiving countries. Kleinman et al's. (1997)

volume on *Social Suffering* complements these views, identifying the social impact of trauma and abuses of power at multiple, and interconnected, levels: "The vicious spiral of political violence, causing forced uprooting, migration, and deep trauma to families and communities, while intensifying domestic abuse and personal suffering, spins out of control across a bureaucratic landscape of health, social welfare, and legal agencies. The gathering cycle churns through domestic and international agendas and threatens both local and global structures of security. At its brutal extremity in the Holocaust, or when it results from the 'soft knife' of routine processes of ordinary oppression, social suffering ruins the collective and the intersubjective connections of experience and gravely damages subjectivity".

5.2 Using a Cultural Competence Approach in Clinical Work with Refugees

As with all other areas of medical practice, approaching psychiatric work with refugees requires the right attitudes, knowledge and skills (ASK model) and a culturally competent approach (Kirmayer et al. 2012; Andermann and Lo 2010; Fung et al. 2008; Lo and Fung 2003). This involves much more than knowledge of PTSD guidelines and treatment algorithms. Clinicians must be to able to understand concerns from the patient's point of view, enquire about explanatory models, recognize cultural variations in the expression of distress, and discuss expectations about the clinical encounter while making culturally valid and acceptable diagnostic formulations and treatment plans. Working cross-culturally with refugees also requires training with emphasis on the full breadth of the Royal College CanMEDS roles[1] (Frank et al. 2005), not only as the more traditional *medical expert* (e.g. writing psychiatric reports for refugee claimants), but also as *health advocate*—having a broad vision of psychosocial aspects of care such as housing and work and ensuring access to primary care; *communicator* (working with interpreters; awareness of issues in cross-cultural communication); and *collaborator*—linking with settlement workers, immigration lawyers, primary care physicians and other community resources to create a support network for clients.

There are now excellent recent guidelines for clinical assessment of mental health of immigrants and refugees, such as the recent and comprehensive review by the Canadian Collaboration for Immigrant and Refugee Health (CCIRH) (Kirmayer et al. 2011). The authors stress the importance of a culturally sensitive enquiry into symptoms as well as migration trajectory; and specifically looking at experiences of adversity before, during and after resettlement in Canada (known as pre-migration, migration and post-migration phases) as being key to modifying or ameliorating certain health problems. Post-migration support, including suitable employment and

---

[1] The seven CanMEDS competencies include: Medical Expert, Communicator, Collaborator, Health Advocate, Manager, Professional and Scholar (Frank et al. 2005). Each role can then be linked to specific learning objectives and evaluation standards.

financial stability can help to maintain the "healthy immigrant effect", whereby newcomers to Canada are found to have somewhat lower rates of mental disorders than the Canadian average. Without a supportive reception, however, these rates can soon increase to match the general population. Refugees, and in particular those who have experienced torture, in addition to their exposure to trauma, war, violence, family separation and forced migration, may be at higher risk than immigrant groups for mental distress and psychiatric disorders. Pain et al. (this volume) present a debate about treatment strategies for refugees, and the use of evidence-based exposure therapy as treatment for PTSD in refugees versus emphasis on psychosocial support and settlement issues. As Hinshelwood (2007) writes, "our Western "culture" of psychotherapy risks being as personally and culturally disorienting as the wider host culture that has just replaced the refugee's taken-for-granted home". Another useful concept pertains to the assessment of post-traumatic growth, now found in a standardized questionnaire used in over 20 countries which has been compared cross-culturally, as a means of capturing survivor's resilience, even though it is acknowledged that "people can experience growth and distress concurrently" (Calhoun et al. 2010).

Because refugee mental health issues are not always adequately addressed in medical training, the development of continuing medical education (CME) and other initiatives is important to have greater numbers of well-trained health care professionals who can work with refugees in a culturally competent way. The postgraduate psychiatry residency program at University of Toronto, which has a fairly extensive cultural psychiatry curriculum (Fung et al. 2008) is now further developing a social responsibility curriculum which will focus on mental health needs of underserved and marginalized populations, including refugees. An excellent online curriculum resource on global health and refugees, which follows the CanMEDS competencies, is available from the Canadian Collaboration for Immigrant and Refugee Health (CCIRH) and the University of Ottawa (Pottie et al. 2012). Another online course specifically addressing refugee mental health, currently offered in two streams for health care providers and settlement workers in Ontario, entitled *E-learning tools and Community of Practice for Refugee Mental Health* encompasses many of the cultural competence principles mentioned above (CAMH 2012). The online course grew out of a Canada-wide study on settlement needs of refugees and factors promoting refugee mental health, resilience and recovery (Vasilevska et al. 2010).

5.3 Clinical Work at CCVT

In my Wednesday afternoon clinic at the Canadian Centre for Victims of Torture (CCVT), where I have been seeing clients for psychiatric assessments for the last several years, I am privileged to witness examples of incredible resilience on a weekly basis. CCVT is a settlement agency that provides trauma counseling and settlement services to refugees and newcomers. The centre was founded 30 years ago by a group of doctors, lawyers and social service professionals in Toronto to deal with the needs of persons who had experienced torture and war in their home countries before coming to Canada as refugees (www.ccvt.org). The workings of the organization are described in more detail as a model of social entrepreneurship by Kidd et al. (this volume). The centre's model of community-based treatment is based partly on the writings and experience of Ignacio Martin-Baro a Jesuit priest and social psychologist who was killed in El Salvador for his political beliefs in 1989. Martin-Baro described the 'circles of silence' that surround communities where torture is practiced, and that allow violence within oppressive societies to continue unchecked. In this model, healing for survivors of torture comes through the establishment of 'circles of solidarity' where suffering can be acknowledged and support systems rebuilt (Simalchik 2013; Chambon et al. 2001).

Physicians at the centre meet regularly at Heath Committee meetings to discuss issues around mental and physical care for refugees, and plan educational events on topics around torture and trauma for the community and the Health and Legal Network of professionals associated with CCVT. Most recently, this has taken the form of a monthly 9-session certificate training course called *"Hope After The Horror"*, which has included sessions on cultural aspects of trauma, torture, stress and resilience, gender and LGBT issues, and impact of trauma among different age groups from children and youth to the elderly (CCVT 2012).

As consultant psychiatrists, we have advocated for a collaborative care approach where the psychiatrist on-site sees clients together with their CCVT counselor for better continuity of care and language support when required, as well as opportunities for in-house clinical sharing and case discussion. This seems to be far superior to having clients come to the foreign and intimidating environment of large downtown teaching hospitals, with crowded elevators and uniformed security guards, to see the psychiatrist. From April 2010-March 2011, over 2,700 clients were seen at CCVT from over 79 countries; 200 of whom were seen by the Psychiatrists or GP's, with 175 seen for either psychiatric reports requested by their lawyers for IRB hearings or treatment (CCVT 2013). For 2012, there were 128 new psychiatric assessments with 94 psychiatric reports provided for the Immigration Review Board (IRB) and close to 400 follow-up visits; and 50 medical reports for IRB done by a family doctor at CCVT (CCVT 2012). Some of the impact of the introduction of in-house psychiatrists to CCVT has been documented in a recent psychiatry residency quality improvement project (Stiglick and Nguyen 2012). At the same time, we have been proceeding with caution so as not to inadvertently medicalize a community-based model of support for refugees that has functioned well for close to 30 years.

Many of the clients who are seen by psychiatrists at the CCVT are referred by their immigration lawyers for psychiatric assessments to support their refugee hearings by the Immigration and Review Board (IRB). This process formally documents their traumatic experiences and past suffering, as well as any fears of future harm or ongoing persecution should they return to their home country. Reports are also supposed to address any reasons that clients might have trouble in the hearing associated with their traumatic experiences, such as level of distress or dissociation, and difficulties with memory for specific dates and events, particularly if detention has been prolonged or there have been numerous traumas over many years. The vast majority of clients have no previous psychiatric history and no experience with counseling or mental health treatment, instead relying, if needed, on other religious or community supports. However, many are also quite isolated, coming to Canada on their own, separated from family members, spouses, children or parents. They may be reluctant to seek out help from their cultural communities because of fears of ongoing persecution, stigma around mental illness, and concerns about confidentiality. They may also be hampered by symptoms of depression or post-traumatic stress including avoidance and hypervigilance. However, we have also seen many young refugees pursuing English as a Second Language and college programs, then finding jobs, and 'landing on their feet'; single mothers with young children getting daycare spots and being able to pursue careers they thought had been left behind in their home countries; and others finding work and being able to send money home to family members, with the hope of one day sponsoring them to come to Canada.

Because of the diversity of the CCVT clients coming from over 79 countries, having a *culturally generic* approach to psychiatric assessment becomes very important (Andermann and Lo 2010). Using principles from the DSM-IV-TR *Outline for Cultural Formulation* for refugee assessments is helpful as it focuses on exploring cultural identity, explanatory models of illness, social and cultural stressors and supports, and cultural factors in the client-clinician relationship (APA 2000; Andermann 2010). Learning approaches to working with interpreters and use of cultural consultants can also be useful in clarifying cultural norms and values (Kirmayer et al. 2011). This also adds to the rationale for seeing clients on-site at CCVT together with their counselors, as they can often serve as both interpreters and cultural consultants.

The period of waiting for a refugee hearing is a time of high anxiety, when it can be difficult to tease out psychiatric symptoms related to past trauma and current worries about the outcome of the process allowing claimants to remain in Canada. Kirmayer writes: "Once future status is decided, resettlement usually brings hope and optimism, which can have an initially positive effect on well-being. Disillusionment, demoralization and depression can occur early as a result of migration associated losses, or later, when initial hopes and expectations are not realized and when immigrants and their families face enduring obstacles in their new home because of structural barriers and inequalities aggravated by exclusionary policies, racism and discrimination" (2011). Again, this highlights the importance of post-migration support in mitigating mental distress that can contribute to the development or perpetuation of PTSD symptoms. Beiser et al. (2011) have eloquently described this type of family and non-family based support as the '*balms of resettlement*' for Sri Lankan Tamil refugees settling in Toronto. When this support is not available, one may find higher rates of PTSD "as the end result of a complex process initiated by catastrophic stress, and reinforced by stresses of passage to a new life, as well as the depletion of internal and external coping resources. Healing should take into account this web of interactions and the potential points of intervention … Sometimes, for example a psychological intervention may be the preferred point of entry, but sometimes it may be more strategic to focus on helping people deal with postmigration stresses, or on developing linkages with settlement and other social services, or on integrating with the receiving society" (Beiser et al. 2011, p. 339).

Writing psychiatric assessments for refugee claimants is an important step in the bigger picture of their psychosocial treatment if it can lead towards improving their sense of safety when approved to remain in Canada. Beginning psychiatric treatment with either trauma therapy or medications during this time can be difficult as the anxiety around the hearing is often so high there is little other focus to the sessions. Supportive counseling is most useful at this time, combined with basic techniques in grounding and relaxation, coping skills, psychoeducation about common responses to trauma and most centrally engagement in their new community with ESL lessons, volunteer or paid work. This counseling is done mainly by the settlement and trauma counselors. Support groups are also very helpful. Advising clients to keep busy outside the home engaging in any healthy activity that helps them become familiar with their new environment in Canada is helpful. Too much time alone at home, ruminating about problems, is not. Not every client requires, or is interested in trying, psychopharmacological treatment. However, if sleep is severely disrupted and daily function is impaired, there is ongoing suicidal ideation, or the waiting period for the hearing has been particularly lengthy and demoralizing, then clinicians could consider a trial of anti-depressant medications with the possible adjunct of a non-addictive (non-benzodiazepine) sleeping medication. Of course, if there is then news of a hearing successfully passed, with sudden remission of depression and anxiety, it is always difficult to know the role played by medication, but it is likely quite small when faced with such intensive psychosocial stressors. Some of these points are illustrated in the following brief examples (with any identifying details removed for confidentiality):

Vignette 1 A young male from Afghanistan came to Canada alone as a refugee after some family members had been killed and his life was threatened. He was very anxious and alone. He was able to pass his IRB hearing successfully, but some time later became depressed and had difficulty functioning at work, in a low-paying job with lots of physical demands. He saw the psychiatrist who started medication and provided a letter for his workplace which allowed him to have a period of short-term disability. During this time, he was able to regroup, find new accommodations and apply to college, and the treatment ended shortly afterwards.

Vignette 2 A West African woman refugee was in Canada alone without her children, having escaped family violence. She presented for a psychiatric assessment in preparation for her refugee hearing with remarkably few symptoms, and busied herself with ESL and church activities. However, more than a year passed between our first appointment and the announcement of her hearing date, and during that time she became progressively more depressed, eventually requiring her to start antidepressant medication. On her first visit back to see the psychiatrist after her positive hearing result, she was beaming, having just wired money to her children in Africa for the first time in over two years, earned from a new job. No further follow-up was needed and medications were tapered and stopped.

Vignette 3 A Tamil male who had spent several periods in detention in Sri Lanka where he experienced torture and violence, was asked to see the psychiatrist for a report by his lawyer to assist with his refugee hearing. Despite his description of multiple abuses and losses, and some mood and anxiety symptoms, he had not lost hope, and having found one person to confide in was sufficient for his stability. We recommended continuing ESL and work, getting more connected with community activities, meeting with his settlement counselor as needed and no psychiatric treatment.

In Vignette 1 and 2, after a brief treatment with the psychiatrist, and lots of good support from their settlement counselors, both of these clients are well on their way to becoming productive new Canadians, and working towards a better future for themselves and their families. Vignette 3 reminds us that not everyone who has experienced trauma will develop PTSD or require formal psychiatric treatment.

In her description of phase-oriented trauma treatment, Judith Herman explains that Phase One is all about safety and stabilization with symptom reduction and attention to basic needs such as housing and finances, making sure that the patient is safe from ongoing traumatization or self-harm, and treating any co-morbid psychiatric conditions such as substance use or depression (Herman 1992). Reinforcing a client's efforts at remaining safe from a return to victimization or to a country where torture has taken place—and could recur at any time after the person's return—would certainly qualify as Phase One work. Phase Two, more typically perceived as trauma treatment—processing traumatic memories and building a cohesive life narrative—can only occur if there are no immediate safety concerns. Certain manualized therapies such as Narrative Exposure Therapy (NET) which combines some elements of evidence-based exposure therapy[2] with testimony therapy[3] in a standardized manual format, have also been shown to be effective in short term use with patients from a variety of cultural backgrounds, in refugee-receiving countries as well as in refugee camps and post-conflict settings (Schauer et al. 2005; www.vivo.org).

Phase Three of trauma treatment is then mostly concerned with the psychosocial rebuilding and reconnecting, encouraging clients to re-engage with their former functional selves and moving on with life after trauma. Although most clients seen at CCVT are refugee claimants awaiting their hearings, the centre keeps an open door for those needing additional support in the months, and sometimes years, after a successful hearing if they continue to have difficulties, even as permanent residents. There are also those clients embroiled in protracted legal issues around their status, sometimes with years of appeals and an ongoing sense of limbo, who require ongoing support.

---

[2] Exposure therapy is a scientifically validated, evidence-based treatment for most anxiety disorders, including PTSD, and recommended as a first-line intervention by many treatment guidelines and algorithms, often even before psychopharmacological treatment (Bisson and Andrew 2007; Foa et al. 2008). Confronting fears and avoidance of the trauma and its' reminders is the hallmark of this approach. These techniques include Trauma-focused cognitive behavior therapy (TF-CBT), Prolonged Exposure (P.E.) and others which may use various combinations of in-vivo and imaginal exposure.

[3] Testimony therapy, initially developed in Chile during a time of political oppression and dictatorship, involves the creation of a written narrative by the client with the help of the therapist, which is then kept by the client as a permanent document. This can be helpful with exposure and can also used for human rights trials or shared with others for witnessing or community awareness (www.vivo.org).

5.4 Conclusion

Working with refugees is rewarding and invigorating, sometimes challenging, and definitely worthwhile. It is an opportunity to get to know intimately, but usually only for a short time, some very determined and brave people, who are trying hard to make a better life for themselves and their families, and want only to live in safety and peace. Most refugees are not psychiatric patients, but people who for the most part have had good families and solid upbringings which have stood them in good stead as they face major adjustments in language and culture in a new, and sometimes unwelcoming, setting with optimism and good grace. Improving post-migration support for refugees, through psychosocial services, education and employment are some of the most important factors in fortifying refugee resilience. Linking with other community agencies, housing providers, ethnocultural community services, religious communities, vocational, legal and medical services completes the "circles of support" which provide a safety net for newcomers and a platform from which to rebuild their lives.

References

Abella, I., & Troper, H. (1983). *None is Too Many: Canada and the Jews of Europe, 1933–1948* (p. 336). Toronto: L. and O. Dennys.

Abella, I. (2013). Canada still has much to learn from None is Too Many. The Globe and Mail, February 26th. http://www.theglobeandmail.com/commentary/canada-still-has-much-to-learn-from-none-is-too-many/article9029037/. Accessed 26 Feb 2013.

Andermann, L. (2010). Culture and the social construction of gender: Mapping the intersection with mental health. *International Review of Psychiatry, 22*(5),501–512.

Andermann, L., & Lo, H.-T. (2010). Cultural competence in psychiatric assessment. In D. Goldbloom (Ed.), *Psychiatric clinical skills* (Revised 1st ed.). Toronto: CAMH. (Originally published by Elsevier Canada (2006))

American Psychiatric Association. (2000). Appendix I: Outline for cultural formulation and glossary of culture-bound syndromes. *Diagnostic and statistical manual of mental disorders* (4th ed.). Arlington: APA Press. (Text Revision (DSM-IV-TR))

Appelfeld, A. (2004). *The story of a life* (p. 198). New York: Schocken Books.

Beder, M., Fung, K., Stergiopoulos, V., Pain, C., Andermann, L., Maggi, J., Munshi, A., & Leszcz, M. (2012). Mental health for all: Why not refugees? Psychiatry Aujoud'hui, Summer issue.

Beiser, M., Simich, L., Pandalangat, N., Nowakowski, M., & Tian, Fu. (June 2011). Stresses of passage, balms of resettlement, and posttraumatic stress disorder among Sri Lankan Tamils in Canada. *Canadian Journal of Psychiatry, 56*(6):333–340.

Bisson, J., & Andrew, M. (2007). Psychological treatment of post-traumatic stress disorder (PTSD). *Cochrane Database System Review, 2005 Apr 18*(2):CD003388.

Calhoun, L. G., Cann, A., & Tedeschi, R. G. (2010). The posttraumatic growth model: Sociocultural considerations. In T. Weiss & R. Berger (Eds.), *Posttraumatic growth and culturally competent practice: Lessons learned from around the world*. Hoboken: John Wiley and Sons.

CAMH Knowledge Exchange. (2012). E-learning tools and community of practice for refugee mental health. Project leads: Agic, B. and Noh, S. http://knowledgex.camh.net/health_equity/immigrants_ethnoracial/Pages/elearning.aspx. Accessed 26 Jan 2013.

Canadian Centre for Victims of Torture. (2012). Hope after the horror: A course series on refugee mental health. www.ccvt.org. Accessed 27 Jan 2013.

Canadian Centre for Victims of Torture. (2013). 2011 and 2012 Annual reports. www.ccvt.org. Accessed 15 March 2013.
Canadian Doctors for Refugee Care. (2013). http://www.doctorsforrefugeecare.ca. Accessed 26 Jan 2013.
Chambon, A. S., McGrath, S., Shapiro, B., Abai, M., Dremetsikas, T., & Didziak, S. (2001). From interpersonal links to webs of relations: Creating befriending relationships with survivors of torture and of war. *Journal of Social Work Research and Evaluation, 2,* 157–171. http://ccvt.org/publications/past-research-projects/from-interpersonal-links-to-webs-of-relations-creating-befriending-relationships-with-survivors-of-torture-and-war/. Accessed 28 Feb 2013.
Chase, S. (2013). New fast-track rules see big drop in refugee asylum claims. Globe and Mail, February 21, 2013. http://www.theglobeandmail.com/news/politics/new-fast-track-rules-see-big-drop-in-refugee-asylum-claims/article8961268/. Accessed 27 Feb 2013.
Cleveland, J., Rousseau, C., & Kronick, R. (2012a). The harmful effects of detention and family separation on asylum seeker's mental health in the context of Bill C-31. Brief submitted to House of Commons Standing Committee on citizenship and immigration concerning Bill C-31, the Protecting Canada's immigration system act. http://www.csssdelamontagne.qc.ca/fileadmin/csss_dlm/Publications/Publications_CRF/brief_c31_final.pdf. Accessed 21 Jan 2013.
Cleveland, J., Rousseau, C., & Kronick, R. (2012b). Bill C-4: The impact of detention and temporary status on asylum seekers' mental health. http://oppenheimer.mcgill.ca/Bill-C-4-The-impact-of-detention. Accessed 21 Jan 2013.
Citizenship and Immigration Canada. (2012). News release: Making Canada's asylum system faster and fairer, December 14th. www.cic.gc.ca. Accessed 14 Dece 2012.
Department of Psychiatry, University of Toronto. (2012). Interim federal health program cuts and bill C31– UofT Psychiatry position statement. http://www.utpsychiatry.ca/bill-c31-uoft-psychiatry-position-statement/. Accessed 21 Jan 2013.
Foa, E., Keane, T. M., Friedman, M. J., & Cohen, J. A. (Eds). (2008). *Effective treatments for PTSD: Practice guidelines from the international society of traumatic stress studies* (2nd ed.). New York: Guilford Press.
Frank, J. R., Gabbour, M., et al. (Eds.). (2005). Report of the CanMEDS phase IV working groups. Ottawa: The royal college of physicians and surgeons of canada. http://www.royalcollege.ca/portal/page/portal/rc/common/documents/canmeds/framework/the_7_canmeds_roles_e.pdf. Accessed 28 Feb 2013.
Fung, K., Andermann, L., Lo, T., & Zaretsky, A. (2008). An integrative approach to cultural competence in the psychiatric curriculum. *Academic Psychiatry, 3,* 272–282.
Health for All. (2013). www.health4all.ca. Accessed 26 Jan 2013.
Herman, J. (1992). *Trauma and recovery: The aftermath of violence from domestic abuse to political terror.* Basic Books.
Hinshelwood, R. D. (2007). Foreword. In A. Alayarian (Ed.), *Resilience, suffering and creativity: The work of the refugee therapy centre.* London: Karnac Books.
Kirmayer, L. J., Nasariah, L., Munoz, M., Rashid, M., Ryder, A. G., Guzder, J., Hassan, G., Rousseau, C., Pottie, K. (2011). Common mental health problems in immigrants and refugees: General approach in primary care. *CMAJ, 183*(12):E959–E967.
Kirmayer, L. J., Fung, K., Rousseau, C., Lo, H. T., Menzies, P., Guzder, J., Ganesan, S., Andermann, L., McKenzie, K. (2012). Guidelines for training in cultural psychiatry. Canadian Journal of Psychiatry 2012 Mar;57(3). A position paper developed by the Canadian Psychiatric Association's Section on Transcultural Psychiatry and the Standing Committee on Education and approved by the CPA's Board of Directors.
Kleinman, A., Das, V., & Lock, M. (1997). Introduction. In A. Kleinman, V. Das, & M. Lock (Eds.), *Social suffering.* Berkeley: University of California Press.
Lo, H. T., & Fung, K. P. (2003). Culturally competent psychotherapy. *Canadian Journal of Psychiatry, Apr; 48*(3):161–70.
Pottie, K., Gruner, D., Ferreyra, M., Ratnayake, A., Ezzat, O., Ponka, D., Rashid, M., Kellam, H., Sun, R., & Miller, K. (2012). Refugees and global health: A global health E-learning

program, Canadian collaboration for immigrant and refugee health (CCIRH) and the University of Ottawa, Canada. http://www.ccirhken.ca/eLearning. Accessed 26 Jan 2013.

Schauer, M., Elbert, T., & Neuner, F. (2005). *Narrative exposure therapy: A short-term intervention for traumatic stress disorders after war, terror or torture* (p. 68). Hogrefe and Huber.

Simalchik, J. (2013) The politics of torture: Dispelling the myths and understanding the survivors. http://ccvt.org/publications/online-publications/the-politics-of-torture-dispelling-the-myths-and-understanding-the-survivors/. Accessed 28 Feb 2013.

Stiglick, A., & Nguyen, H. P. (2012). The effects of regular-visiting psychiatry at CCVT: A quality improvement project. Grand Rounds Presentation at Mount Sinai Hospital, Toronto, June 15th.

Vasilevska, B., Madan, A., & Simich, L. (2010). *Refugee mental health: Promising practices and partnership building resources*. Toronto: Centre for Addiction and Mental Health.

Victim's Voice. (2013). www.vivo.org. Accessed 26 Feb 2013.

Chapter 6
Personal and Social Forms of Resilience: Research with Southeast Asian and Sri Lankan Tamil Refugees in Canada

Morton Beiser

Abstract Despite pre-migration assaults such as persecution, escape, and internment, and despite the challenges of resettling in a strange country, only a minority of refugees become mental health casualties. Stress process theory provides a useful framework for understanding what happens to refugees and how they respond. Personal characteristics, pre- and post-migration risk and protective factors, both at the psychological and social levels interact to affect mental health. Pre- and post-migration stresses jeopardize mental health while personal and social resources not only enhance mental health directly but also buffer the effects of stress. This chapter focuses on two dimensions of resilience among refugees: time perspective as a personal resource and social resources based in family, like-ethnic community, and the larger society.

Keywords Psychological resilience · Social resilience · Time perspective · Like-ethnic community · Bridging social network · Bonding social network · Connecting network · PTSD · Depression · Southeast Asian refugee · Tamil refugee

Despite pre-migration assaults such as persecution, escape, and internment, and despite the challenges of resettling in a strange country, only a minority of refugees become mental health casualties (Beiser 1999; Vaage et al. 2010). In the making of mental disorders, stress counts, but only as part of a more complex story. Using stress process theory (Beiser 1999; Pearlin et al. 1981) as a conceptual framework, Fig. 6.1 proposes that personal characteristics, pre- and post-migration risk factors, and protective factors—both psychological and social—interact to affect mental health. Pre- and post-migration stresses jeopardize mental health while personal and social resources not only enhance mental health directly but also (as indicated by broken arrows) buffer the effects of stress.

M. Beiser (✉)
Ryerson University, Toronto, Canada
e-mail: mail@mortonbeiser.com

Keenan Research Centre and Li Ka Shing Knowledge Institute,
St. Michael's Hospital, Toronto, Canada

Cultural Pluralism and Health, University of Toronto, Toronto, Canada

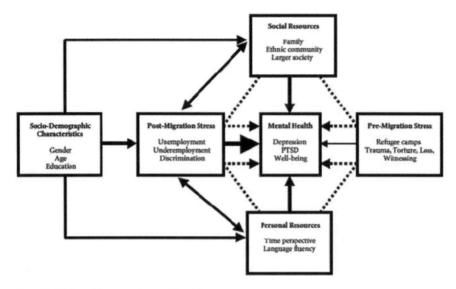

Fig. 6.1 Risk, resilience and mental health

This chapter focuses on two dimensions of resilience extracted from Fig. 6.1: (i) Time perspective as an example of a personal resource and (ii) Social resources, primarily family, like-ethnic community, and the larger society. Data and inferences about handling time as a psychological coping mechanism derive from the Refugee Resettlement Project (RRP) a longitudinal study of Southeast Asian refugees in Vancouver, British Columbia. Illustrations concerning the role of social resources as a source of resilience derive from both the RRP and the Community in Distress (CID), a study of mental health among the Sri Lankan Tamil community in Toronto, Ontario.

6.1 Two Refugee Communities in Canada

1. The Refugee Resettlement Project (RRP)

In 1978, several years after the fall of Saigon, the Hanoi government expelled ethnic Chinese living in Vietnam. Ethnic Vietnamese, unhappy about living under the communist regime, took advantage of the confusion surrounding the massive expulsions to escape along with the Chinese. At roughly the same time, Vietnamese raids on Cambodia destabilized the country's government, creating an opportunity for Cambodians to escape Pol Pot's tyranny. Raids on Laos prompted Laotians who feared retaliation because of previous alliances with the west to flee their homeland. More than one million people poured out of the Southeast Asian peninsula only to be met with, at best, a cold reception in nearby countries, and, at worst, outright refusal of sanctuary. Prompted by sympathetic media coverage and world-wide sympathy for the refugees, North America, Australia, Israel, and a number of European countries eventually offered the refugees sanctuary and the opportunity of permanent resettlement. During the period 1979 to 1981, Canada admitted 60,000 "Boat People." After setting what was, at the time, an exceptionally high admission quota, the government of the day encouraged individuals as well as organizations such as church groups to become private sponsors. Eventually, 40,000 refugees came to Canada under private sponsorship, 20,000 under government sponsorship (Beiser 1999). Approximately 5,000 of Canada's admission complement of 60,000 refugees were resettled in and around Vancouver, British Columbia, where the RRP was carried out between the years 1981 and 1991.

The Southeast Asian (SEA) refugees taking part in the study constituted a one in three community-based probability sample of 1,348 adults, 18 years of age and older. After an initial survey, in 1981, the participants were subsequently re-interviewed in 1983 and then again in 1991. As the RRP Principal Investigator, I personally interviewed a subsample of 120 study participants, half of whom, according to the quantitative data, had developed significant mental distress, and half of whom, according to various community agencies, were adapting particularly successfully.

2. A Community in Distress (CID)

Sri Lanka's declaration of independence from British rule in 1948 opened the door to a half century of conflict between the Sinhalese majority and the Tamil minority. Tensions began with the enactment of the Citizenship and Official Languages Act, which Tamils experienced as a direct threat to the survival of their language. In 1983, the inter-ethnic hostilities erupted into violence that was to persist for the next quarter century. Tens of thousands on both sides of the conflict lost their lives, and, between 1983 and 1996, 11,513 others "disappeared" (UN Commission 1999). With one million internally displaced people and more than 900,000 seeking refuge abroad, Sri Lanka became one of the world's leading sources of refugees.

Canada offers permanent resettlement to refugees through two possible routes. The first, much preferred by government, relies on immigration officials to select refugees from refugee camps and holding facilities in countries of initial asylum. This was the Southeast Asian refugees' route of entry. The second route is for a candidate to somehow find the means to reach Canada on his or her own, and claim refugee status. Claimants judged to conform to the UN convention definition of "refugee" will be granted permanent resident status and may eventually sponsor other members of the family left behind in refugee camps or in the home country. Most Sri Lankan Tamils used the second route to establish residence in Canada. Tamils soon became one of Canada's fastest growing ethnic communities (Hyndman 2003). By the year 2010, Toronto's Tamil population—approximately 200,000—was the largest urban concentration of Tamils outside Sri Lanka. Successful in many ways, Toronto's Sri Lankan Tamils were also a community in distress. In early 2001, Toronto newspapers ran the shocking story of a young Tamil father, his child in his arms, who leaped to his death from a subway platform. Like other incidents of despair, the story initially excited media coverage and public dismay, only to quickly fade from public consciousness. This time, however, a group of community leaders decided they needed information to help avert future tragedies. These leaders approached me with a request to carry out a community study of mental health, and of service needs. With funding support from Canada's Institutes of Health Research, the Community in Distress—a mental health survey of 1,603 Tamil adults living in Toronto, Canada—was initiated in 2001.

6.1.1 Mental Distress Among Refugees

Theory, clinical lore and common sense would predict that refugees—survivors of violence, (Westermeyer et al. 1983a; Hollifield et al. 2002), torture and abuse of human rights (Mollica 2006; Mollica et al. 1998), perilous flight followed by incarceration in refugee camps (Beiser et al. 1989), and further challenged by a new country and a new culture—should have high rates of mental disorders (Pedersen 1949; Baskauskas 1981; Goldfield and Lee 1982). Study data offer mixed results. In 1981, when most of the refugees in the RRP sample had been in Canada between one and two years, the rate of depression was 7.5 %. The rate for a community sample of native-born Vancouverites studied at the same time was 8.9 % (Beiser 1999). Three to four years after arrival, depression among the SEA refugees had fallen to a rate of 4.4 %, and after 10 years, to 2.3 %.

Post-traumatic stress disorder (PTSD) yields a different picture. The rate of lifetime PTSD in the general population is about 2 % (ESEMeD/MHEDEA 2000 Investigators 2004). By comparison, according to a comprehensive meta-analysis (Fazel et al. 2005), PTSD affects about 10–12 % of refugees. The RRP estimate for PTSD was 7 % (Beiser 1999), somewhat lower than the average for refugees in general, but still much higher than general population estimates. The PTSD rate among the CID sample was 12 % (Beiser et al. 2011). A much higher proportion—about one third—had experienced the traumas that commonly give rise to PTSD.

The discrepancy between the rate of traumatic experience and the substantially lower rate of PTSD illustrates that stress matters, but that it is far from the whole story concerning mental health. Resilience, both personal and social, matters too.

6.2 Personal and Social Sources of Resilience

6.2.1 Psychological Resilience

Under conditions of extreme adversity, human beings resort to time splitting, substituting what Thomas Cottle (1976) called "Atomistic" perception for the more usual psychological set in which past, present, and future are connected. Having split the three spheres of time apart, victims of overwhelming stress concentrate on the present, to the relative exclusion of past and future. Dissociating painful memories from consciousness can be an effective coping strategy, rather than a neurotic defence mechanism.

Early in 1980, I visited Bangkok which, at the time, was the site of several refugee camps from which people were selected for permanent resettlement in other countries, Canada among them. In one of these camps, I interviewed "Nong", a wiry, watchful, thirty-five year old man who was slated to leave for Canada the following day. After covering all the material that interested me, I asked Nong my usual wind-up questions, "Do you have anything you would like to ask me? Is there anything you've been wondering about Canada, or about Vancouver?" Like everyone else I had interviewed, Nong had no questions. Other refugees in the camp had evidenced a similar lack of curiosity and it was a puzzle that was beginning to bother me. I said, "I find that hard to believe. You're scheduled to leave tomorrow afternoon. You and your family are going to live in a place you know nothing about. I come from that place. I don't understand why you don't take this opportunity to ask me some questions." Fortunately, our interpreter didn't censor Nong's reply. "You can ask that question," he said, "because you've never been a refugee. You don't understand how we think. *If* I get on that aeroplane tomorrow and *if* I see that we're really flying over an ocean, then I might allow myself to think we're going to Canada. When you live as we have for the past few years, never knowing what will happen, you live day by day. We do not think about the past. We cannot let ourselves think about the future."

Part of the explanation for the unexpectedly low risk of psychopathology during the early years of resettlement is that many of the SEA refugees used dissociation of traumatic memories (a concept similar to "suppression") to cope. The strategy was effective, at least for the short and medium term. By contrast, people who admitted the past into consciousness experienced a concomitant increase in risk for depression.

Several months after I returned from Bangkok to Vancouver, a community mental health agency called to tell me about "Li Wuchin," a former Vietnamese industrialist who attempted suicide. Wuchin's attempt to cut the jugular vein in his neck was gruesome; he did not succeed in killing himself, but he had undoubtedly meant to.

Li Wuchin tried to kill himself with an old wooden-handled ice pick he found in the basement of the church in which he worked as a janitor. By that time, he and his family had been living in Vancouver for about one year. Hoping to establish as favourable rapport as possible before asking about his suicide attempt, my interpreter and I began the interview by focusing on his family's life in Vietnam and their escape to Thailand. A rich industrialist in pre-1975 Saigon, Li Wuchin automatically became a special object for the new regime's attention. Taking away his factories, his house and his servants apparently was not enough. To deal with his potential threat to the regime, the authorities sent him to a re-education camp. A man who slept in the bed next to Li's was undergoing his third re-education. One morning, Li woke to an incessant creaking sound. When he looked to the side of his bed, he saw his neighbour hanging by his neck from one of the ceiling rafters.

Li did not adopt much communist doctrine in camp, but he did realize that escape was imperative. After his release, he banded his family together for a difficult overland trip through Laos. The Mekong River, separating Laos from Thailand, was the last barrier on their ten day exodus. Li chose a crossing point in the river heavily guarded by Thai soldiers whose job was to drive refugees away from the border. To divert the guards' attention, Li jumped into the Mekong, making as loud a splash as he could. While the sentries fired at him, the rest of the family crossed the river at a point now left unguarded. Miraculously, everyone survived. At the time of Li Wuchin's suicide attempt, he and his family were living in a crowded but clean basement apartment whose rent consumed most of a janitor's salary. Li's wife, who supplemented the family income by working as a seamstress, sat in on our interview. She agreed with her husband that the children were becoming Canadianized too quickly. Perhaps she was a little less concerned than he was. Their son's long hair bothered her, but not to the point of preoccupation, and she turned a blind eye to their daughter's dating—something she knew about, but that her husband only suspected.

A traditional East Asian man, Li Wuchin was concerned that his daughter was jeopardizing their family's face by going out without a chaperone. Dating a young man would be out of the question. Li was upset about more than family face. He was worried about his own. In place of the authority he used to exert over workers and servants, he now took orders from others. Instead of the absolute obedience he could have expected from his family in Vietnam, he had to contend with his children's half-hidden disobedience, a situation that his wife's apparent complicity made even worse. As the months went by, Li Wuchin began to think more and more about his houses, his factories and his servants in the old world. Soon his sleep became disturbed. Walking around the house in the early morning while his family still slept, he had more and more time for reminiscence. He lost his appetite, began to feel tired all the time and was troubled by bouts of constipation. Although it was hard for him to admit, there were many times when he felt like crying.

The interpreter for my interviews with Li Wuchin was a wonderfully sensitive mental health worker from Hong Kong. Ordinarily, she was an excellent interpreter, waiting for, rather than prompting my questions or the interviewee's responses, translating everything as idiomatically as possible, patiently repeating questionable phrases or nuances until we could be reasonably sure all three parties shared a common understanding. This time, the mental health professional in her became impatient with the interview's pace. She couldn't resist breaking in with a question of her own, that she later translated to me, "Why, after all you've been through—all the suffering and the fear—did you do this? You're safe now, your family's together. Why would you try to kill yourself?" Li replied: "I was thinking then about the past just as you are now. I still do. But when I consider the past, I don't think of myself in the re-education camp, or in the middle of the Mekong River. I think about life when it was at its best. Compared to that, I have nothing now, and I never will again."

To convert the idea of time splitting into an operational measure that could be used for a community survey, I developed a culture-free, easily understandable task based on T. Cottle's (1967, 1969, 1976) well-known "circles test" to measure the relative focus on past, present and future. The refugees' performance on the test, supplemented by qualitative data from the intensive interviews during the study's decade-long course, described the constructive use of suppression to get on with life in the short and medium-term, the ineluctability of memory over longer periods, and the factors predicting whether or not recovery of the past would lead to mental disorder (Beiser 1987, 1999; Beiser and Hyman 1997).

The data showed that it may be possible to leave dreadful things behind, at least in the short and medium-term aftermath of catastrophe. Rather than the neurotic defence mechanism depicted in psychoanalytic lore, suppression can buffer the impact of damaging memory, and thereby reduce the risk for depression (Beiser et al. 1989; Beiser and Hyman 1997; Beiser 1999).

Time heals, according to the ever-popular popular apothegm. RRP data suggest this is only partly true. Suppression of traumatic memory may be an effective coping strategy in the short and medium term aftermath of trauma but the reintegration of past memories into consciousness is probably an ineluctable process, and one that becomes more pressing with the passage of time (see Beiser and Wickrama 2004; Beiser 1999; Friedlander 1979; Ellenberger 1993; Kirmayer 1996; Antze and Lambek 1996).

Recovered memory brings with it increased risk of mental disorder (Beiser and Wickrama 2004), a finding that bears testimony to the continuing power of a disturbing past. At the end of the first decade in Canada, refugees taking part in the RRP were just beginning to admit the past into consciousness and experiencing concomitant mental health risk.

Intensive case studies with 60 refugees who seemed to be adapting well, and 60 who developed mental health problems during the early years of resettlement, made up an important component of the RRP. The RRP intensive case studies provided insights about the trends appearing in the quantitative data. The interviews revealed that it is not just isolated incidents involving suffering which are kept out of awareness. Large swatches of personal history, including memories of happy times, were also kept from awareness. Recognizing loss was part of the pain of remembering, and part of the process of risk for depression and possibly other mental disorders.

Whether time heals or not depends on the conditions of its passage. Although many refugees might benefit from professional help in recovering and dealing with dissociated memory, timing and context are all-important. According to the RRP's quantitative longitudinal data, the longer the SEA refugees were in Canada (and the older they became), the more likely they were to begin admitting the past into consciousness. The process of recall created a definite risk for developing depression. However, involvement in a stable work situation, and in a stable relationship helped protect individual mental health during the process of temporal reintegration. Interestingly, neither job satisfaction nor the quality of one's relationship made a difference. As moderators of mental health risk, job stability trumped satisfaction, and relational durability trumped affection.

6.2.2 Social Sources of Resilience: Significant Others, the Like-ethnic Community, and the Larger Society

Simple formulas explaining human behaviour have a great deal of appeal. Small wonder then that, although it was based on a small number of uncontrolled observations in clinical situations, "disillusionment" was the dominant model about refugees and their mental health for half a century (Grinberg 1984; Holmes and Masuda 1973; Tyhurst 1951, 1977). The disillusionment model is straightforward, easy to understand, and seems to have direct applicability to quotidian experience. According to the model, the psychological process of adapting to a new country follows predictable phases. During the initial, "euphoria of arrival" phase, immigrants and refugees are relieved, hopeful, and in good spirits. The second phase, inevitably overtaking the first, is a phase of disillusionment with the receiving society, and nostalgia for what people feel they lost in leaving home. During this phase, immigrants and refugees are at high risk for developing psychiatric disorders. Eventually, adaptation to the new environment takes place. New settlers begin to think and act more and more like people in the majority population and their mental health improves. The unfortunate few who do not manage to resolve the issues of the disillusionment phase develop chronic psychiatric disorders.

Tested against data, the disillusionment model proves too simplistic. The RRP is one of several studies (Beiser 1988; Bagheri 1992; Rumbaut 1985, 1998) that have tested the validity of the disillusionment model with community-based surveys. Consistent with the model, the community studies identify a period of high risk for the development of depressive symptoms between 10 and 24 months post-arrival. However, the RRP results also challenge the model's emphasis on interiority and inevitability. The three-phase process, with elevated mental health risk a feature of the second phase, is not universal. Only those refugees taking part in the RRP who lacked personal and social supports suffered an increased risk of depression 10–12 months after arrival in Canada. People with a significant other and/or a supportive like-ethnic community did not show the time-dependent spike in mental health risk (Beiser 1988).

The RRP results are consistent with many other studies in demonstrating the importance of social connection as a source of resilience. Researchers (Putnam 2000; Granovetter 1973; DeRose 2008; Kim et al. 2006) have made a useful conceptual distinction between three different forms of social connection: bonding (with family and co-ethnics), bridging (connections with other communities) and linking (with institutions of society and the state).

Bonding Networks

Family, marital and like-ethnic relationships contribute to a sense of belonging (Ager and Strang 2008), and marriage can act as a buffer against adversity, such as losing a job (Ross 2000; Ritsner et al. 2000). Consistent with the RRP results, other studies have shown that married refugees have a mental health advantage over singles (Berry and Blondel 1970; O'Campo et al. 2009; Beiser 1999). RRP results both confirmed these cross-sectional study results, and provided an additional dimension. Because the RRP was a longitudinal investigation, the team was able to demonstrate that a sustained relationship has positive effects, not only during early stages of resettlement, but at subsequent stages as well. Thus, the availability of a significant other not only seemed to mitigate the disillusionment that affects the mental health of some newcomers during the early years of resettlement (Beiser 1988), but also later in the resettlement process, when the emergence of suppressed memory threatened well-being. Consistent work was also a protective factor. These observations recall Freud's famous formulation that mental health consists of "Lieben and arbeiten," love and work. But there is an interesting twist. Love had less to offer as a coping capacity than longevity, and work satisfaction was trumped by stability. The critical element in confronting the past was stability—the longevity of an intimate relationship and the permanency of work (Beiser and Wickrama 2004).

Citizenship and Immigration Canada's Longitudinal Study of Immigrants in Canada (LSIC) expands the scope of social connectivity by demonstrating that, in addition to kinship networks (family and relatives), friendship and organizational networks (including community organizations, religious groups and ethnic associations) affect health (Zhao et al. 2010; Levitt et al. 2005). CID results demonstrating that non-kin support reduce the risk for developing PTSD, but kin support does not, is particularly striking. Although social support is multi-dimensional, interpretations of its effects usually center on emotional support, a focus implying that would lead to the expectation that intimate relationships would be a more powerful buffer against PTSD than relationships outside the family (Stewart et al. 2008) However, kin groups may not always be as supportive as might be supposed (Harris 1992) New settlers may perceive non-family social resources as more supportive than family-based resources because they entail less mutual obligation and associated burden (Simich et al. 2003). Furthermore, non-family social relations may be important for reasons other than emotional support. Reestablishing life and social order in a new place—as refugees and their communities must do—calls for the establishment of links to the wider community.

The RRP illuminated the importance of the like-ethnic community as a social resource, particularly during the early years of resettlement (Beiser 1999; Canadian Task Force 1988). During the initial years in a new country, the search for a like-ethnic community exerts a stronger pull on refugees than the search for jobs (Simich et al. 2003). The presence of a large like-ethnic community, which some researchers (Murphy 1973, 1977) have conceptualized as "critical mass" and others (Becares et al. 2009; Georgiades et al. 2007; Boyle et al. 2007) as neighbourhood ethnic density protects mental health (Beiser 1999; Murphy 1973, 1977; Boyle et al. 2007; Georgiades et al. 2007).

Explaining the advantage of a like-ethnic community is not straightforward. It seems plausible that the like-ethnic community provides instrumental support, for example as an avenue towards finding employment. According to RRP results, however, this potential advantage was negligible. A small number of the marginally employable were able to find work in like-ethnic businesses, but there was a potential down-side since many of the jobs were poorly paid and offered little or no chance for advancement (Johnson 1988). The inner life of the refugee offers a more likely route to explanation. Having someone with whom to share memories of the sights, sounds and smells of home provides emotional support for people trying to find their way in a new country. Aside from friendship, the like-ethnic community probably provides affirmational support (Stewart 2000; Stewart and Lagille 2000; Stewart et al. 2008), by nurturing one's inner life. Major life disruptions, such as becoming a refugee in a strange country, challenge basic assumptions about self-worth and its relationship to the past. North America offers little reassurance to immigrants and refugees from other places that their cultural histories make them worthwhile people. Ethnic enclaves probably offer a partial remedy for self-doubt. The language, institutions and patterns of social interaction within the ethnic enclave provide a bridge between present and past, and a sense of continuity that affirm the value of one's historical identity within a radically new environment.

The benefits of the like-ethnic community appear to be time-dependent. According to the RRP, the like-ethnic community made a powerful contribution to maintaining mental health during the immediate post-arrival period, but by the end of the first decade of resettlement, refugees who were initially disadvantaged by lack of an ethnocultural community presence were more likely than the others to have learned English and to have established contacts with the wider society (Beiser 1999). The RRP results are consistent with the LSIC in suggesting the mental health salience of network diversity—having a foot firmly implanted in a heritage community, while at the same time making new friends and participating in larger organizational networks (Levitt et al. 2005).

Putnam (2000) opines that bonding and bridging are not either-or categories, but, instead that simultaneous bonding along some social dimensions and bridging across others is both common and helpful, but others (Eastmond 1998, 2011; Beiser and Johnson 2003) caution that overly exclusive within ethnic group bonding creates a risk of missing out on the benefits of building bridging relationships.

Bridging Networks

Newcomers don't always have ready-made like-ethnic communities waiting for them. After all, someone has to be the first to arrive. The way in which Canada chose to admit SEA refugees created an "experiment in nature" that the RRP investigators used to test the idea that private sponsors might potentially provide the support refugees typically look for in like-ethnic communities. The federal government resettled the SEA refugees throughout Canada's ten provinces and two territories. Like all citizens and permanent residents of Canada, the refugees were entitled to provincially administered, insured health care. Many received language training in federally funded programs, and their children attended schools supported by provincial tax dollars.

On the whole, privately sponsored refugees received a little extra support. Sponsors were obliged to provide financial support for the person or family they sponsored for a period of one year, or until the person or family had achieved financial stability, whichever came first. Moved by the horrors of the Southeast Asian experience, most private sponsors did more: they helped refugees find jobs, schools for their children, doctors and dentists. Assuming that the level of welcome the privately sponsored group received would give them an advantage over the government sponsored, whose only official guide to the new society was a usually overworked civil servant, the RRP investigators predicted that privately sponsored refugees would enjoy better mental health than the government sponsored. In the short run, the prediction proved wrong. There were no mental health differences between the two groups in 1981 or in 1983. In retrospect, government and academics were more impressed with the virtues of private sponsorship than the refugees themselves. Most people, including the RRP investigators, predicted that the private sponsors' willingness to commit their time and personal resources to newcomers could be nothing but an advantage.

A survey of the refugees, conducted a few years after they came to Canada, offered some insights. Half of all privately sponsored Southeast Asian refugees and almost all the government sponsored said that government sponsorship was preferable to private (Woon 1987). Intrusiveness was one of the downsides of private sponsorship. Feeling they were acting as good, concerned hosts, private sponsors called the refugees at all hours and insisted on taking them to activities. Sometimes they forgot that refugee families, like all other families, need and value privacy. There were other well-intentioned sponsor actions that proved insensitive to the refugees' situations. For example, they often found housing that the refugees could not afford once the sponsorship period terminated, or they looked for housing close to them rather than to the ethnic communities in which the refugees would have preferred to live. Inequity was another source of discontent. Government sponsored refugees all got the same treatment, whereas, in the words of one refugee, "With private sponsorship, sometimes it depended on luck whether you met a nice group or not" (Woon 1987, p. 141).

A sub-group of privately sponsored refugees in the RRP was, in fact, at greater risk for depression than the government sponsored (Beiser 1999). These were refugees whose religions did not match their sponsors. Most of the sponsors were Christian or non-denominational, most of the refugees either Christian, Buddhists or members of one of the smaller Southeast Asian religious groups. Non-Christian refugees sponsored by Christian groups developed very high rates of depression.

Overt attempts to proselytize the refugees took place, but the psychological pressures the refugees experienced were often at a more subtle level. The refugees had difficulty understanding the concept of voluntary sponsorship. Since the sponsors were not family, but strangers, many reasoned that something was required in return. Virtually all the sponsoring groups had been organized through a network of multi-faith religious institutions. Since religious institutions provided the context for sponsorship, the refugees came to believe that they were expected to adopt their sponsors' religions. Some did and regretted it. Others did not, but felt they were being ungrateful. In these circumstances, the risk of depression increased (Beiser et al. 1989; Beiser 1999).

The difficulties with Canada's large-scale experiment with private sponsorship by no means suggests that Canada or other countries should abandon hosting or sponsorship programs. First of all, there were successes that offset some of the difficulties, even in the short run. For example, the privately sponsored refugees were quicker than the government sponsored to adopt constructive financial practices such as opening savings accounts and buying insurance, presumably because of their sponsors' tutelage (Johnson 1988). Over the longer term, some sponsor relationships turned into long-term friendships, from which the refugees benefited (Woon 1987; Westermeyer et al. 1983b). Furthermore, RRP findings deriving from the end of the refugees' first decade in Canada (Beiser and Johnson 2003) strongly suggest that private sponsorship promoted integration, including learning to speak English and obtaining long-term employment.

The RRP's quantitative results direct attention to trends and associations. They do not explain, and explanation is badly needed. For example, although the data suggest that private sponsorship helped the refugees adapt, they do not explain how this type of support helped. According to Neuwirth and Clark (1981), private sponsors may have exposed refugees to a broader range of services than government settlement workers were able to, for example, helping the refugees find their way to language training classes, helping them find schools for their children and helping them find places to live. These authors do, however, point out that still more might have been accomplished: "Sponsors act, as it were, as the direct representatives of the new society: apart from providing material help, they, ideally should also guide the refugees in their initial social and cultural adjustment" (Neuwirth and Clark, p. 139). In some cases, according to these authors, private sponsors fulfilled this role in whole or in part and, in the process, helped the refugees deal with feelings of isolation, and of social inferiority. Since sponsorship is a potentially powerful tool to facilitate both refugee admission and integration, the topic requires more research attention. Future studies should investigate how factors such as the actual length of contact between refugees and their sponsors, the kinds of help proffered by sponsorship groups, and how non-instrumental aspects of the sponsorship role may affect long-term success.

Linking Networks

There is surprisingly little interaction between refugees and formal helping agencies in the post-arrival period, even though services do apparently help (Beiser 1999; Rutter et al. 2007). Language training is one example: although it is, in theory, available to all newcomers, women and the elderly are notably less likely to receive it than other refugees (Beiser 1999), despite the fact that, in the job market, women benefit more from such training than men (Beiser and Hou 2001).

Without language one can never really enter a new society. Two years after their arrival in Vancouver, 17 % of the refugees in the RRP sample spoke English well, 67 % had moderate command of the language, and 16 % spoke no English. Ten years later, 32 % had good language skills, 60 % moderate skills, and 8 % still spoke no English (Hou and Beiser 2006). For a country committed to equal opportunity, it is troubling that, as long as a decade after arriving in Canada, a small, but significant number of newcomers had not acquired one of the most basic tools for integration. This shortfall highlights the need for research to illuminate the respective effects of disadvantage, incentive, and opportunity on language acquisition.

During the initial period of resettlement, English-speaking ability had no effect on depression or on employment. However, by the end of the first decade in Canada, English language fluency was a significant predictor of depression and employment, particularly among refugee women and among people who did not become engaged in the labor market during the earliest years of resettlement (Hou and Beiser 2006). Language and employment had a reciprocal relationship over time. Language not only helped ensure job advancement, but steady employment in non-ethnic settings proved a powerful predictor of language acquisition.

Young, well educated male refugees were the most likely to learn English during the first year or two in Canada. In comparison with their young male counterparts, females and elderly refugees tended to be less well educated and less likely to have had any prior exposure to English, and their level of language fluency was correspondingly lower (Beiser 1999). The initial linguistic disadvantages of women and the elderly were compounded by lack of opportunity. For example, because English as a Second Language (ESL) classes were primarily directed to persons deemed likely to enter the labour force, women and the elderly were less likely to receive such instruction (Beiser 1999; Beiser and Hou 2001, Hou and Beiser 2006). More recent developments such as Canada's Language Instruction for Newcomers to Canada programmes have been developed in order to reach previously neglected groups, but there is evidence that women are still underserviced by language-training programmes (Boyd 1992). This is ironic in view of the fact that, according to RRP data, women derived more benefit from ESL classes than men (Beiser and Hou 2001).

Elderly Chinese were one of the groups least likely to learn English. Although a large like-ethnic community provides many advantages for new settlers (Beiser 1999), RRP study findings suggest that, unless balanced by integrative efforts, the strands of what was initially a safety net can knit together into a cocoon. Although linguistic segregation may be an option for newcomers who become part of large, established communities, the elderly who opt for this type of adaptation are at risk of becoming isolated from their grandchildren as well as the larger society (Beiser 1999).

Taking a cue from the criteria used by the British Council & Migration Policy Group (MPG) ratings of countries according to policies and institutions likely to promote the integration of newcomers, the Community in Distress (CID) focused on the role of linking networks in predicting successful integration. The opportunity to pursue education is one of the MPG criteria. According to CID results, the opportunity to obtain education in Canada—whether this consisted of job re-training, or the pursuit of higher education—created a definite advantage.

According to Ryan (2010), religious participation contributes to building relationships with the larger society, and other research demonstrates that religious institutions can help communities mobilize in order to address refugee unemployment (Channel 2000; Fenta et al. 2004). According to CID results, religious belief was an advantage for women, albeit not for men. The importance of religious faith for women resettling in new countries has been documented in other studies. For example, in a study of Latin American migrants in Europe, Kirchner and Patino (2010) found an inverse relationship between religiosity and depression among women, but not among men.

6.3 Focusing on Resilience: Implications for Practice and for Policy

Data suggesting that the way in which refugees handle time perspective is a component of their psychological resilience has important implications for clinical practice. The data suggest that the question, "Does psychological intervention mitigate distress or impede recovery from the effects of trauma? (Deahl 2000)" is too simplistic. Evidence suggests that interventions based on the premise that it is always better for survivors of trauma to reveal than to conceal their experiences are either not effective or can be harmful (Deahl 2000; McNally et al. 2003). In addition to individual needs, which can vary from survivor to survivor, approaches to care should take timing and context into account. In the immediate or medium-term aftermath of catastrophe, it may prove most effective to support individual attempts to suppress the past and focus on the present and future. Helping refugees address issues such as employment, housing, and effective parenting rather than focusing on prematurely tearing away the scar tissue of forgetting is one important way to support resilience.

The CID results contribute to a growing literature portraying PTSD as the end result of a complex process initiated by catastrophic stress, and reinforced by stresses of passage to a new life, as well as the depletion of internal and external coping resources. Healing should take account of this web of interactions and of potential points of intervention that the findings suggest. Sometimes, for example, a psychological intervention to help individuals deal with index trauma may be the preferred point of entry, but sometimes it may be more strategic to focus on helping individuals deal with post-migration stresses, or on developing linkages with settlement and other social services, or on integrating with the receiving society (Peisker and Tilbury 2003).

Health care providers should, however, be vigilant about the possibility that years, or even decades after refugees have resettled and apparently effected a satisfactory adjustment, mental health risk based on past experience may resurface, and that resurfacing may be tied to significant adult developmental periods. Context affects mental health risk. Earlier attempts to help refugees achieve occupational success and to establish and maintain an enduring relationship provides a supportive context for mental health intervention when the apparently ineluctable process of retrieving memory is set in motion.

Although a considerable amount is known about social networks as a source of resilience, much remains unknown. It is, for example, important to explore and establish why non-kin social networks appear to be more powerful than kin-based networks in protecting against the emergence of mental disorders such as PTSD, and in promoting integration. The mental health effects of linking networks and societal institutions such as the health care system, education, and religious institutions are at best poorly understood.

National policy has been too exclusively preoccupied with adjudicating the legitimacy of refugee claims, and with developing selection procedures to ensure that Canada admits healthy people. Too little policy and practice are directed to ensuring that refugees stay healthy. This neglect is wrong-headed: ensuring that new settlers not only are healthy when they get here, but that they stay that way is just, humane, and consistent with national self-interest.

References

Ager, A., & Strang, A. (2008). Understanding integration: A conceptual framework. *Journal of Refugee Studies, 21*(2), 166–191.
Antze, P., & Lambek, M. (Eds.). (1996). *Tense past: Cultural essays in trauma and memory*. New York: Routledge.
Bagheri, A. (1992). Psychiatric problems among Iranian immigrants in Canada. *Canadian journal of psychiatry. Revue canadienne de psychiatrie, 37*(1), 7–11.
Baskauskas, L. (1981). The Lithuanian refugee experience and grief. *International Migration Review, 15*(1), 276–291.
Becares, L., Nazroo, J., & Stafford, M., (2009). The buffering effects of ethnic density on experienced racism and health. *Health and Place, 15*(3), 700–708.
Beiser, M. (1987). Changing time perspective and mental health among Southeast Asian refugees. *Culture, Medicine and Psychiatry, 11*, 437–464.
Beiser, M. (1988). Influences of time, ethnicity, and attachment on depression in Southeast Asian refugees. *The American journal of psychiatry, 145*(1), 46–51.
Beiser, M. (1999). *Strangers at the gate. The "Boat People's" first ten years in Canada*. Toronto: University of Toronto Press.
Beiser, M., & Hou, F. (2001). Language acquisition, unemployment and depressive disorder among Southeast Asian Refugees: A 10-year study. *Social Science & Medicine, 53*, 1321–1334.
Beiser, M., & Hyman, I. (1997). Refugees' time perspective and mental health. *American Journal of Psychiatry, 154*, 996–1002.
Beiser, M., & Johnson, P. (2003). Sponsorship and resettlement success. *Journal of International Migration and Integration, 4*(2), 203–216.
Beiser, M., & Wickrama, K. A. S. (2004). Trauma, time and mental health: A study of temporal reintegration and depressive disorder among Southeast Asian Refugees. *Psychological Medicine, 34*(5), 899–910.
Beiser, M., Turner, R. J., & Ganesan, S. (1989). Catastrophic stress and factors affecting its consequences among Southeast Asian refugees. *Social science & medicine (1982), 28*, 183–195.
Beiser, M., Johnson, P. J., & Turner, R. J. (1993). Unemployment, underemployment and depressive affect among Southeast Asian refugees. *Psychological medicine, 23*, 731–743.
Beiser, M., Simich, L., Pandalangat, N., Nowakowski, M., & Fu, T. (2011). Stresses of passage, balms of resettlement, and posttraumatic stress disorder among Sri Lankan Tamils in Canada. *Canadian Journal of Psychiatry, 56*(6), 333–340.
Berry, J. W., & Blondel, T. (1970). Psychological adaptation of Vietnamese refugees in Canada. *Can J Community Mental Health, 1*, 81–88.
Boyd, M. (1992). Gender issues in immigration and language fluency. In B. R. Chiswick (Ed.), *Immigration, language, and ethnicity: Canada and the United States* (pp. 305–372). Washington, D. C.: The AEI Press.
Boyle, M. H., Georgiades, K., Racine, Y., & Mustard, C. (2007). Neighbourhood and family influences on educational attainment: Results from the Ontario child health study follow-up 2001. *Child Development, 78*(1), 168–189.
Canadian task force on mental health issues affecting immigrants and refugees. (1988). *After the door has been opened: Mental health issues affecting immigrants and refugees in Canada*. (No. Ci96-38/1988E). Ottawa: Ministry of Supply and Services Canada.
Channel, K. (2000). The social mobilization approach: A participatory model for local resources mobilization. *Canadian Journal of Development Studies, 21*(4), 479–494.
Cottle, T. J. (1967). The circles test: An investigation of perceptions of temporal relatedness and dominance. *Journal of Projective Techniques and Personality Assessment, 31*, 58–71.
Cottle, T. J. (1969). The location of experience: A manifest time orientation. *Acta Psychological (Amst), 28*, 129–149.
Cottle, T. J. (1976). *Perceiving time. A psychological investigation of men and women*. New York: Wiley.

Deahl, M. (2000). Psychological debriefing: Controversy and challenge. *Australian and New Zealand Journal of Psychiatry, 34,* 929–939.
Derose, K. P. (2008). Do bonding, bridging, and linking social capital affect preventable hospitalizations? *Health Services Research (October 2008), 43*(5p1), 1520–1541.
Eastmond, M. (1998). Bosnian Muslim refugees in Sweden. *Journal of Refugee Studies, 11*(2), 161–181.
Eastmond, M. (2011). Egalitarian ambitions, constructions of difference: The paradoxes of refugee integration in Sweden. *Journal of Ethnic and Migration Studies, 37*(2), 277–295.
The ESEMeD/MHEDEA 2000 Investigators. (2004). Prevalence of mental disorders in Europe: Results from the European study of the epidemiology of mental disorders (ESEMeD) project. *Acta Psychiatrica Scandinavica 2004, 109*(Suppl. 420), 21–27.
Ellenberger, H. F. (1993). The pathogenic secret and its therapeutics, in Beyond the Unconscious: Essays of Henri F. Ellenberger. In M. Micale (Ed.), *The History of Psychiatry.* Princeton: Princeton University Press.
Fazel, M., Wheeler, J., & Danesh, J. (9 April 2005). Prevalence of serious mental disorder in 7000 refugees resettled in western countries: A systematic review. *The Lancet, 365,* 1309–1314.
Fenta, H., Hyman, I., & Noh, S. (2004). Determinants of depression among Ethiopian refugees in Toronto. *Journal of Nervous and Mental Disease, 192,* 363–372.
Friedlander, S. (1979). *When memory comes.* Toronto: McGraw-Hill.
Georgiades, K., Boyle, M., & Duku, E. (2007). Contextual influences on children's mental health and school performance: The moderating effects of family immigrant status. *Child Development, 78*(5), 1572–1159.
Goldfield, N., & Lee, W. (1982). Caring for Indochinese refugees. *American family physician, 26*(3), 157–160.
Granovetter, M. S. (1973). "The Strength of Weak Ties." American. *Journal of Sociology, 78*(6), 1360–1380.
Grinberg, L. (1984). A psychoanalytic study of migration: Its normal and pathological aspects. *Journal of the American Psychoanalytic Association, 32,* 13–38.
Harris, T. O. (1992). Some reflections on the process of social support; and nature of unsupportive behaviours. In H. O. F. Veiel & U. Bumann (Eds.), *The meaning and measurement of social support* (pp. 171–189). New York: Hemisphere Publishing Corp.
Hollifield, M., Warner, T. D., Lian, N., Krakow, B., Jenkins, J. H., Kessler, J., et al. (2002). Measuring trauma and health status in refugees. A critical review. *JAMA: the journal of the American Medical Association, 288*(5), 611–621.
Holmes, T. H., & Masuda, M. (1973). Life change and illness susceptibility. In J. P. Scott & E. C. Senay (Eds.), *Separation and Depression: Clinical and Research Aspects.* Washington, DC: American Association for the Advancement of Science.
Hou, F., & Beiser, M. (March 2006). Learning the language of a new country: A ten-year study of english acquisition by Southeast Asian Refugees in Canada. *International Migration, 44*(1), 135–165.
Hyndman, J. (2003). Aid, Conflict and Migration: The Canada Sri Lanka Connection. The Canadian Geographer, *47,* 251–258.
Johnson, P. J. (1988). The impact of ethnic communities on the employment of Southeast Asian refugees. *Amerasia, 14*(1), 22.
Kim, D., Subramanian, S. V., & Kawachi, I. (2006). Bonding versus Bridging Social Capital and Their Associations with Self-Rated Health: A Multilevel Analysis of 40 US Communities. *Journal of Epidemiology and Community Health, 60,* 116–122.
Kirchner, T., & Patio, C. (2010). Stress and depression in Latin American immigrants: The mediating role of religiosity. *European Psychiatry, 25,* 479–484.
Kirmayer, L. J. (1996). Landscapes of memory: Trauma, narrative, and dissociation. In P. Antze & M. Lambek (Eds.), *Tense past: Cultural essays in trauma and memory* (pp. 173–198). New York: Routledge.

Levitt, M., Lane, J., & Levitt, J. (2005). Immigration stress, social support, and adjustment in the first postmigration year: An intergenerational analysis. *Research in Human Development, 2*(4), 159–177.

McNally, R. J., Bryant, R. A., & Ehlers, A. (2003). Does early psychological intervention promote recovery from posttraumatic stress? Psychological Science in the. *Public Interest, 4*(2), 45–79.

Mollica, R. (2006). *Healing invisible wounds. Paths to hope in a violent world*. Orlando: Harcourt.

Mollica, R. F., Poole, C., & Tor, S. (1998). Symptoms, functioning and health problems in a massively traumatized population: The legacy of the Cambodian tragedy. In B. P. Dohrenwend (Ed.), *Adversity, stress and psychopathology*. New York: Oxford University Press.

Murphy, H. B. M. (1973). Migration and the major mental disorders: A reappraisal. In C. Zwingmann & M. Pfister-Ammende (Eds.), *Uprooting and After* (pp. 204–220). New York, NY: Springer-Verlag.

Murphy, H. B. M. (1977). Migration, culture and mental health. *Psychological medicine, 7*(4), 677–684.

Neuwirth, G., & Clarke, L. (1981). Indochinese refugees in Canada: Sponsorship and adjustment. *International Migration Review, 15*(131), 140.

O'Campo, P., Salmon, C., & Burke, J. G. (2009). Neighbourhoods and mental well-being: What are the pathways? *Health and Place, 15*, 56–68.

Pearlin, L., Lieberman, M. A., Menaghan, E. G., & Mullan, O. T. (1981). The stress process. *Journal of Health and Social Behavior, 22*, 337–356.

Pedersen, S. (1949). Psychopathological reactions to extreme social displacements (refugee neuroses). *Psychoanalytic Review, 36*, 344–354.

Peisker, V. C., & Tilbury, F. (2003). Active and passive resettlement: the influence of support services and refugees' own resources on resettlement style. *International Migration, 41*(5), 61–89.

Putnam, R. D. (2000). *Bowling alone: The collapse and revival of American Community*. New York: Simon & Schuster.

Ritsner, M., Modai, I., & Poniszovsky, A. (2000). The stress-support patterns and psychological distress of immigrants. *Stress Medicine, 16*(3), 139–147.

Ross, C. D. (2000). Neighbourhood disadvantage and adult depression. *Journal of Health and Social Behavior, 41*, 177–187.

Rumbaut, R. G. (1985). Mental health and the refugee experience: A comparative study of Southeast Asian refugees. In T. Owan, B. Bliatout, K. M. Lin, et al. (Eds.), *Southeast Asian mental health: Treatment, prevention, services, and research*. Rockville: National Institute of Mental Health.

Rumbaut, R. G. (1998). Portraits, patterns and predictors of the refugee adaptation process: A comparative study of Southeast Asian refugees. In D. W. Haines (Ed.), *Refugees and immigrants: Cambodians, Laotians, and Vietnamese in America*. Totowa: Rowman and Littlefield.

Rutter, J., Colley, L., Reynolds, S., & Sheldon, R. (2007). From refugee to citizen: "Standing on my own two feet," a research report on integration, "Britishness" and citizenship. Refugee Support Trust and the Institute of Public Policy Research.

Ryan, A. (2010). The bonding and bridging roles of religious institutions for refugees in a non-gateway context. *Ethnic and Racial Studies, 33*(6), 1049–1068.

Simich, L., Beiser, M., & Mawani, F. (2003). Social support and the significance of shared experience in refugee migration and resettlement. *Western Journal of Nursing Research, 25*(7), 872–891.

Stewart, M. (2000). *Chronic conditions and caregiving in Canada: Social support strategies*. Toronto: University of Toronto Press.

Stewart, M. J., & Lagille, L. (2000). A framework for social support assessment and intervention in the context of chronic conditions and caregiving. In M. J. Stewart MJ (Ed.), *Chronic conditions and caregiving in Canada: Social support strategies (pp. 3–28)*. Toronto, Canada: University of Toronto Press.

Stewart, M., Anderson, J., & Mwakarimba, E. et al. (2008) Multi-cultural meanings of social support among immigrants and refugees. *International Migration, 46*(3), 123–159

Tyhurst, L. (1951). Displacement and migration: A study in social psychiatry. *The American journal of psychiatry, 107,* 561–568.
Tyhurst, L. (1977). Psychological first aid for refugees. *Mental Health and Society, 4,* 319–431.
UN commission on human rights. (1999) report of the working group on enforced or involuntary disappearances: Civil and political rights, including questions of disappearances and summary executions. Report on the visit to Sri Lanka by a member of the working group on enforced or involuntary disappearances, E/CN.4/Add.1/2000/64.
Vaage, A. B., Thomsen, P. H., Silove, D., Wentzel-Larsen, T., Ta, T. V., & Hauff, E. (2010). Long-term mental health status of Vietnamese refugees in the aftermath of trauma, The British. *Journal of Psychiatry, 196,* 122–125.
Westermeyer, J., Vang, T. F., & Neider, J. (1983a). Migration and mental health among Hmong refugees: Association of pre- and postmigration stress with self-rating scales. *Journal of Nervous and Mental Disease, 171,* 86–91.
Westermeyer, J., Vang, T. F., & Neider, J. (1983b). Refugees who do and do not seek psychiatric care: An analysis of pre-migratory and post-migratory characteristics. *Journal of Nervous and Mental Disease, 171,* 92–96.
Woon, Y. (1987). The mode of refugee sponsorship and the socio-economic adaptation of Vietnamese in Victoria: A three-year perspective. In K. B. Chan & D. M. Indra (Eds.), *Uprooting, loss and adaptation: The resettlement of Indochinese in Canada* (pp. 132–146) Ottawa: Canadian Public Health Association.
Zhao, J., Xue, L., & Gilkinson, T. (2010). Health status and social capital of recent immigrants in Canada: Evidence from the longitudinal survey of immigrants to Canada. In T. McDonald, E. Ruddick, A. Sweetman, & C. Worswick (Eds.), *Canadian immigration: Economic evidence for a dynamic policy environment. Montréal and Kingston* (Chapter 12, pp. 311–340). Canada: McGill-Queen's University Press.

Chapter 7
Social Support in Refugee Resettlement

Miriam J. Stewart

Abstract Refugees face challenges in resettlement countries, including language difficulties, acculturative stress, societal prejudice, and loneliness that jeopardize their integration. They have been exposed to violent conflicts and acute traumatic incidents, including forced separation from family members. Social support has the potential to decrease refugees' isolation and loneliness, enhance their sense of belonging and life fulfillment, mediate the stress of discrimination and facilitate integration into a new society. Differences among refugees reinforce the need to elucidate the role of ethnicity in the design of culturally-relevant social support interventions. The studies described in this chapter explicate African refugees' support needs, support resources and preferences for ethno-culturally based support interventions and their impacts.

Keywords Refugee · Africa · Isolation · Social support · Support intervention

7.1 Research Approach and Conceptual Foundation

Refugees face challenges in resettlement countries, including language difficulties, acculturative stress, societal prejudice, and loneliness that jeopardize their integration (Beiser et al. 2011a, b; Ellis et al. 2010; McMichael and Manderson 2004; Karunakara et al. 2004; Stewart et al. 2010a, b). Refugees have been exposed to violent conflicts, and acute traumatic incidents, including forced separation from family members (Jaranson et al. 2004).

Social support has the potential to decrease refugees' isolation and loneliness (Bhui et al. 2006; Jaranson et al. 2004); enhance their sense of belonging and life fulfillment; mediate the stress of discrimination (Brooker and Eakin 2001; Din-Dzietham et al. 2004); and, facilitate integration into a new society (Stewart et al. 2008a, b). Our previous Canadian research revealed refugees' belief that social support can enhance health and reduce loneliness and isolation

M. J. Stewart (✉)
Faculty of Nursing, University of Alberta, Edmonton, Canada
e-mail: miriam.stewart@ualberta.ca

(Stewart et al. 2010a, b; Stewart et al. 2008a, b). However, several factors obstruct newcomers' ability to mobilize social support in their countries of resettlement, including intergenerational conflicts, struggle for employment, inadequate knowledge of resources, language difficulties, and lack of transportation (Guerin et al. 2003). The loss of social support has detrimental impacts for refugees (Reynolds 2004; Simich et al. 2004). Loss of social support through migration and diminished social networks exert detrimental impacts on integration (Reynolds 2004; Merry et al. 2011; Simich et al. 2004). Lack of social support has a detrimental effect on mental health (Beiser et al. 2011a, b; Gottlieb and Bergen 2010). Separation from family exacerbates the severity of psychological problems. Newcomers with extensive social support are more likely to access professional services (Alegria et al. 2004). Social support can reduce refugees' isolation and loneliness (Beiser et al. 2011a, b; Beiser et al. 2010; Bhui et al. 2006; Jaranson et al. 2004); enhance their sense of belonging and life satisfaction; mediate the stress of discrimination (Brooker and Eakin 2001; Din-Dzietham et al. 2004); and, facilitate integration into a new society (Stewart et al. 2008a, b).

Migration, with attendant lack of support from extended kin, may compromise the adaptation of refugee new parents and their children (Foss et al. 2004; Schweitzer et al. 2006; Warner 2007). Social isolation is amplified by restrictions on travel to home countries, and barriers to family reunification. Social relations that provide meaning in the country of origin are often disrupted in the new country (McMichael and Manderson 2004). Migration can alter the customary patterns of parenting and family care giving (Drummond et al. 2011; Merry et al. 2011). Recent migration can negatively affect children's social development (Anne Casey Foundation 2006; Foss et al. 2004). Sole responsibility for family support, family composition, and length of time in the new country influence refugees' experiences and perceptions of social support (Davies and Bath 2001; Simich et al. 2004). Newcomer mothers experience loss of supportive networks (Foss et al. 2004; Merry et al. 2011; Murray et al. 2010). Types of sources (Harrison et al. 1995; Morrison et al. 1997) and appraisal (Moon-Park and Dimigen 1994) of social support may differ cross-culturally and social support yields differing adaptive results for migrants from different source and host countries (Simich et al. 2010).

African refugees' perceptions of their support needs and of interventions that could strengthen support have not been solicited. Despite the demonstrable importance of social support for refugees, research focused on culturally appropriate social-support interventions is rare (Barrio 2000) and the interaction between support and ethnicity has been neglected in social support intervention research (Gottlieb 2000). Although recent research suggests the potential beneficial effects of social support in ameliorating acculturative challenges, isolation, and resource deprivation (Beiser 1999; Davies and Bath 2001; Stewart et al. 2008a, b; Warner 2007), no support interventions for refugees have been designed and tested. Our review of research published from 1996 to 2011 revealed no social support intervention studies focused on African refugees. Differences among refugees reinforce the need to elucidate the role of ethnicity in the design of culturally-relevant social support interventions for refugees. Consequently, the studies described in this chapter explicate African refugees' support needs, support resources and preferences for ethno-culturally based support interventions and the impacts of support interventions.

7.1.1 Conceptual Foundation

Social support is a resource for *coping* with stressful situations (Gottlieb and Bergen 2010) (e.g., immigration, resettlement, stressful new parenthood). Social support is defined as interactions with family members, friends, peers, and professionals that communicate information, affirmation, practical aid, or understanding (Stewart 2000). Social networks provide varied types of support functions (Gottlieb and Bergen 2010; Stewart 2000), which should be specific to stressful situations (Cutrona 1990). As most social relationships have positive and negative elements (House et al. 1988; Thoits 1986), the supportive and non-supportive elements of interactions and relationships should be appraised (Gottlieb and Bergen 2010). Support can either endure or dissipate over time in stressful situations (Lawrence and Kearns 2005; Stewart et al. 2008a, b) (e.g., migration). *Support-seeking* as a coping strategy for managing stressful situations has been linked to greater provision of support, whereas people who use distancing and avoidance coping strategies tend to have fewer support resources (Thoits 1995). Social support and coping have bi-directional effects (House et al. 1988). For example, the ways refugees cope can provide clues to potential supporters about support needed. Conversely, the amount and type of support received can influence refugees' choice of coping strategies. Variables that influence social support include community size, socioeconomic status, age, gender, marital status, and ethnicity (Maton et al. 1996; Gottlieb and Bergen 2010). Three social processes (social exchange, social comparison, social learning) can emerge within support groups and/or dyads in social support interventions. As close relationships develop between refugee parents and peers, reciprocity would be evident in dyadic and group interactions (social exchange theory) (House et al. 1988; Thoits 1995). According to social comparison theory, individuals compare themselves and affiliate with others (e.g. peers in dyads or groups who share language and culture) who have first-hand experiential knowledge of the stressful situation (House et al. 1988). Self-efficacy and communal efficacy, concepts integral to social learning theory (Thoits 1995), can be enhanced through support interventions. Peer support, based on personal 'experiential knowledge', is a critical source of social learning for vulnerable people and can supplement professional support derived from professional knowledge (Caputo et al. 1997; Health Canada 1996; Miller 1992).

7.1.2 Design/Methods

Consistent with principles of participatory research (Stewart et al. 2010a, b; Ahmed et al. 2004), participants specified their support needs and preferred type and substantive content of a support intervention in the studies described in this chapter. Support interventions have typically not been informed by participants' assessment of their support resources, needs, and preferences (Gottlieb 2000; Gottlieb and Bergen 2010). Advisory committees composed of partners from public, practice, program, and policy domains were created in each city to provide advice and feedback on: the selection, screening and training of research staff; amendment of interview guides and measures; culturally appropriate recruitment strategies; design of the intervention; and, knowledge mobilization. Organizations serving African refugees participated in these community advisory committees. Moreover, use of experienced peers (former African refugees) to conduct interviews and provide support enhanced the credibility and acceptability of the studies.

The studies employed a multi-method research design (Ahmed et al. 2004; Stewart et al. 2008a, b) to address complex research problems (Tashkkori and Teddlie 2003). Qualitative and quantitative methods were used (Stewart et al. 2008a, b; Tashkkori and Teddlie 2003) to corroborate, elaborate, and illuminate understanding of the phenomena under study, thereby enhancing validity, transferability, and confidence (Beazley and Ennew 2006). Qualitative methods were employed to enhance understanding of sensitive issues and meanings, perceptions, beliefs, values, and behaviours of refugee new parents (Gottlieb and Bergen 2010; Tashakkori and Teddlie 2003). An interpretive critical perspective within ethnography (Carpecken 1996) emphasizes the cultural and structural context. Qualitative data on intervention processes helped to elucidate the "black box" (who, what, where, when, why, how) of this psycho-social intervention (Stewart et al. 2008a, b; Tashkkori and Teddlie 2003). Quantitative measurements were used to test psycho-social outcomes of the support intervention (Stewart et al. 2008a, b); elucidate distinctions among pertinent variables; extend, refine, and cross-check qualitative data; and, potentially enable generalization to other refugee populations(Beazley and Ennew 2006; Tashkkori and Teddlie 2003). Qualitative data are emphasized in this chapter.

Participants were given information and consent forms translated into their preferred language and were asked for permission to audiotape their confidential interview for later transcription and analysis. Peer interviewers were matched to participants by gender (wherever possible), language and ethnicity, and interviews were conducted in each participant's preferred language, in sites accessible and acceptable to participants. Semi-structured interview guides for individual interviews and group interviews were translated into relevant languages including Shona, Ndebele and Arabic. Group interviews were conducted in the predominant language of group participants. All interviews were taped and transcribed for analysis. *The demographic characteristics of participants and data collection strategies for the five studies are summarized in Table 7.1.*

Table 7.1 Four Refugee Social Support Studies. (Source: Stewart et al. 2010a, b; Anderson et al. 2010; Stewart et al. 2008a, b; Makwarimba et al. 2013; Stewart et al. in press; Stewart et al. 2012; Stewart et al. 2011)

Focus and Funder	Objectives	Participants	Methods
Study 1 *Multicultural Meanings of Social Support among Immigrants and Refugees* (1,2,3) Social Sciences and Humanities Research Council	*Assessment of support needs* Describe the *meanings* of social support from the perspective of immigrants and refugees; Sources and types of support in Canada compared to homeland; Appraisal of support in Canada compared to homeland; Duration and changes in support over residency in Canada; Perceived impact on health, health behaviour, and use of health services. Identify immigrants and refugees' *methods* of accessing/seeking social support. Determine *mechanisms* to strengthen support for immigrants and refugees by identifying:	Somalia refugees (n= 60) Chinese immigrants/refugees (n= 60) Urban centers in Ontario, British Columbia, & Alberta	*Qualitative, participatory* Qualitative individual interviews conducted in participants' language by trained community research assistants
Study 2 *Assessment of African Refugees Support Needs and Support Intervention Preferences* (4) Social Sciences and Humanities Research Council	*Assessment of support needs and support intervention preferences* Assessment of support needs and preferences for support intervention Design a pilot support intervention in partnership with refugee-serving community partners for Somali and Sudanese refugees, their families, and communities	Somali refugees (n= 39) Sudanese refugees (n=29) Urban centers in Ontario & Alberta	*Multi-method participatory;* Qualitative individual interviews conducted in participants' language by trained community research assistants
Study 3 *Social Support Program for African Refugees* (5,6) Social Sciences and Humanities Research Council	*Support intervention* Evaluate the impact and benefits of the pilot support intervention on health, functioning, and resilience of refugees	Somali refugees(n= 27) Sudanese refugees (n=32) Peer and professional facilitators (Somali and Sudanese former refugees who had settled in Canada for more than 10 years). Urban centers in Ontario & Alberta	*Qualitative, participatory;* Post-test qualitative group interviews conducted in participants' language by trained community research assistants

Table 7.1 (continued)

Focus and Funder	Objectives	Participants	Methods
Study 4 *Mental Health of Sudanese and Zimbabwean First Time Parents and Children: Assessing the Support Needs and Intervention Preferences* (7) Alberta Centre for Child, Family & Community Research	*Assessment of support needs and support intervention preferences* Identify the 1) support needs, informal and formal support resources, and access and barriers to support for Sudanese and Zimbabwean refugees who are new parents; 2) their experiences of loneliness, social isolation, and attendant mental health challenges requiring support; 3) culture-specific and intracultural variations in support-seeking and support needs among these new refugee parents; 4) preferences for relevant social support interventions for refugee children and parents	Sudanese refugees (n=36) Zimbabwean refugees (n=39) Urban centers, 2 provinces, Ontario & Alberta	*Multi-method participatory;* Assessment of support needs and preferences for support; Qualitative interviews conducted in participants' language by trained community research assistants
Study 5 *Service Providers (from mainstream and refugee-serving organizations) and Policymakers* (7) Alberta Centre for Child, Family & Community Research	Determine *mechanisms* to strengthen support for refugees by: Including perspectives of immigrants/refugees and immigrant/refugee serving organizations on needed programs and policies Identifying implications for policies and programs	Service providers and policy influencers (n=22) Urban centers, 2 provinces, Ontario & Alberta	*Qualitative, Participatory,* Group interviews with service providers and with policy makers

7.2 Related Research Findings

7.2.1 Study 1 Assessment of Support Resources and Needs of Somali Refugees

We interviewed Somali refugees across three urban sites in three Canadian provinces—Ontario, British Columbia, and Alberta. Many Somali interviewees lived in poverty. They contrasted the notions of social support based on traditional norms of interdependence and reciprocity with norms and practices of a fragmented and impersonal service bureaucracy in Canada. Interviews with Somali refugees reveal a view of social support based primarily on historical cultural experiences of informal social networks. Influenced by norms of family connectedness and a deep sense of obligation to kin, Somali refugees continued to hold the same expectations for support that they did in their homeland, but circumstances forced them to rely on formal institutions. The Somali community in Canada is small and has limited social networks. These Somali refugees valued self-reliance, but coped independently primarily because of the relative lack of supports. Somali refugees revealed that culture influenced their support-seeking behaviors. They were guided by and found comfort in religious beliefs. This study revealed that social networks of newcomers and attendant supports dwindled upon immigration, particularly for Somali refugees. These findings complement McMichael and Manderson's (2004) study of Somali women in Australia, which revealed that problematic social networks restricted the women's capacity to use and create social capital in their new country. In our study, Somali refugees found it hard to support each other because of their poor financial standing, and the need to send money back to Somalia.

Our research revealed that Somali refugees experience unmet support needs, depleted social support networks, separation from families, difficulty establishing new ties in new communities, inadequate access to services, and lack of linguistically and culturally-appropriate support services. These newcomers described pathways through which social support influenced physical, mental, spiritual, and mental health. They emphasized the significant effects of social networks on health outcomes. In their view, social support facilitated their ability to meet basic needs; reduced stress; and, improved physical and mental health. Moreover, these newcomers believed that inadequate support exerted a negative influence on their health and use of health-related services, and conversely that poor health had a detrimental effect on their ability to seek or offer support. Our study demonstrated needs for support from ethnic peers and professionals. The major support needs and desires identified informed the design of a peer support intervention.

7.2.2 Study 2 Support Interventions for Somali and Sudanese Refugees- Assessment of Support Needs & Intervention Preferences

Somali and Sudanese refugees wanted assistance to enlarge and strengthen their existing networks and create new social networks. These newcomers faced difficulties establishing and maintaining social networks which impeded their integration in Canada. Participants reported experiencing many challenges including multiple low-paying jobs, lack of child care, family conflict, cramped living quarters in unsafe neighborhoods, financial worries, and language difficulties. These refugees wanted to explore ways to cope with their difficult circumstances and to access support. They desired culture-friendly programs encompassing other refugees from their cultural community. They recognized that there were many untapped resources in the community, and needed to know how to use these resources.

> At arrival one is completely confused and does not know where to begin. The second stage is during the period of settling, this is the period when crises usually crop up and without adequate support a family can easily disintegrate.

> Now the most needed support is at crisis time where frustrations have build up and expectations may not be up to one's hopes. This is the tempting time where families break apart easily. This is when true love and genuine relationship is put to the test. Without adequate support or intervention it becomes very fluid.

Some challenges prolonged integration into the Canadian system and support was needed to overcome these challenges. Language difficulties encountered with service providers inhibited access to services. Many service providers did not speak these refugees' languages.

Many participants lacked knowledge of the Canadian work culture and described discrimination manifested in job insecurity, poor treatment by employers, and inconsistent wages. Most participants perceived stigma about their religion and refugee status. Some reported humiliation when seeking services because they were treated as foreigners. Most participants faced difficulties navigating services such as education, health care, child care, legal aid, translation, community support, employment, recreation, and transportation. Lack of familiarity with these services, coupled with language barriers, made these refugees hesitant to approach service providers. These refugees reported loneliness and isolation which they attributed to discrimination and depleted social networks.

> How do we integrate if we are isolated to our confines of either refugees or low income families?

Spousal conflicts also emerged as a significant challenge. Conflicts and tensions within participants' families made it difficult for them to establish a new life in Canada. Conflicts arose when one spouse was dependent on the other for finances, language, and transportation. Moreover, changes in gender roles and responsibilities contradicted their culturally established husband-wife roles.

> When I first arrived I was desperately in need of many of the supports but at the same time after staying for a little while challenges ... arose in the house and this is the dangerous time where families can break apart. I think support is most needed on arrival but also at critical few months down the road when real issues begin to arise and the conflict in culture begins to take effect.

Refugees were often separated from their families for long periods of time. Participants were concerned about challenges facing family members left in their home country; their inability to communicate with their kin; and the prolonged process of family reunion. Some participants indicated that they had limited contact with their parents, children, or siblings who still lived in the home country or neighboring countries. They wanted to learn more about coping with the stresses of family separation and expediting the reunification process.

> I would like to know why family reunion takes so long. There are many refugees who left their loved ones behind and feel incomplete without those loved ones. Does the Government care so much that this is part of the support that the refugee is desperate to have in a limited time frame?

Refugees who had personal problems preferred one-to-one support because their issues were sensitive and confidential. Participants believed they could share personal information related to their problems with individual support providers and work together to find the best remedy.

> The one-on-one-support is more important for me. It gives me the opportunity to express myself without fear. Sometimes we are scared of sharing our challenges with our own community members for fear of being talked about or laughed at.

Participants who preferred group support noted that some common problems are faced by refugees. Groups can save time and resources, provide opportunities for participants to share coping strategies, and promote networking. They thought that group support was appropriate for dealing with issues in general terms and for receiving information.

Face-to-face support was the preferred mode of support delivery as participants believed that there would be no barrier between them and the support provider. Moreover, face-to-face support offered an opportunity to explain their needs with the help of body language and other cues. They believed they would be more comfortable asking some questions in person rather than via the telephone or internet. Face-to-face meetings offered lonely and isolated newcomers opportunities to socialize and receive human contact.

> In face-to-face type of service, I can try to explain what I need even if it is by gesture or by asking someone who knows my language to translate for me.

Participants preferred connecting with refugees who shared the same cultural background. For some participants, refugees shared similar experiences, while for others specific nationality was a distinguishing factor. Some, however, thought that culture-specific groups limited opportunities to learn from and integrate with people representing different backgrounds and cultures.

Many refugees from Sudan and Somalia were not proficient in English. In their view, common language should be the first consideration in creating support groups to enable newcomers to share experiences and learn from peers. Language was described as the key to effective support groups because refugees want to express themselves fully and seek answers without feeling self-conscious.

> Group [members] ... need to communicate or express their views to one another so they need to understand and speak [a] common language. Language is important in group support, for example I don't understand French or English but if anyone in our group speaks such languages I cannot understand and at the same time there will be no communication.

Refugees in different age groups experience different challenges, aspirations and expectations. Although older newcomers may be more concerned about health, children, and retirement, younger refugees may be preoccupied by education, work, and entertainment. While older generation refugees based behaviors and roles on their past, younger refugees were more focused on the future and less ingrained in their country of origin's traditions.

Peer and professional helpers who speak their language were considered particularly important to ensure that refugees' concerns received serious consideration and their support needs were communicated. Peer and professional helpers could offer potential solutions to challenges and enable refugees to discuss settlement challenges.

As accessibility to support programs was very important to these refugees, they recommended community venues close to their place of residence, free transportation, or home visits. Provision of child care was needed to increase accessibility and acceptability of support programs.

7.2.3 Study 3 Support Interventions for Somali and Sudanese Refugees

The support intervention gave refugees opportunities to meet new people and socialize with peers. Participants reported that they shared their problems within their support group and received different perspectives on potential solutions. Support groups were a source of informational support. Peer facilitators noted that some challenges faced by newcomers could have been avoided if they had information on support resources and services. The intervention promoted information exchange among refugee group members.

In addition to facilitating mutual exchange of support among group members, peer and professional facilitators provided translation and interpretation. Peer helpers enabled participants to complete immigration documents and facilitate reunion with family members from their home country. They provided information on available services to expedite reunification. Practical support offered included resume writing, job interview skills, and cooking. Peer and professional facilitators explained workers' rights and labor relations in Canada and provided information on conflict management, financial counseling, addressing spousal conflicts, supporting children with school work, dealing with discrimination, accessing services, and seeking optimum employment.

Participants shared stories of challenges at home and workplace, and suggested strategies to cope with these challenges. Participants had the opportunity to converse in their mother tongue with other refugees who shared the same cultural or ethnic background. Support sessions offered relief to participants who craved reconnection to their ethnic community. Prior to the intervention, they had no opportunity to meet with their peers. Refugees felt encouraged because they could bring their problems to the group and seek support. This social support intervention resulted in increased social integration, decreased loneliness, and expanded repertoire of coping strategies (Stewart et al. 2011).

Some participants indicated that support group sessions were not sufficiently long to discuss complex issues. Scheduling was challenging because most refugees worked multiple low-paying jobs, faced pressing issues, and had insufficient time. Although child care was provided in this support group intervention, it was not always convenient to travel with children to meeting venues, particularly for people who relied on public transit. For participants who did not prefer to bring their children to group meetings, finding trusted babysitters was sometimes challenging. A few participants mentioned that groups were intimidating for shy people, particularly when other participants had more education or better paying jobs.

7.2.4 Study 4—Support Needs and Support Intervention Preferences of Zimbabwean and Sudanese Refugee New Parents

Seventy-two new mothers and fathers from Sudan and Zimbabwe who came to Canada in the past five years and who had a first baby born in Canada under 12 months old, were interviewed individually. Support needs identified in interviews included isolation, loneliness, lack of culturally sensitive support, and information gaps regarding parenting skills, marital challenges, family disintegration, cultural conflict, employment, gender roles, and upgrading education. Following individual interviews, four group interviews were conducted with Sudanese ($n = 18$) and Zimbabwean ($n = 15$) new parents to seek information on support intervention preferences.

These new refugee parents were isolated and lonely. They lacked traditional family support during pregnancy, birth, and early postpartum and many had little contact with people from similar cultural backgrounds. Developing supportive networks is difficult because Sudanese and Zimbabwean family members were geographically dispersed. These interviews revealed significant needs for information about culturally appropriate services, more supportive service providers, and peer support to supplement professional support.

Some participants reported unprofessional attitudes from nurses and physicians. Many Sudanese female participants believed that their rights were violated when they had to sign hospital papers, without proper explanation in their own language. Refugee participants believed that their signatures were just a routine to protect hospital staff without considering their own preferences.

> I felt ignored at the hospital because I could not express myself in English. I was speaking [to] my husband. I told him—I feel pain and please tell the nurses. I didn't even have painkillers because the baby already came, because they hadn't really believed me because I wasn't crying or speaking for myself (Sudanese woman).

Men from both cultural communities expressed concerns regarding cultural family dynamics that threatened or disrupted newcomer homes. Access to supportive counseling and cultural sensitiveness by service providers was seen as essential. They reported that there is need for support programs that help families stay together. Some men believed that many programs were geared to support women at the expense of men and children. They noted that agencies should include settlement workers who are informed about the background and cultural context of family challenges.

> These elders could counsel families or couples and tell them, "my children what you are doing in your marriage is not part of our culture, this foreign behavior is ruining you, this is how you should treat your wife and this is how a man is treated." (Zimbabwean man)

Zimbabwean male participants discussed division of work at home. Some men felt that the circumstances in Canada warranted that spouses assume equal roles in the home. Others, however, believed men should take a helping role when they see the need but housework should remain the domain of the wife.

Refugee communities need outside support to address challenges such as marital conflicts and reconcile cultural differences. Suggested solutions include the use of peers in initiating dialogue around sensitive topics such as sharing household chores and family budgets.

7.3 Implications for Refugee Mental Health Practice and Policy

7.3.1 Study 5 Insights of Service Providers and Policy Influencers Regarding Refugee Support Needs

Group interviews with service providers and with policy makers revealed that services are disjointed and refugees do not have the knowledge or skills to find culturally appropriate supports. Both service providers and policy makers agreed that informal cultural networks were most effective in helping newcomers to navigate the systems and reduce isolation. Developing peer support and mentoring skills within refugee communities has the potential to build sustainable capacity. Services providers noted that research and evaluation focused on support programs is critical. Some service providers reported that loneliness was a major issue for refugee new parents. Service providers highlighted the need for family support at the time of giving birth. One way of dealing with loneliness for refugees was to create little villages in apartments. Although this approach has been criticized for creating ghettos, some participants thought that it was an effective strategy to deal with loneliness. In their view, hospitals could improve support for patients with language barriers by hiring more qualified interpreters. Inability to speak English was considered a major problem for many refugees. Participants noted that language barriers prevail in hospitals, physician offices, and clinics. Language was also cited as a barrier to giving consent.

Some participants reported that the system was too complex for most refugees to understand. Information and education on how the system operated is needed, starting from arrival in Canada, to "settling in" and then accessing other services once settled. Participants reported that some available services were not well coordinated. Information was scattered and difficult to access and intra-agency communication was rare.

7.3.2 Implications for Practice and Programs

- The experiential knowledge and credibility of ethnic peers can supplement and interpret the professional knowledge of service providers in health and social sectors.
- Peer support interventions can diminish African refugees' loneliness and enhance their social integration, factors influencing health.
- Peer support interventions can improve African refugees' support seeking skills for coping with social and health- related challenges.
- Culturally and linguistically appropriate and gender-sensitive support programs could be adapted and tested in community-based intervention trials prior to integration in social and health services for vulnerable refugees.

References

Ahmed, S. M., Beck, B., Maurana, C. A., & Newton, G. (2004). Overcoming barriers to effective community-based participatory research in US medical schools. *Education for Health, 17*(2), 141–151.

Alegría, M., Takeuchi, D., Canino, G., Duan, N., Shrout, P., Meng, X., et al (2004). Considering context, place and culture: The National Latino and Asian American Study. *International Journal of Methods in Psychiatric Research, 13*, 208–220.

Anderson, J. M., Reimer, J., Khan, K. B., Simich, L., Neufeld, A., Stewart, M., & Makwarimba, E. (2010). Narratives of "dissonance" and "repositioning" through the lens of critical humanism, exploring the influences on immigrants' and refugees' health and well-being. *Advances in Nursing Science, 33*(2), 101–112.

Asgary, R., & Segar, N. (2011). Barriers to health care access among refugee asylum seekers. *Journal of Health Care for the Poor and Underserved, 22*(2), 506–522.

Barrio, C. (2000). The cultural relevance of community support programs. *Psychiatric Services, 51*(7), 879–884.

Beazley, H., & Ennew, J. (2006). Participatory methods and approaches: Tackling the two tyrannies. In V. Desai & R. Potter (Eds.), *Doing development research* (pp. 189–199). London: Sage Publications.

Beiser, M. (1999). *Strangers at the gate: A 10 year study of refugee settlement in Canada*. Toronto: University of Toronto Press.

Beiser, M., Wiwa, O., & Adebajo, S. (2010). Human-initiated disaster, social disorganization and post-traumatic stress disorder above Nigeria's oil basins. *Social Science and Medicine, 71*(2), 221–227.

Beiser, M., Simich, L., Pandalangat, N., Nowakowski, M., & Tian, F. (2011a). Stresses of passage, balms of resettlement, and posttraumatic stress disorder among Sri Lankan Tamils in Canada. *Canadian Journal of Psychiatry, 56*(6), 333–340.

Beiser, M., Zilber, N., Simich, L., Youngmann, R., Zohar, A. H., Taa, B., & Hou, F. (2011b). Regional effects on the mental health of immigrant children: Results from the New Canadian. *Health and Place, 17*(3), 822–829.

Bhui, K., Craig, T., Mohamud, S., Warfa, N., Stansfeld, S. A., Thornicroft, G., et al (2006). Mental disorders among Somali refugees: Developing culturally appropriate measures and assessing socio-cultural risk factors. *Social Psychiatry and Psychiatric Epidemiology, 41*(5), 400–408.

Brooker, A., & Eakin, S. (2001). Gender, class, work-related stress and health: Toward a power centred approach. *Journal of Community and Applied Social Psychology, 11*, 97–109.

Caputo, T., Weiler, R., & Anderson, S. (1997). *The street lifestyle study*. Ottawa: Health Canada.

Carpecken, P. F. (1996). *Critical ethnography in education research: A theoretical and practical guide*. London: Routledge.

Citizenship and Immigration Canada. (2009). Facts and figures: Immigration overview: Permanent and temporary residents 2008. http://www.cic.gc.ca/english/pdf/research-stats/facts2008.pdf. Accessed 10 Oct 2009.

Coker, E. B. (2004). "Traveling pains": Embodied metaphors of suffering among Southern Sudanese Refugees in Cairo. *Culture, Medicine and Psychiatry, 28*, 15–39.

Cutrona, C. (1990). Stress and social support: In search of optimal matching. *Journal of Social and Clinical Psychology, 9*(1), 3–14.

Davies, M. M., & Bath, P. A. (2001). The maternity information concerns of Somali women in the United Kingdom. *Journal of Advanced Nursing, 36*(2), 237–245.

Din-Dzietham, R., Nembhard, W. N., Collins, R., & Davis, S. K. (2004). Perceived stress following race-based discrimination at work is associated with hypertension in African-Americans. the Metro Atlanta Heart Disease Study, 1999–2001. *Social Science & Medicine, 58*(3), 449–461.

Drummond, P. D., Mizan, A., Brocx, K., & Wright, B. (2011). Barriers to accessing health care services for West African refugee women living in Western Australia. *Health Care for Women International, 32*(3), 206–224.

Ellis, B. H., MacDonald, H. Z., Klunk-Gillis, J., Lincoln, A., Strunin, L., & Cabral, H. J. (2010). Discrimination and mental health among Somali refugee adolescents: The role of acculturation and gender. *The American Journal of Orthopsychiatry, 80*(4), 564–575.

Finch, B. K., & Vega, W. A. (2003). Acculturation stress, social support, and self-rated health among Latinos in California. *Journal of Immigrant Health, 5*, 109–117.

Foss, G. F., Chantal, A. W., & Hendrickson, S. (2004). Maternal depression and anxiety and infant development: A comparison of foreign-born and native-born mothers. *Public Health Nursing, 21*(3), 237–246.

Fozdar, F. (2009). "The golden country": Ex-Yugoslav and African refugee experiences of settlement and depression. *Journal of Ethnic and Migration Studies, 35*(8), 1335–1352.

Goodman, J. H. (2004). Coping with Trauma and Hardship among Unaccompanied Refugee Youths from Sudan. *Qualitative Health Research, 14*(9), 1177–1196.

Gottlieb, B. (2000). "Accomplishments and challenges in social support intervention research". In M. Stewart (Ed.). *Chronic conditions and caregiving in Canada: Social support strategies*. Toronto: University of Toronto Press.

Gottlieb, B., & Bergen, A. E. (2010). Social support concepts and measures. *Journal of Psychosomatic Research, 69*(5), 511–520.

Guerin, B., Abdi, A., & Guerin, P. (2003). Experiences with the medical and health systems for Somali refugees living in Hamilton. *New Zealand Journal of Psychology, 32*(1), 27–32.

Harrison, A., Stewart, R., Myambo, K., & Teeraishe, C. (1995). Perceptions of social networks among adolescents from Zimbabwe and the United States. *Journal of Black Psychology, 21*(4), 382–407.

Health Canada. (1996). *Peer helper initiatives for out-of-the-mainstream youth: A report and compendium*. Ottawa: Health Canada.

House, J., Umberson, D., & Landis, K. (1988). Structures and processes of social support. *Annual Review of Sociology, 14*, 293–318.

House, J. S., Landis, K. R., & Umberson, D. (1999). Social relationships and health. In I. Kawachi, B. P. Kennedy, & R. Wilkinson (Eds.), *The Society and population health reader: Income inequality and health*. New York: The New Press.

Jaranson, J. M., Butcher, J., Halcon, L., Johnson, D. R., Robertson, C., Savik, K., Spring, M., & Westermeyer, J. (2004). Somali and Oromo refugees: Correlates of torture and trauma history. *American Journal of Public Health, 94*(4), 591–598.

Jorden, S., Matheson, K., & Anisman, H. (2009). Supportive and unsupportive social interactions in relation to cultural adaptation and psychological distress among Somali refugees exposed to collective or personal traumas. *Journal of Cross-Cultural Psychology, 40*. doi:10.1177/0022022109339182.

Karunakara, U. K., Neuner, F., Schauer, M., Singh, K., Hill, K., Elbert, T., & Burnha, G. (2004). Traumatic events and symptoms of post-traumatic stress disorder amongst Sudanese nationals, refugees and Ugandans in the West Nile. *African Health Sciences, 4*(2), 83–93.

Khawaja, N. G., White, K. M., Schweitzer, R., & Greenslade, J. (2008). Difficulties and coping strategies of Sudanese refugees: A qualitative approach. *Transcultural psychiatry, 45*(3), 489–512.

Lawrence, J., & Kearns, R. (2005). Exploring the 'fit' between people and providers: Refugee health needs and health care services in Mt Roskill, Auckland, New Zealand. *Health & Social Care in the Community, 13*(5), 451–461.

Letcher, A. S., & Perlow, K. M. (2009). Community-based participatory research shows how a community initiative creates networks to improve well-being. *American Journal of Preventative Medicine, 37*(6, Suppl. 1), S292–S299.

Makwarimba, E., Stewart, M., Simich, L., Makumbe, K., & Shiza, E. (2013). Sudanese and Somali refugees in Canada: Support needs and intervention preferences. *International Migration, 51*(5), 106–119.

Maton, K., Teti, D., Corns, K., Viera-Baker, C., Lavine, F., Gouze, K., & Keating, D. (1996). Cultural specificity of support sources, correlates and contexts: Three studies of African American and caucasian youth. *American Journal of Community Psychology, 24*(4), 551–587.

Maximova, K., & Krahn, H. (2010). Health status of refugees settled in Alberta: Changes since arrival". *Canadian Journal of Public Health, 101*(9), 322–326.

McKenzie, K., Hansson, H., Tuck, A., Lam, J., Jackson, F., Chodos, H., et al. (2009). *Improving mental health services for immigrant, refugee, ethno-cultural and racialized groups: Issues and options for service improvement*. Ottawa: Mental Health Commission of Canada.

McMichael, C., & Manderson, L. (2004). Somali women and well-being: Social networks and social capital among immigrant women in Australia. *Human Organization 63*(1), 88–99. http://www.findarticles.com/p/articles/mi_qa3800/is_200404/ai_n9392916. Accessed 1 Feb 2009.

Merry, L. A., Gagnon, A. J., Kalim, N., & Bouris, S. S. (2011). Refugee claimant women and barriers to health and social services post-birth. *Canadian Journal of Public Health, 102*(40), 286–290.

Miller, F. J. (1992). Enhancing Self-Esteem. In J. F. Miller (Ed.), *Coping with chronic illness Ch.16*. Philadelphia: F.A. Davis Company.

Moon-Park, E., & Dimigen, G. (1994). Cross-cultural comparisons of the social support system after childbirth. *Journal of Comparative Family Studies, 25*(3), 345–352.

Morrison, J. D., Howard, J., Johnson, C., Navarro, F., Plachetka, B., & Bell, W. T. (1997). Strengthening neighbourhoods by developing community networks. *Social Work, 42*(5), 527–534.

Murray, L., Windsor, C., Parker, E., Tewfik, O. (2010). The experiences of African women giving birth in Brisbane, Australia. *Health Care for Women International, 31,* 458–472.

Neufeld, A., Harrison, M. J., Stewart, M. J., Hughes, K. D., & Spitzer, D. (2002). Immigrant women: Making connections to community resources for support in family caregiving. *Qualitative Health Research, 12,* 751–768.

Nicado, E. G., Hong, S., & Takeuchi, D. T. (2008). Social support and the use of mental health services among Asian Americans: Results from the national Latino and Asian American study. *Research in Sociology of Health Care, 26,* 167–184.

Okpewho, I., & Davies, C. B. (1998). *The African diaspora: African origins and new world identities.* Wayne: Indiana University Press.

Reynolds, R. (2004). "We are not surviving, we are managing": The constitution of a Nigerian diaspora along the contours of the global economy. *City & Society, 16*(1), 15–37.

Schweitzer, R., Melville, F., Steel, Z., & Lacherez, P. (2006). Trauma, post migration living difficulties, and social support as predictors of psychological adjustment in resettled Sudanese refugees. *Australian and New Zealand Journal of Psychiatry, 40,* 179–187.

Simich, L., Hamilton, H., Baya, B. K., & Neuwirth, G. (2004). The study of Sudanese settlement in Ontario: Final report. Ottawa: Citizenship and Immigration Canada, Settlement Directorate, Ontario, May 28. http://settlement.org/downloads/atwork/Study_of_Sudanese_Settlement_in_Ontario.pdf.

Simich, L., Beiser, M., Stewart, M., & Makwarimba, E. (2005). Providing social support for immigrants and refugees in Canada: Challenges and directions. *Journal of Immigrant Health, 7*(4), 259–268.

Simich, L., Este, D., & Hamilton, H. (2010). Meanings of home and mental well-being among Sudanese refugees in Canada. *Ethnicity & Health, 15*(2), 199–212.

Stewart, M. J. (2000). Social support, coping, and self-care as public participation mechanisms. In M. J. Stewart (Ed.), *Community nursing: Promoting Canadians' health* (2nd ed, pp. 83–104). Toronto: W. B. Saunders Company.

Stewart, M., Anderson, J., Beiser, M., Makwarimba, E., Neufeld, A., Simich, L., & Spitzer, S. (2008a). Multicultural meanings of social support among immigrants and refugees. *International Migration, 46*(3), 123–159.

Stewart, M., Makwarimba, E., Barnfather, A., Letourneau, N., & Neufeld, A. (2008b). Researching reducing health disparities: Mixed methods approaches. *Social Science & Medicine, 66,* 1406–1417.

Stewart, M., Letourneau, N., & Kushner, K. (2010a). Participatory pilot interventions for vulnerable populations. *Social Science & Medicine, 71*(11), 1913–1915.

Stewart, M., Makwarimba, E., Beiser, M., Neufeld, A., Simich, P., & Spitzer, D. (2010b). Social support and health: Immigrants' and refugees' perspectives. *Diversity in Health and Care, 7*(2), 91–103.

Stewart, M., Makumbe, K., Kariwo, M., Makwarimba, E., Letourneau, N., Kushner, K., Shizha, E., Williamson, D., Dennis, C. L., & Siziba, C. (2011, September 8). *Supporting the Mental Health of African Refugee Children and New Parents: Experiences of Zimbabwean And Sudanese Refugees.* ACCFCR research report, Social Support Research Program, University of Alberta.

Stewart, M., Simich, L., Beiser, M., Makumbe, K., Makwarimba, E., Shizha, E., Anderson, S. (in press). Impacts of a social support intervention for Somali and Sudanese refugees in Canada. *Ethnicity and Inequalities in Health and Social Care.*

Stewart, M., Simich, L., Shiza, E., Makumbe, K., & Makwarimba, E. (2012). Supporting African refugees in Canada: Insights from a support intervention. *Health & Social Care in the Community, 20*(5), 516–527. doi:10.1111/j.1365-2524.2012.01069.x.

Tashakkori, A., & Teddlie, C. (Eds.) (2003). *Handbook of mixed methods in the social and behavioral research*. Thousand Oaks: Sage Publications.

The Anne E. Casey Foundation, Canadian Council on Social Development and Red Por Los Derechos De La Infancia En Mexico. (2006). *Growing up in North America: Child well-being in Canada, The United States, and Mexico*. Baltimore: The Anne E. Casey Foundation.

Thoits, P. A. (1986). Social support as coping assistance. *Journal of Consulting & Clinical Psychology, 54*(4), 416–423.

Thoits, P. A. (1995). Stress, coping, and social support processes: Where are we? What's next? *Journal of Health & Social Behavior, 35*, 53–79.

Warner, F. R. (2007). Social support and distress among Q'eqchi refugee women in Maya Tecun, Mexico. *Medical Anthropology Quarterly, 21*(2), 193–217.

Chapter 8
Newcomer Youth Self-Esteem: A Community-Based Mixed Methods Study of Afghan, Columbian, Sudanese and Tamil Youth in Toronto, Canada

Nazilla Khanlou, Yogendra B. Shakya, Farah Islam and Emma Oudeh

Abstract Self-esteem is recognized as an important correlate of youth mental wellbeing and, by extension, supportive of individual resilience. While an extensive body of literature exists on self-esteem of mainstream youth, less is known about self-esteem experiences of immigrant youth, and in particular newcomer and refugee youth. Applying a community-based participatory research approach, and using mixed methods, the aim of the study presented was to understand social determinants of newcomer youth's mental wellbeing, and recognize both their challenges and resilience. The chapter focuses on the self-esteem of newcomer youth from four ethnic backgrounds (Afghan, Colombian, Sudanese, and Tamil).The study findings can contribute to mental health promotion strategies in multicultural and immigrant-receiving community settings.

Keywords Canada · Community-based participatory research · Gender · Mental Health · Mixed methods · Newcomer · Self-esteem · Youth

Self-esteem is recognized as an important aspect of youth mental wellbeing. It refers to the self-evaluative component of one's sense of self, and entails a sense of self-worth. While an extensive body of literature exists on self-esteem of mainstream youth in immigrant receiving countries, less is known about self-esteem experiences of migrant youth, and in particular newcomer and refugee youth. In the mental health field, existing conceptions of youth self-esteem have often regarded it as a personal attribute (such as individual personality trait), with limited links to youth's social context. Yet, we argue that, as with a system's approach to understanding

N. Khanlou (✉)
Women's Health Research Chair in Mental Health, Faculty of Health,
Associate Professor, School of Nursing, York University, HNES 3rd floor,
4700 Keele Street, Toronto, ON M3J 1P3, Canada
e-mail: nkhanlou@yorku.ca

Y. B. Shakya
Access Alliance Multicultural Health and Community Services, Toronto, Canada

F. Islam · E. Oudeh
York University, Toronto, Canada

youth's resilience (Barankin and Khanlou 2007), youth's self-esteem is also more accurately considered in the context of multiple systems, interacting with each other in youth's individual and social environmental context (such as their relationships with their family and peers, and in the case of newcomer youth also their experiences of resettlement).

In this chapter we consider the self-esteem of newcomer refugee youth by drawing from a community-based participatory research (CBPR) project we conducted with four newcomer groups in Toronto, Canada. We first start with an overview of our CBPR approach and then outline the migration context for these youth in Canada. We present what the literature says about newcomer youth self-esteem and we then report on our findings in order to fill the gap in the extant literature.

8.1 Conducting Community-Based Participatory Research with Refugee Youth

Community-based participatory research requires the collaboration of community and academic partners in conducting research that is of use for the communities of interest. In this case the community partner was Access Alliance Multicultural Health and Community Services in Toronto (http://accessalliance.ca/). One of the co-authors of this chapter, Y. Shakya, was the community Principal Investigator on the study. The author of the chapter, N. Khanlou, was the academic Principal Investigator. In the early phases of the project the partners discussed their interests, expertise and intent in studying the mental health of newcomer youth in Canada. The community partner identified interest in learning more about mental health concerns among newcomer youth from Afghanistan, Columbia, Sri Lanka, and Sudan who were between the ages of 14–18 and who had come to Canada within the last five years. The four target communities reflected the key priority groups for the community partner and provided a cross-cultural regional diversity. Together the partners wrote a grant application and submitted it to be considered for funding. We were successful in achieving funding from the Provincial Centre of Excellence for Child and Youth Mental Health at CHEO in Ontario, Canada.

The overall aim of our study was to understand the social determinants of newcomer youth's mental wellbeing, and recognition of both their challenges and resilience (Khanlou et al. 2011). Its specific objectives were to explore the newcomer youth's: (1) conceptualizations of mental health and illness; (2) their reported needs and help-seeking behaviours; (3) access barriers to services; and to (4) propose policies and practices to remove barriers; and (5) actively engage newcomer youth in the research process. In this chapter we focus on our findings related to newcomer youth self-esteem, as this was one of the specific areas of attention for the study, and given that self-esteem is linked to mental health and physical health outcomes and, therefore, an important concept to focus on in the mental health promotion field.

8.2 Migration Context in Canada for Youth from Afghanistan, Colombia, Sri Lanka, and Sudan

Although relatively small in number, Colombia, Sri Lanka, Afghanistan, and Sudan all contribute to Canada's immigration population. In 2010, 4,796 Colombians, 4,181 Sri Lankans, 1,549 Afghanis, and 618 Sudanese immigrated to Canada. Of these four countries, Afghanistan, Sri Lanka, and Sudan have seen decreasing numbers while Colombia has seen an increase in the number of immigrants (CIC 2011).

Afghanistan According to the UNHCR Country Profile (2011a), security, protection of civilians, and poverty continue to be the biggest threats to life and progress for Afghan civilians. According to the 2006 Census 36,165 immigrants were born in Afghanistan. This population has grown steadily since 1991. Before 1991, 4,215 Afghanis had emigrated to Canada. Between 2001 and 2006, 16,420 Afghanis emigrated to Canada (Statistics Canada 2009). However, although the total number of Afghan immigrants has increased over the past twenty years, as a percentage of the total immigrant population, Afghanistan's immigration trend is on the decline. The total number of Afghan immigrants entering Canada has decreased by 50 % in the last ten years, from 3,182 in 2001 to 1,549 in 2010 (CIC 2011).

Colombia According to the UNHCR, Colombia's long-lasting conflict between the government and several guerrilla organizations has resulted in 3.4 million internally displaced persons (IDPs). IDPs suffer from precarious living conditions, the absence of long-lasting solutions, and threats and selective killings. As a result, there are currently 115,000 Colombian refugees and asylum seekers continuing to seek international protection outside the country (UNHCR 2011b). As of 2006, 39,145 Colombian-born immigrants were living in Canada. Since 1991, the total number of Colombian-Canadians has risen steadily. Between 1996 and 2000, 5,240 Colombians emigrated to Canada. This number rose drastically between 2001 and 2006 when 25,305 Colombians emigrated to Canada (Statistics Canada 2009). Canada admitted between 2,966 and 6,031 Colombian immigrants to enter between 2001 and 2011. Furthermore, the percentage distribution of total Colombian immigrants to Canada increased between 2001 and 2011 from 3.7 to 7.4 % (CIC 2011).

Sri Lanka In May 2009 the 26-year war between the Tamil Tigers and government forces ended. Nonetheless, displacement remains an issue. The UNHCR is attempting to find mutually agreeable and durable solutions for the 212,000 internally displaced persons (UNHCR 2011c). Sri Lanka has experienced civil war since 1983, resulting in large-scale displacement. The death toll exceeds 60,000 and there are more than 800,000 internally displaced persons in Sri Lanka—of which 78 % are Tamil. As a result of the decades of war, a large Tamil diaspora emerged in many countries, including Canada (Hyndman 2003). Canada's Sri Lankan population was 105,670 as of the 2006 Census. Between 1991 and 1995, 35,390 Sri Lankans emigrated to Canada. This is in contrast to 1996 to 2000 and 2001 to 2006 where 23,280 and 22,305 Sri Lankans emigrated to Canada, respectively (Statistics Canada 2009). Yearly trends from Statistics Canada over the last decade also show a decline in

Sri Lankan immigrations. In 2001, Canada admitted 5,520 Sri Lankans to enter the country and in 2011 Canada admitted only 4,181 (CIC 2011).

Sudan The people of Sudan, specifically in the western region of Darfur, are suffering from a genocide and humanitarian crisis. According to the UN, since fighting broke out in 2003, at least 2 million Sudanese have been displaced from their homes and more than 200,000 people are estimated to have died (United Nations and Darfur 2007). According to United Human Rights Council five thousand die every month and over 4.7 million Darfuris rely on humanitarian aid (United Human Rights Council 2011). Atrocities such as the murder and rape of civilians have been widespread and continue (United Nations and Darfur 2007). Despite the hardships of life in Sudan, the acceptance of Sudanese immigrants has traditionally been low. According to the 2006 Census, there were 8,745 Sudanese-born Canadians living in Canada (Statistics Canada 2009). Yearly trends indicate a decrease in Sudanese immigrants, even though the crisis in Darfur began in 2003. Between 2001 and 2009 the number of Sudanese immigrants steadily decreased 1,179 to 455, yet did see a spike to 618 immigrants in 2010 (CIC 2011). Upon coming to Canada, many Sudanese find it difficult to integrate into Canadian society. In their study, Simich et al. (2006) found that the majority of Sudanese refugees thought life would be easier and they would have better opportunities, but that was not the case as they struggled with the cost of living and finding employment.

Statistics on total refugees from 2001 to 2010 were found only for Colombia and Sri Lanka. Although the yearly numbers fluctuate, the total number of Colombian refugees has remained relatively high over the past ten years as compared to Sri Lanka, Afghanistan, and Sudan. In only four of the last ten years has the number of Colombian refugees fallen below 2,000 refugees per year. The number was as high as 3,924 in 2004 (CIC 2011). Comparing two five year time spans, 2001–2006 and 2006–2010, the number of Colombian refugees has remained steady. Between 2001 and 2006, 11,526 Colombian refugees entered Canada and between 2006 and 2010, 11,394 Colombian refugees entered Canada. The number of Sri Lankan refugees has fallen sharply in the last ten years. In 2001 2,820 Sri Lankan refugees entered Canada, the highest number in the past ten years (CIC 2011). Numbers may be higher for previous years but no data was available. Between 2001 and 2005, 7,635 Sri Lankan refugees entered Canada. In contrast, between 2006 and 2010, only 4,654 refugees entered Canada, a decrease of nearly 40 %.

8.3 Refugee Mental Health and Self-Esteem: Current Knowledge

Self-esteem contributes to youth resilience and both impact one's mental wellbeing. As described above we are influenced by a systems approach to understanding self-esteem and resilience. Elsewhere we have discussed the importance of recognizing refugee populations' resilience and agency (Hajdukwoski-Ahmed et al. 2008), thus avoiding the further marginalization of "refugees". In this section we draw upon a significant body of literature that examines the particular challenges faced by refugees, which can lead to specific threats to their psychosocial wellbeing. Others have noted that refugees are a vulnerable population that experience isolation, a lack of social support, racism and poor treatment (Khawaia et al. 2008). Salient challenges that refugees face acutely include forced migration, life trauma experiences (such as war, violence, and torture), protracted situations of precarious immigration status and living in under-serviced refugee camps, and exclusion from education, labour market and political participation. These factors can result in low literacy and education levels, low fluency in 'host language,' limited work/professional skills and experiences, family separation and fracturing, and less than optimal physical health and mental health concerns.

During the initial years of resettlement and as newcomers, both refugee youth and adults may face difficulty assimilating into individualistic cultures in the post-migration context. However, some studies show that immigrant children and youth are better at coping with the psychosocial transition than adults (Hyman et al. 1996). Despite their ability to better transition from collectivist to individualistic cultures, children and youth are not immune to mental illnesses and can suffer from depression, anxiety and PTSD (Crowley 2009). Refugees often emigrate from collectivist to individualistic cultures and this transition has been shown to have psychosocial and mental health implications.

Community ties function as a preventative factor of mental health problems for refugees (Weine 2011). Although research on mental health determinants in refugees is mainly focused at the individual level, family and community support has shown to positively influence their cultural transition and mental health (Weine 2011). Mels et al. (2008) studied social support in unaccompanied asylum-seeking boys and found that the asylum centre staff and community were the most important resources for support, highlighting the importance of a supportive community network for refugees. For youth refugees, school was found to be a helpful community support (Crowley 2009). Social support has also been found to increase self-esteem in younger refugee populations (Mels et al. 2008).

Religion is another prevalent form of community support for refugees and is relied upon as a common coping strategy when faced with mental health problems. Religion was found to work in conjunction with other social support networks such as communities of friends, family and neighbours from home (Khawaia et al. 2008). In a study examining resilience among Sudanese refugees, researchers found that religious beliefs helped them regain some control and meaning in life to cope with the unhappiness and loneliness they felt post-migration (Schweitzer et al. 2007).

Self-esteem is a significant predictor of mental health and cumulative adult adjustment. However, research examining mental health in immigrant populations is focused mainly on PTSD, anxiety and depression to the exclusion of self-esteem (Weine 2011; Trzesniewski et al. 2006). When self-esteem was compared in collectivist and individualistic countries, the most collectivist cultures had higher levels of self-liking and lower levels of self-competence while the most individualistic cultures had higher levels of self-competence and lower levels of self-liking (Allik and

Schmitt 2005). Self-competence was defined as "the instrumental feature of the self as causal agent, the sense that one is confident, capable, and efficacious" (Allik and Schmitt, p. 625). The same study also found that self-esteem functions in a similar manner across cultures; it was associated with low levels of neuroticism and high levels of extraversion (Allik and Schmitt 2005).

Although there are differences in the degree of influence and effect self-esteem has across cultures, studies have shown that adolescents with lower self-esteem have more issues with mental illness and physical health in adulthood compared with adolescents who had higher self-esteem (Trzesniewski et al. 2006). For example Trzesniewski et al.'s (2006) study results showed that adolescents with low self-esteem were "1.6 times more likely to develop an anxiety disorder, 1.32 times more likely to be dependent on tobacco during adulthood, and 1.26 times more likely to develop major depression disorder" (p. 384). The researchers also found that adolescents with low self-esteem had more physical health problems in adulthood compared to adults who had higher self-esteem as adolescents. Study participants who had lower adolescent self-esteem had higher BMI's and systolic blood pressures in adulthood (Trzesniewski et al., p. 384). In addition, adolescents with low self-esteem in Trzesniewski et al.'s study were 1.48 times more likely to be convicted of a crime and 2.13 times more likely to leave school early (p. 384). In the same study, 56 % of adolescents with low self-esteem had multiple problems in adulthood compared to adolescents with higher self-esteem of which only 17 % had multiple problems as adults (p. 385). Therefore, in order to cultivate a more holistic picture of the factors influencing mental health post migration, it is necessary to include the role of self-esteem.

8.4 Migration and Self Esteem

There are mixed results concerning the effect that length of time in a new country has on self-esteem. Driscoll et al. (2008) found that self-esteem was influenced by generation. Their findings support the idea that third generation youth have higher self-esteem compared to second and first generation immigrants. In contrast, Jaret and Reitzes (2009), who also studied first, second, and third generation youth found that there was no significant difference in self-esteem between generations.

Research supports the idea that both the physical and mental health of immigrants is often affected after resettlement. Omeri et al. (2006) studied health, related resettlement issues, and barriers that 4,695 Afghan refugees faced in New South Wales, Australia. They found that the Afghan refugees struggled with emotions such as anger, guilt, sadness, lack of belonging, and alienation. These feelings resulted from their loss of sense of belonging, country, and identity; discrimination from members of their new community; an inability to earn money (many qualifications earned in Afghanistan were not recognized in Australia) and provide adequate housing for the family; and isolation from family and friends back home. A common theme identified in this study was the frustration associated with learning a new language.

A 2006 Canadian study of 220 Sudanese refugees (Simich et al. 2006) found results similar to those of Afghan refugees. Overall, Sudanese refugees believed that immigrating to Canada would allow them to lead a better life. Their expectations were not met and many found their lives harder as 85 % of respondents had trouble finding employment. Furthermore, many Sudanese refugees also felt increased psychological distress because of economic hardships and unmet expectations that prevented them from living a productive life and taking care of their families.

Compared to other influences on immigrant and refugee mental health, there is little relevant research on self-esteem. Research concerning the mental health of immigrants is mostly focused on PTSD, anxiety and depression. There is also little research examining the mental health of Colombian and Tamil refugees. To help fill the gap, this study applied a community-based participatory approach to examine conceptions of mental health and wellbeing among newcomer refugee youth.

8.5 Youth Participants in the Newcomer Youth Mental Health Project

To best meet our study's objectives, a mixed methods approach entailing qualitative and quantitative methods was applied. In line with CBPR, a Youth Advisory Committee (YAC) was formed and included 7 youth. Youth Peer Researchers (PRs) were also hired (1 from each of the 4 groups) and assisted with youth recruitment into the study. Regular meetings were organized by the Project Coordinator with the YAC and PRs groups. The youth provided valuable insights on how to make data collection instruments more youth-friendly. They assisted and participated with knowledge exchange activities through a one-day Youth Conference focusing on newcomer youth mental health. The youth also received training on topics such as CBPR; the social determinants of mental health; and anti-racism and anti-oppression.

As outlined in Table 8.1 (Study Participants), qualitative data was attained through 7 focus groups (2 Afghan youth focus groups, 2 Colombian, 1 Sudanese, 1 Tamil, 1 service providers) and 16 in-depth interviews (2 Afghan youth, 4 Sudanese youth, 4 Sudanese parents, 1 Colombian parent, 5 service providers).

Quantitative data was attained through questionnaires, 56 questionnaires were administered to youth of which 52 (27 male; 25 female) were completed and used for analysis. All youth participants in the qualitative portion of the study, save for three, also participated in the questionnaire portion. Table 8.2 (Profile of Youth Participants) provides information on gender, age, and ethnicity of participants.

All youth who participated in this study were born outside of Canada. Lack of strong connections with Sudanese and Tamil community in Toronto hindered our ability to recruit more participants from these two communities. The four most commonly identified places of birth were: Colombia, Afghanistan, Sri Lanka, and India. Half of the Tamil participants were born in Sri Lanka and the other half in India. All of the 4 Sudanese participants were born outside of Sudan (majority in Saudi Arabia) while their mothers were born in Sudan. Many participants had gone through

Table 8.1 Study Participants

	Focus Group	Interview	Total
Afghan	2 FGs		
Male	4	1 (youth)	5
Female	6	1 (youth)	7
Colombian	2 FGs		
Male	9		9
Female	8	1 (mother)	9
Sudanese	1 FG		
Male	3	1	4
Female	2	7 (3 youth, 4 mothers)	9
Tamil	1 FG		
Male	2		2
Female	6		6
Service Providers	1FG		
Male	2	2	4
Female	5	3	8
TOTAL qualitative sample	47	16	59[a]

[a] While the total of Focus Group and Interview participants is 63, four participants from the focus groups were the same as in the interviews. Thus the actual number of participants is 59

Table 8.2 Profile of Youth Participants

Sociodemographic variables	
Gender n (%)	
Male	27 (52 %)
Female	25 (48 %)
Age (mean, SD)	16, 1.4
Ethnicity n (%)	
Afghan/Pashto	18 (35 %)
Colombian	21 (40 %)
Sudanese	4 (8 %)
Tamil	8 (15 %)
Missing	1 (2 %)
TOTAL quantitative sample	52

SD standard deviation

multiple migrations before coming to Canada. Almost half of the Colombian youth came to Canada through United States. For Afghan youth, the country of residence before coming to Canada varied and included Pakistan, Iran, Tajikistan, Uzbekistan, and Kazakhstan.

The average length of stay in Canada was 2 years. The majority of participants spoke one language at home (48 %), while 33 % spoke 2 languages, 10 % spoke 3 languages, and 4 % spoke 4 languages at home. About one third (30.1 %) of the participants had 3 or more siblings; 13 % had no siblings. Majority of Sudanese participants (75 %) and Colombian participants (61 %) were in grade 11 and 12.

All participants' parents were also born outside of Canada. The top four most commonly identified ethnic backgrounds of both mothers and fathers were: Colombian,

Afghan, Sri Lankan Tamil, and Sudanese. Two indicators of socioeconomic status (SES), parental education level and parental employment status were considered for the sample. Respondents' mothers and fathers had similar levels of education. While 6 % of mothers and fathers had no education, 18 % of mothers and fathers had completed high school, 67 % of mothers and 64 % of fathers had college/university education, and lastly 4 % of fathers had postgraduate level education. In our sample, 32 % of participants' mothers were currently working in Canada, and 62 % were currently not working (remaining 6 % were missing responses). Similar current employment levels were found for fathers as well, with 38 % of respondents' fathers were working and 51 % were currently unemployed.

8.6 How Self-Esteem was Considered in the Newcomer Youth Mental Health Project

Newcomer youth self-esteem was considered both in the qualitative and quantitative components of the study. In the focus groups youth were asked about what self-esteem meant to them. For example, "What does self-esteem mean to you?"; and What are some of the things that affect your self-esteem?" In the interviews, youth were asked about self-esteem in the context of their mental health help-seeking behaviors. For example, "When you are feeling sad or down, what do you usually do to make yourself feel better?"; "When you are feeling lonely or isolated, what do you usually do to make yourself feel better?"; and "Who do you talk to first when you are feeling sad or lonely?"

In the questionnaire, two self-esteem scales, the Rosenberg Self-Esteem Scale (1965) and the Current Self-Esteem Scale (Khanlou 2004; Khanlou and Crawford 2006), were used to examine self-esteem and strategies for mental health promotion. The Current Self-Esteem Scale is a 4-item self-report scale that includes a visual analogue scale and three open-ended questions, developed by Khanlou through her work with immigrant youth from diverse cultural backgrounds. The Rosenberg Self-Esteem Scale (1965) is a 12 question, 4-point Likert self-report scale that examines self-esteem and has been used widely across study populations, including youth, ethno-cultural groups, and geographic settings. Two measures were used as the Rosenberg Self-Esteem Scale is a composite measure based on multiple indicators for overall self-esteem; and the Current Self Esteem is based on a single visual analogue scale to measure current self-esteem (i.e. over the course of the past). In addition it contains open-ended items through which youth narrate what factors promote or challenge their self-esteem (See Appendix A: Current Self-Esteem Scale).

In the following sections we refer to existing literature on youth self-esteem and share findings from our study.

Table 8.3 Global Self-Esteem Scores by Gender

	Male	Female
High	67 %	52 %
Medium	33 %	48 %
Low	0 %	0 %

8.7 Newcomer Youth Self-Esteem and Gender

Research suggests mixed results concerning the effects of gender on youth self-esteem. Some studies found that males had higher self-esteem (Khanlou 2004; Moksnes et al. 2010), others found that gender did not affect self-esteem (Jaret and Reitzes 2009). Research examining the effect of gender differences on stress, depression, anxiety and self-esteem found that boys had markedly higher self-esteem than girls and self-esteem was inversely correlated with anxiety and depression (Moksnes et al. 2010). Also, self-esteem moderated the association between stress related to peer pressure, romantic relationships, school performance and anxiety; girls had significantly higher stress scores than boys (Moksnes et al. 2010).

School and grades also predicted self-esteem for newcomer adolescent females in Toronto as academic success played a large role in their sense of self-worth; the participants were conscious of the link between academic success and broader career options (Khanlou and Crawford 2006). In the same study, self-esteem was negatively influenced by the loss of friendship and difficulty with the language in the post-migration context, resulting in a sense of lack of belonging to Canadian culture (Khanlou and Crawford 2006).

Others have noted that the self-esteem of women affected by conflict is lower than men's because they associate feelings of helplessness with the loss of their status in society (Palmer and Zwi 1998). In a study of Sudanese women in a refugee camp in Kenya, the refugee women expressed feelings of lower self-esteem because they no longer took care of the family and household as they traditionally did (Russell and Stage 1996). Women were also frustrated by the wasted time in refugee camps and the disruption of traditional gender roles caused by the dependency on relief agencies (Russell and Stage 1996).

Our study findings using data from the questionnaire indicate that youth participants enjoyed good self-esteem. Table 8.3 (Global Self-Esteem Scores by Gender) summarizes the participants' global self-esteem scores by gender, using the Rosenberg Self-Esteem Scale (RSE). Most participants fell into the high or medium range of global self-esteem.[1]

Table 8.4 (Current Self-Esteem Scores by Gender) summarizes the participants' current self-esteem scores by gender, using the Current Self-Esteem Scale (CSE).

---

[1] When ethnic group averages were used to substitute for missing cases, 60 % of participants scored in the highest tercile of Global Rosenberg Self-Esteem Scale scores (GL-RSE score 30–40), while 40 % scored in the medium self-esteem level tercile (GL-RSE score 20–29), and 0 % in the lowest self-esteem tercile (GL-RSE score 10–19). Male and female youth both had an average GL-RSE score of 31. When GL-RSE were subdivided into high, medium, and low self-esteem terciles, 33 % of males fell into the medium GL-RSE score range, while 67 % fell into the highest self-esteem bracket. The trend was more of an even distribution for females with 48 % of females falling in the medium self-esteem range and 52 % in the high self-esteem range.

Table 8.4 Current Self-Esteem Scores by Gender

	Male	Female
High	54 %	68 %
Medium	11 %	12 %
Low	0 %	12 %

Most participants fell into the high current self-esteem range and there was no statistically significant gender difference.[2]

8.8 Newcomer Youth Self-Esteem, Migration and Culture

For minority groups residing in a new country other than their country of birth, ethnic identity and identification with the majority group are predictors of self-esteem (Gong 2007; Cavaos-Rehg and Waack 2009). Consequently, immigrants who experience a cross-cultural geographical move in childhood can experience cultural homelessness. They can experience lower self-esteem because of low sense of cultural identity, whereas individuals who have a strong sense of cultural identity can have higher self-esteem (Hoersting and Jenkins 2011); however the long-term age effect of immigration on self-esteem remains inconclusive. Acceptance and recognition of cultural diversity and identity are also predictors of self-esteem for cross-cultural immigrants (Verkuyten 2009). Lam (2007) found that higher collective self-esteem creates a stronger sense of coherence; those who have a strong sense of collective identity with their ethnic group are less prone to distress.

Although predictors of self-esteem may be similar for individuals and groups who have emigrated, some research shows that there is a difference between collectivist and individualistic predictors of self-esteem. In a study of self-esteem and social comparison in middle childhood, Guest (2007) compared two communities. One was a Chicago public-housing development and the other was in refugee camps near Luanda, Republic of Angola. While both communities were in relative poverty and received interventions from external agencies, conceptions of childhood varied. Accelerated childhood into adult attributes was associated with high self-esteem and highly competitive social comparison in the Chicago community. In the Angolan community, childhood was conceived as being different from adulthood, resulting in integrative social comparison and placing more emphasis on role achievement over self-esteem. However, others have alluded to the move away from a binary distinction

---

[2] The average Current Self Esteem score (CU-SE) for the participants was 7.8 (SD = 2.1). In our sample, 17 % of respondents had the highest CU-SE score of 10. Males and females both had an average score of 8. CU-SE scores were classified into three groups: high current self-esteem (7–10), medium current self-esteem (scores 5–6), and low current self-esteem (scores 1–4). In our youth sample, 75 % of participants fell in the highest current self-esteem bracket, 12 % in the medium bracket, and 6 % in the lowest bracket. While 54 % of males scored in the highest current self-esteem bracket, 11 % scored in the medium bracket, and no males scored in the lowest bracket. Females followed a similar trend for the highest (68 %) and medium brackets (12 %), however, 12 % of females fell in the lowest current self-esteem bracket.

Table 8.5 Global Self-Esteem Scores by Ethnicity

	Afghan/Pashto	Colombian	Sudanese	Tamil
High	39 %	68 %	100 %	62 %
Medium	61 %	32 %	0 %	38 %
Low	0 %	0 %	0 %	0 %

Table 8.6 Current Self-Esteem Scores by Ethnicity

	Afghan/Pashto	Colombian	Sudanese	Tamil
High	67 %	77 %	100 %	75 %
Medium	17 %	17 %	0 %	–
Low	6 %	9 %	0 %	–

* 25 % of the Tamil participants did not fill out the current self-esteem visual analog scale

between individualism and collectivism, in achieving autonomy and relatedness, and toward recognition of variations within individuals and cultures among parents' developmental goals for their children (see Tamis-LeMonda et al. 2008).

We also considered self-esteem differences between the four youth groups. Due to the small number of participants in two of the groups (Sudanese and Tamil), *across groups findings need to be interpreted with caution*. In general, however, all groups enjoyed good self-esteem, with scores in the medium to high range.[3] Table 8.5 (Global Self-Esteem Scores by Ethnicity) summarizes the participants' global self-esteem scores by ethnicity, using the RSE scale.

Table 8.6 (Current Self-Esteem Scores by Ethnicity) summarizes the participants' current self-esteem scores by ethnicity, using the CSE scale. Most participants fell into the high current self-esteem.

The four groups did not significantly differ in CU-SE scores. When CU-SE were divided into terciles, 67 % of the Afghan/Pashto participants scored in the highest current self-esteem bracket, 17 % in the medium bracket, and 6 % in the lowest bracket. Colombian participants followed a similar trend: 77 % fell in the highest bracket, 17 % in the medium bracket, and 9 % in the lowest bracket. 100 % of our Sudanese sample fell into the highest current self-esteem tercile, while 75 % of the Tamil participants were in the highest bracket. When the terciles were analyzed, there was no significant difference between ethnocultural groups in current self-esteem levels (Pearson chi square test $p > 0.05$). These results are summarized in Table 8.6.

---

[3] The GL-RSE scores differed between ethnic groups (Afghan/Pashto mean = 28, SD = 5.9; Colombian mean = 31, SD = 4.6; Sudanese mean = 39, SD = 0.88; Tamil mean = 32, SD = 3.8). When GL-RSE were subdivided into high, medium, and low self-esteem terciles, 61 % of Afghan/Pashto sample scored in the medium self-esteem bracket, while 39 % scored in the highest GL-RSE tercile. For the Colombian sample, 32 % of youth fell in the medium self-esteem range, while 68 % scored in the highest self-esteem bracket. All of the Sudanese participants scored in the highest self-esteem bracket. For the Tamil group, 38 % of youth scored in the medium self-esteem range, while 62 % fell in the highest self-esteem tercile.

8.9 Newcomer Youth Self-Esteem, Perception of Parent and Peer Support, and Relationships

An important contributor to adolescent self-esteem is perceived family and peer support (Khanlou 2004). Perceived discrimination and parent-adolescent conflict are significant predictors of adolescent internalizing problems and low self-esteem (Smokowski and Bacallao 2007). While adolescents who experienced high levels of parental conflict internalized issues that resulted in lower self-esteem, adolescents who had strong, supportive family relationships internalized fewer problems and had higher self-esteem. Consequently, supportive family relationships are cultural assets associated with higher self-esteem (Smokowski and Bacallao 2007). In another study, Driscoll et al.(2008) found that teenagers who had disengaged mothers had lower levels of self-esteem.

Perceived discrimination negatively influences self-esteem. However, supportive familial relationships and friendships can mediate the influence of perceived discrimination (Smokowski and Bacallao 2007). Smokowski and Bacallao, (2007) found that "Familism" is the strongest factor associated with self-esteem; and that parent-adolescent conflict led to lower self-esteem for youth (Smokowski et al. 2010). Individuals who have emigrated cross-culturally often have limited relationships with those outside their family, demonstrating that parents and their relationships with their children influence self-esteem.

In our study, youth perception of parental social support was assessed using three Likert scale items of the Health Behaviour in School-Aged Children (HBSC) items included in the questionnaire. In response to the question: "How easy is it for you to talk to your father about things that really bother you?" 23 % of respondents answered difficult-very difficult, while 62 % said easy-very easy. Participants had an easier time talking with their mothers. When asked, "How easy is it for you to talk to your mother about things that really bother you?" 10 % of participants said difficult-very difficult, while 82 % of respondents answered with easy-very easy. When asked how much they agreed/disagreed with the statement "My parents understand me." 4 % strongly disagreed, 8 % disagreed, 12 % neither agreed nor disagreed, 40 % agreed, and lastly, 37 % strongly agreed.

Other items from the HBSC measured perception of peer support using four Likert scale questions. Among the youth participants, 86 % agreed-strongly agreed that they could talk to their friends about things that were important to them, while only 14 % disagreed-strongly disagreed. When participants were asked how easy it was to talk to their friends about things that really bothered them, about 80 % of youth felt their best friend was easy-very easy to talk to, while 73 % of participants said their friends of the same sex were easy-very easy to approach. Youth had a more difficult time connecting with friends of the opposite sex. Just less than half of the participants (49 %) found friends of the opposite sex easy to talk to about issues that bothered them.

Findings from the open ended items of the CSE also indicated that relationships played an important role in the self-esteem of youth. To conduct the analyses of responses, the theme and sub-theme categories developed in previous studies

Table 8.7 Rank Order of First Current Self-Esteem Influences and Strategies by Gender

Current self-esteem	Response	Overall	Male	Female
Promoting influences	1st	Relationships	Relationships	Relationships
Challenging influences	1st	Relationships	Self	Relationships
Promoting strategies	1st	Lifestyle	Lifestyle	Relationships

(Khanlou 2004; Khanlou and Crawford 2006) were applied and further modified for the data of this study. Responses to CSE's "What things made you feel GOOD about yourself?" are identified as *Promoting Influences*. Responses to "What things made you feel NOT GOOD about yourself?" are identified as *Challenging Influences*. Responses to "What things can you DO TO FEEL GOOD about yourself?" are identified as *Promoting Strategies*.

As presented in Table 8.7 (Rank Order of First Current Self-Esteem Influences and Strategies by Gender), when the first response of participants' was analyzed, the theme that was most commonly listed first for the overall group was Relationships (e.g., parents, friends as Relationships' sub-themes) for Promoting Influences, Relationships for Challenging Influences, and Lifestyle (e.g., exercise) for Promoting Strategies. While males and females both indicated Relationships related responses for Promoting Influences, their first response patterns were different for Challenging Influences and Promoting Strategies. Self-related responses (e.g., appearance, personality attributes as Self's sub-themes) were most common first responses for males for as Challenging Influences, and for females it was Relationships. For Promoting Strategies, males most commonly referred to Lifestyle first, while females again referred to Relationships. If first order ranking of themes can be used as a means to assess what themes youth placed importance on, relationships were ranked in greater importance for females than males, while self and lifestyle were more important to males than females.

8.10 Self-Esteem Narratives of Newcomer Youth

The qualitative narratives from focus groups and interviews with newcomer youth closely resonate with the results from the questionnaire. They also provide nuanced insights on the everyday lived experiences of how newcomer youth understand, navigate and engage with the factors that affect their self-esteem. In line with results from the questionnaire, youth participants from focus groups and interviews emphasized the important role that friends, parents and social 'environment' play in shaping self-esteem. For example, a 15 year old Sudanese boy highlighted how having many friends helps to boost his self-esteem and that lack of good friends can lower self-esteem:

> Friends, many friends. I never feel like I'm left out. That's why I feel that my self-esteem is very high…The people around you. It seems to be hard to know them. Some people are hard to get to know. And sometimes you can become easily friends with other people. If

you have people easily become your friends and stuff, then they can help you build up your self-esteem and make you feel good about yourself. Otherwise, if they're not open to talk to, not easy to talk to, not easy to become friends with, it's going to be hard for you to think that of yourself. That's why they lower your self-esteem. So, that's why environment plays a big role; (Sudanese boy, age 15).

Many youth echoed that parents "do a big part in building self-esteem." Another youth noted how self-esteem and self-confidence is impacted by how you are treated by people around you:

It's usually the people around them. If you get a group of people tell someone, you look ugly, your dress looks ugly they try to change themselves and then they keep changing until the people around them likes them. That lowers the respect for themselves (Afghan youth).

Several youth spoke about how broader systemic factors impact self-esteem including discrimination, linguistic barriers, and economic difficulties. When asked about the impact of discrimination, a young Tamil girl shared how in addition to creating sadness, the experience can undermine a person's confidence to interact with society:

You become sad and you don't feel comfortable enough to talk to people more often. So you try to avoid talking to different people. So you ask yourself why, they're only making fun of you. So you stop talking to them; (Tamil girl, age 14).

A slightly older Tamil girl mentioned that while discrimination can test self-esteem, having high self-esteem can enable youth to challenge discrimination:

I think the word self-esteem relates to the words harassment and discrimination based on race and color and ethnicity and whatnot. So, say you walk into a group of people who are considered the cooler, popular ones and you walk outside. It really depends on how much self-esteem you have for yourself. So say they look down on you and they say 'look at your skin color' and 'look how ugly you look' right? So it really depends on your self-esteem that gives you the answer to reply to them. So, if you have low self-esteem, then you would walk away saying 'I'm sorry, I won't come here again'. But, if you have a high self-esteem, then you would say 'cut it out' and they would treat you the way you want to be treated; (Tamil girl, age 16).

At the same time, some youth were not familiar with the term "self-esteem." As one Afghan youth put it "I have heard about self-esteem but don't know what it means exactly." During the focus groups, youth identified comparable terms to self-confident in their language (for example, *Etamod-benafs* in Dari; *Alta estema* in Spanish).

Youth with low English language fluency shared about how facing linguistic barrier had immediate and acute impact on their self-esteem. In the words of one Colombian youth:

I think self-esteem in this situation of us changed. In Colombia it was always easy because you could talk with everybody and you can do everything you want but here you have another, because you can't do something because the people don't care if you don't speak English. I think it's a change here, it's strong, something feel bad so we need to get used to the situation; (Colombian boy, age 15).

Youth narratives from focus group and interviews indicate that unemployment and labour market barriers faced by parents appear to have negative impacts on youth's self-esteem and mental wellbeing. Many youth spoke about feeling "depressed" and "hopeless" due to labour market and other systemic barriers that their parents are facing in Canada. The following quote comes from a service provider participant in the study:

> For a lot of new immigrants may be well educated and had a high profession back in their own country. Many cannot find a profession here that would equate with their previous profession back home and this is what would break up the family. So the clients that I work with, work in shifts. This changes the family dynamics. The newcomer youth feel isolated and not being accepted. When at home, they cannot talk to their parents because the parents are not there. The kids begin to skip school and the parents become extremely angry, saying that they spend a fortune to come here in Canada so that the kids could go to school. There are a lot of conflicts with the kids in terms of mental health issues and in turn the parents also go through a lot of issues such as racism and discrimination at work; (Service provider).

Similar to results in the questionnaire about what promotes self-esteem, focus group participants discussed a range of factors related to relationship, lifestyle, self, and achievement. Male participants talked more about lifestyle related factors such as sports (particularly soccer) and music while female participants focused more on relationship based factors such as going to parties and knowing more people.

The following quote from an Afghan male participant embeds the overlap between self-esteem, resilience, relationships and the importance of social networks in the resettlement context:

> When I came first, I didn't have immediate family in Canada. The good thing about me is that I am shameless. I am outgoing. I am not shy, I go out and talk to people. What I'm saying is that if it was hard for me, which I am not shy, imagine how hard it would be for someone who is a different person from me. I tried to make different friends and contact the Afghan society and see if they could help me in my immigration case. And also as a newcomer to settle in Canada. It kind of helped. It showed that there are people like me in Canada who don't know what to do and where to start from. Then I realized to myself, it might take a while;" (Afghan male participant).

8.11 Newcomer Youth Self-Esteem, Resettlement Policies, and Future Search

Our findings point toward and support the application of a systems approach in understanding and promoting newcomer youth self-esteem. Good relationships and communication with friends is an important predictor of high self-esteem for newcomer youth. And yet newcomer youth report acute difficulties making friends in the initial years in Canada. This has policy/service implications in connection with the need for more youth-focused programs and youth spaces that build positive youth to youth friendships/linkages for newcomer youth and decrease their isolation/exclusion. The need for more youth-to-youth peer mentoring programs (which can include online based programs) and overcoming barriers to making friends (such as reducing linguistic barriers through ongoing ESL classes and support) are areas to be considered by policy makers and program planners.

In the resettlement context, some newcomer youth may be more likely to have difficulties communicating with their fathers about things that bother them than they do communicating with their mothers. Post-migration challenges can have negative impacts on parent-child relationships and communications, through shifts in family power (for example, when children assume primary responsibility for translating communication to their parents across service sectors). Resultant policy/service implications are that more programs promote good family/intergenerational relationships and communication between parents and children within the post-migration context are needed as are, yet again, reduction of linguistic barriers.

Finally, youth's appraisal of their self-worth (their self-esteem) does not take place in a void. In this chapter, we highlighted the importance of relationships in connection with newcomer youth self-esteem. However, self-esteem is also connected to other domains and has the potential to be influenced by prevailing policies in the resettlement context. For example, Berry et al. (2006) conducted a large international study of the acculturation and adaptation of immigrant youth in thirteen countries and proposed solutions to effectively incorporate immigrant youth into the larger society. They concluded that there is positive psychological and sociocultural adaptation among immigrants when governments support integration. Integration includes immigrants maintaining their own cultural heritage and traditions while at the same time participating in the life of the larger society. Berry et al. (2006) suggested that governments promote the ethnic identity of immigrants and develop "policies and programs to encourage the participation of immigrants in the daily life of the national society," (p. 328).

In future studies, an understanding of how newcomer refugee youth negotiate their identities and its impact on their self-esteem would help inform policies and practices that focus on refugee populations in particular. While a number of studies exist that have looked at immigrant youth in this context, the literature on refugee youth, self-esteem and identity is scant. Our study recruited newcomer youth some of who, if not many, had refugee status in Canada. However, the youth did not explicitly refer to themselves as refugees, as they may have perceived this a stigmatized identity, and therefore, we chose to identify the participating youth as newcomers in this chapter. Future studies can benefit from incorporating a number of proximal and distal measures to determine refugee or immigrant status of youth.

Acknowledgements This study was made possible through funding provided by the Provincial Centre of Excellence for Child and Youth Mental Health at CHEO, Ontario, Canada (Research Grant # 122). We are grateful for the assistance of our research personnel during the different phases of the study: our Project Coordinator, Tahira Gonsalves, and our Research Assistants: Michelle Lee, Lauren Glassen, Emma Oudeh, and Farah Islam. Emma and Farah are co-authors of this chapter. We also acknowledge the research administrative support provided by Alliance Multicultural Health and Community Services in Toronto, Faculty of Nursing (University Toronto) and Faculty of Health (York University). We worked with an energetic and passionate group of youth as part of the study's Youth Advisory Committee and Peer Researchers and acknowledge all their efforts and support.

APPENDIX A

CURRENT SELF-ESTEEM INSTRUMENT

(Khanlou 2004)

1. On the following scale, please **circle** the number that shows how you have felt about yourself over the course of the **pastweek**. The bigger the number, the more positive you have felt about yourself. **1** means you **didn't feel good about yourself. 10** means you **felt great** about yourself.

      1   2   3   4   5   6   7   8   9   10

Didn't feel good   Felt great

about myself   about myself

2. What things made you feel **GOOD** about yourself?

3. What things made you feel **NOT GOOD** about yourself?

4. What things can you **DO TO FEEL GOOD** about yourself?

References

Allik, J., & Schmitt, D. P. (2005). Simultaneous administration of the Rosenberg self-esteem scale in 53 nations: Exploring the universal and cultural-specific features of global self-esteem. *Journal of Personality and Social Psychology, 89*(1), 623–642. doi:10.1037/0022-3514.89.4.623.

Barankin, T., & Khanlou, N. (2007). *Growing up resilient: Ways to build resilience in children and youth.* Toronto: Centre for Addiction and Mental Health.

Berry, J. W., Phinney, J. S., Sam, D. L., & Vedder, P. (2006). Immigrant youth: Acculturation, identity, and adaptation. *Applied Psychology: An International Review, 55*(33), 303–332.

Canada's Engagement in Afghanistan. (2011, October 12). *Canada's Engagement in Afghanistan.* http://www.afghanistan.gc.ca/canada-afghanistan/index.aspx?lang=eng&view=d.

Cavazos-Rehg, P. A., & DeLucia-Waack, J. L. (2009). Education, ethnic identity, and acculturation as predictors of self-esteem in Latino adolescents. *Journal of Counseling and Development, 87,* 47–54. http://web.ebscohost.com.ezproxy.library.yorku.ca/ehost/.

Citizenship and Immigration Canada. (2011, August 30). *Facts and figs. 2010–Immigration overview: Permanent and temporary residents.* http://www.cic.gc.ca/english/resources/statistics/facts2010/index.asp.

Crowley, C. (2009). The mental health needs of refugee children: A review of literature and implications for nurse practitioners. *Journal of the American Academy of Nurse Practitioners, 29*(1), 322–331. doi:10.1111/j.1745-7599.2009.00413.x.

Driscoll, A. K., Russell, S. T., & Crockett, L. J. (2008). Parenting styles and youth well-being across immigrant generations. *Journal of Family Issues, 29*(2), 185–209. doi:10.1177/0192513X07307843.

Gong, L. (2007). Ethnic identity and identification with the majority group: Relations with national identity and self-esteem. *International Journal of Intercultural Relations, 31,* 503–523. doi:10.1016/j.ijintrel.2007.03.002.

Guest, A. M. (2007). Cultures of childhood and psychosocial characteristics: Self-esteem and social comparison in two distinct communities. *ETHOS, 35*(1), 1–32. doi:10.1525/ETH.2007.35.1.1.

Hajdukowski-Ahmed, M., Khanlou, N., & Moussa, H. (2008). Introduction. In M. Hajdukowski-Ahmed, N. Khanlou, & H. Moussa (Eds.), *Not born a refugee woman: Contesting identities, rethinking practices* (pp. 1–23). Oxford: Berghahn Books (Forced Migration Series).

Hoersting, R. C., & Jenkins, S. R. (2011). No place to call home: Cultural homelessness, self-esteem and cross-cultural identities. *International Journal of Intercultural Relations, 35*(1), 17–30. doi:10.1016/j.ijintrel.2010.11.005.

Hyman, I., Beiser, M., & Vu, N. (1996). The mental health of refugee children in Canada. *Refuge, 15*(5), 4–8.

Hyndman, J. (2003). Aid, conflict and migration: The Canada-Sri Lanka connection. *The Canadian Geographer,47*(3), 251–268. http://journals2.scholarsportal.info.ezproxy.library.yorku.ca/details-sfx.xqy?uri = /00083658/v47i0003/251_acamtclc.xml.

Jaret, C., & Reitzes, D. C. (2009). Currents in a stream: College student identities and ethnic identities and their relationship with self-esteem, efficacy, and grade point average in an urban university. *Social Science Quarterly, 90*(2), 345-367. http://journals1.scholarsportal.info.ezproxy.library.yorku.ca/details-sfx.xqy?uri=/.

Khanlou, N. (2004). Influences on adolescent self-esteem in multicultural Canadian secondary schools. *Public Health Nursing, 21*(5) 404-411. http://journals1.scholarsportal.info.ezproxy.library.yorku.ca/details-sfx.

Khanlou, N., & Crawford, C. (2006). Post-migratory experiences of newcomer female youth: Self-esteem and identity development. *Journal of Immigrant and Minority Health, 8*(1), 45–56. doi:10.1007/s10903-006-6341-x.

Khanlou, N., & Wray, R. (2010). *Resilience and the promotion of protective factors among children and youth: Review of concepts, promising practices and public health roles in mental health promotion.* Ottawa: Public Health Agency of Canada. (Unpublished).

Khanlou, N., Shakya, Y., & Gonsalves, T. (2011). Mental health services for newcomer youth: Exploring needs and enhancing access. In: Building Equitable Partnerships: Tools and Lessons Learned-A Resource for Individuals and Organizations (pp. 16–18). Toronto: Centre for Addiction and Mental Health.

Khawaja, N. G., White, K. M., Schweitzer, R., & Greenslade, J. (2008). Difficulties and coping strategies of Sudanese refugees: A qualitative approach. *Transcultural Psychiatry, 45*(3), 489–512. doi:10.1177/1363461508094678.

Lam, B. T. (2007). Impact of perceived racial discrimination and collective self-esteem on psychological distress among Vietnamese-American college students: Sense of coherence and mediator. *American Journal of Orthopsychiatry, 77*(3), 370–376. doi:10.1037/0002-9432.77.3.370.

Mels, C., Derluyn, I., & Broekaert, E. (2008). Social support in unaccompanied asylum-seeking boys: A case study. *Child: Care, Health, and Development, 1*(1), 757–762. doi:10.1111/j.1365-2214.2008.00883.x.

Moksnes, U. K., Moljord, I. E., Espnes, G. A., & Byrne, D. G. (2010). The association between stress and emotional states in adolescents: The role of gender and self-esteem. *Personality and Individual Differences, 49,* 430–435. doi:10.1016/j.paid.2010.04.012.

Omeri, A., Lennings, C., & Raymond, L. (2006). Beyond asylum: Implications for nursing and health care delivery for Afghan refugees in Australia. *Journal of Transcultural Nursing, 17*(1), 30–39. doi:10.1177/1043659605281973.

Peace and Security Section of the United Nations Department of Public Information. (2007, August). United Nations and Darfur Fact Sheet. http://www.un.org/News/dh/infocus/sudan/fact_sheet.pdf.

Russell, R. V., & Stage, F. K. (1996). Leisure as burden: Sudanese refugee women. *Journal of Leisure Research, 28*(2), 108–121.

Schweitzer, R., Greenslade, J., & Kagee, A. (2007). Coping and resilience in refugees from the Sudan: A narrative account. *Australian and New Zealand Journal of Psychiatry, 41*(1), 282–288. http://web.ebscohost.com.ezproxy.library.yorku.ca/ehost/pdfviewer/pdfviewer?vid=3& hid=12 3&sid=bf952de6-0793-4029-aa10-f385f92cdb75%40sessionmgr110.

Simich, L., Hamilton, H., & Baya, B. K. (2006). Mental distress, economic hardship and expectations of life in canada among sudanese newcomers. *Transcultural Psychiatry, 43*(3), 418–444. doi:10.1177/1363461506066985.

Shakya, Y., Khanlou, N., & Gonsalves, T. (2010). Determinants of mental health for newcomer youth: Policy and service implications. *Canadian Issues/Thèmes canadiens, Summer,* 98–102.

Smokowski, P. R., & Bacallao, M. L. (2007). Acculturation, internalizing mental health symptoms, and self esteem: Cultural experiences of Latino adolescents in north Carolina. *Child Psychiatry Human Development, 37,* 273–292. doi:10.1007/s10578-006-0035-4.

Smokowski, P. R., Rose, R. A., & Bacallao, M. (2010). Influence of risk factors and cultural assets on Latino adolescents' trajectories of self-esteem and internalizing symptoms. *Child psychiatry and human development, 41*(1), 133–155. doi:10.1007/s10578-009-0157-6.

Statistics Canada. (2009, March 27). Place of birth for the immigrant population by period of immigration, 2006 counts and percentage distribution, for Canada, provinces and territories-20 % sample data. http://www12.statcan.gc.ca/census-recensement/2006/dp-pd/hlt/97-557/T404-eng.cfm?Lang=E&T=404&GH=4&GF=1&SC=1&S=1&O=D.

Tamis-LeMonda, C. S., Way, N., Hughes, D., Yoshikawa, H., Kalman, R. K., & Niwa, E. Y. (2008). Parents' goals for children: The dynamic coexistence of individualism and collectivism in cultures and individuals. *Social Development, 17*(1), 183–209. doi: 10.1111/j.1467-9507.2007.00419.x.

Trzesniewski, K. H., Donnellan, M. B., Moffitt, T. E., Robins, R. W., Poulton, R., & Caspi, A. (2006). Low self-esteem during adolescence predicts poor health, criminal behaviour, and limited economic prospects during adulthood. *Journal of Developmental Psychology, 42*(2), 381–390. doi:10.1037/0012-1649.42.2.381.

United Human Rights Council. (2011). *Genocide in Darfur.* http://www.unitedhumanrights.org/genocide/genocide-in-sudan.htm.

United Nations High Commissioner for Refugees. (2011a). *2011 UNHCR Country Operations Profile-Afghanistan.* http://www.unhcr.org/cgi-bin/texis/vtx/page?page=49e486eb6&submit=GO.

United Nations High Commissioner for Refugees. (2011b). *2011 UNHCR Country Operations Profile-Colombia.* http://www.unhcr.org/cgi-bin/texis/vtx/page?page=49e492ad6&submit=GO.

United Nations High Commissioner for Refugees. (2011c). *2011 UNHCR Country Operations Profile-Sri Lanka.* http://www.unhcr.org/cgi-bin/texis/vtx/page?page=49e4878e6&submit=GO.

Verkuyten, M. (2009). Self-esteem and multiculturalism: An examination among ethnic minority and majority groups in the Netherlands. *Journal of Research in Personality, 43,* 419–427. doi:10.1016/j.jrp.2009.01.013.

Weine, S. M. (2011). Developing preventive mental health interventions for refugee families in resettlement. *Family Process, 50*(3), 410-430. http://web.ebscohost.com.ezproxy.library.yorku.ca/ehost/pdfviewer/pdfviewer?vid=4&hid=123&sid=bf952de6-0793-4029-aa10-f385f92cdb75%40sessionmgr110.

Chapter 9
Newcomer Refugee Youth as 'Resettlement Champions' for their Families: Vulnerability, Resilience and Empowerment

Yogendra B. Shakya, Sepali Guruge, Michaela Hynie, Sheila Htoo, Arzo Akbari, Barinder (Binny) Jandu, Rabea Murtaza, Megan Spasevski, Nahom Berhane and Jessica Forster

Abstract Due to experiences of forced migration, a large proportion of resettled refugee families arrive in resettlement countries with low levels of education, limited official language fluency, fractured family relationships, and less than optimal physical and mental health. These pre-migration determinants intersect with systemic barriers in ways that make it extremely difficult for refugees to secure employment/income security, access health and settlement services, and pursue their educational and other goals. This chapter discusses the role that newcomer refugee youth play in helping their families resettle in response to systemic post-migration barriers.

Keywords Refugee · Newcomer youth · Resettlement · Youth leadership · Health · Access barriers · Resilience

9.1 Introduction

> My parents cannot speak English. So I teach them. As they cannot travel on their own, I help them go to and from to recognize the ways. I teach my siblings in learning their school lessons. I help read all the mail letters that come to my parents in English (Participant from Karen Male Focus Group, age 16–19).

> When my father came here, he doesn't know English and neither does my mother. Before when we were in another country, my father knew their language, and he was almost responsible for everything. But here, because I and my brother know English more and better

Y. B. Shakya (✉) · S. Htoo · A. Akbari · B. Jandu · R. Murtaza · M. Spasevski · N. Berhane · J. Forster
Access Alliance Multicultural Health and Community Services, Toronto, Canada
e-mail: yshakya@accessalliance.ca

S. Guruge
Ryerson University, Toronto, Canada

M. Hynie
York University, Toronto, Canada

than my father, then our responsibility increases as well. We have to take our grandmother and our father to doctors' appointments and also solve the problems at home. Here the responsibilities fall more on the children because they learn English much faster. (Participant from Afghan Female Focus Group, age 16–19)

In our community based research project on determinants of health for newcomer refugee youth, our refugee youth "peer researchers"[1] took a leadership role in steering our research towards an appreciative inquiry framework.[2] Instead of exclusively documenting negative impacts of forced migration and resettlement we decided to focus on examining the role that refugees play in their own resettlement process. More specifically, our research question investigated what family roles and responsibilities refugee youth undertake during resettlement. This refocusing of research was not to underplay the powerful forces of forced migration and resettlement but rather to better understand its complexities through examining how refugee youth and their families engage with these forces. We conducted focus groups and interviews with newcomer refugee youth (between the ages of 16–24 who had arrived in Canada within the last 5 years) from Afghan, Karen and Sudanese communities in Toronto.

As captured in two quotes above, refugee youth shared with us the significant reconfiguration and intensification of their responsibilities to their family and community after coming to Canada. Responsibilities youth mentioned include navigating services, doing interpretation, taking care of family sponsorship applications, earning income, finding housing, sending money back home, mentoring siblings, as well as caretaking responsibilities and giving emotional support. To this extent, we argue that refugee youth are serving as "resettlement champions" in Canada for their families. However, a closer look at youth narratives reveal a tenuous and ambivalent relationship between empowerment and vulnerability within these shifts: refugee youth articulate a sense of self-initiative and empowerment in their roles in resettlement while at the same time being concerned about the burdens from imposed responsibilities, and from the powerful systemic conditions that shape and necessitate these responsibilities.

Drawing on youth narratives, this chapter discusses the dimensions and implications of the resettlement responsibilities that refugee youth assume. In particular, we are interested in the following questions. How do refugee youth articulate, negotiate or contest post-migration stressors and their resettlement responsibilities? How do the resettlement responsibilities youth take on affect their own mental wellbeing, particularly their self-esteem, sense of self, capacity for self-care, and capacity to

---

[1] 'Peer researchers' are members of the community of interest who are involved in a community based research project as co-researchers.

[2] We use 'appreciative inquiry framework' broadly to refer to parallel bodies of work that depart from "deficit" "problem" or "needs" focused methods of inquiry towards documenting sources and agency of positive change within people, organizations, and communities. This includes appreciative inquiry framework promoted by Cooperider and Srivastav (1987) about organizational change and the 'asset mapping' approach put forth by Kretzmann and McKnight's (1993). Our use of this framework is particularly grounded on Paulo Friere's work on critical dialogical inquiry that seek to recognize and build on subversive capacities of marginalized people specifically to transform systemic inequalities, including inequities in asset distribution and impediments to change.

handle stress? In the numerous resettlement responsibilities that refugee youth take on, what policy and service gaps do they reflect? We draw on bio-politics literature and post-colonial critiques of immigration policy to reveal the systemic causes and political implications of these transformations that refugee youth go through.

Refugees occupy what Babha (2003) calls "historically and temporally disjunct and ambivalent subjectivities" and what critical scholars of refugee issues call "liminal spaces" (see for example, Simich et al. 2010). These disjunct subjectivities and liminal spaces continually push sacredly protected national boundaries of citizenship and belonging. Governments struggle to accommodate the tensions and contradictions in citizenship caused by forced migrants/diasporas that traverse these liminal spaces. Most policy makers and public view refugees as "second class migrants" and "helpless victims" that only need what Agamben refers to as "bare life" existence (Nyers 1999); consequently, supports for refugees tend to be limited and often mixed with policies that seek to control, contain, detain, and exclude them. Rather, what is needed is to transform these disjunct and liminal spaces that refugees occupy from sites of oppression and vulnerability to catalysts for creating more inclusive public policies related to immigration, resettlement, and citizenship.

Within resettlement studies, there is an emerging body of literature on resilience. In the words of Fergus and Zimmerman (2005, p. 399), resilience "refers to the process of overcoming the negative effects of risk exposure, coping successfully with traumatic experience, and avoiding the negative trajectories associated with risks." Youth in particular are viewed as intrinsically having stronger resilient capacities compared to adults. There is value to understanding and building on people's capacity for resilience, self-reliance and positive coping strategies. For example, Magro (2009, p. 82) found that refugee youth in Canada had resilient attitudes and approaches to challenges, demonstrating "remarkable tenacity, patience, self-reliance, and an openness to new experience." Researchers in other countries have also documented positive outcomes of resilient capacities among refugee youth. See, for example, research by Brough et al. (2003) on refugee youth in Australia, Raghallaigh and Gilligan (2010) on unaccompanied minors in Ireland, and Rana et al. (2011) on unaccompanied Sudanese minors in the U.S. In our study as well, refugee youth talked about numerous coping strategies they use to deal with stressors.

However, the concept of resilience has recently come under criticism for being symptom focused and ignoring the root causes of negative stressors. Scholars like Bottrell, (2009), Vanderbilt and Shaw (2008), and Portes and Rumbaut (2001) have highlighted how resilience itself is shaped by systemic factors and that individuals' capacity for resiliency and coping can vary significantly depending on conditions. Moreover, being resilient to and learning to cope with systemic marginalization may serve to maintain the root causes of marginalization. As Bottrell (2009, p. 335) aptly questioned "at the policy level there needs to be a question of limits—to what extent will adversity be tolerated, on the assumption that resilient individuals can and do cope? How much adversity should resilient individuals endure before social arrangements rather than individuals are targeted for intervention?"

What is needed is a more transformative understanding of resilience. Unlike static conceptions of resilience, transformative resilience (i) is firmly critical of the systemic conditions that shape or limit resilience; and (ii) recognizes and builds political agency of marginalized people to not just cope with stressors and injustices but also to contest, subvert, reshape and transform them. As highlighted by Walter Benjamin, Paulo Friere, Gayatri Spivak, and other critical scholars, promoting progressive counter discourse and semantics is as important as direct action for overcoming oppressive systems and policies. Researchers and policy makers preoccupied with documenting or portraying refugees in a passive light as suffering or merely coping with marginalization may inadvertently be complicit in reproducing patronizing, exclusionary, and depoliticized refugee resettlement policies. Undoing this requires reframing our views about refugees as agents of change and involving them in developing equity-informed and empowering policy solutions. Our repositioning of refugee youth as "resettlement champions" seeks to highlight the transformative capacity within their resilience and political agency.

9.2 Forced Migration and Refugee Resettlement: Current Knowledge

There is now a wealth of literature on the experiences and consequences of forced migration and protracted refugee situations. Studies by the UNHCR and other researchers have documented that, unlike economic migrants, most refugees may have experienced brutal and protracted armed conflicts, targeted persecution, and violence (some have witnessed the death of family members or massacre of entire community) (Geltman et al. 2005; Wenzel et al. 2007). Many refugees have been forcibly uprooted from their home, have had to flee or be in "hiding" often without legal status, and/or lived in refugee camps with deplorable living conditions and minimal services and rights (Fazel and Stein 2002; Goodman 2004; Heptinstall et al. 2004; Lustig et al. 2004; Morris et al. 2009). These experiences can result in detrimental impacts on mental health including post-traumatic stress disorder (PTSD), depression, anxiety disorders (Anstiss et al. 2009; Beiser 2005; Hyman et al. 2000; Rousseau et al. 2004; Soroor and Popal 2005), sleep disturbance (Montgomery and Foldspang 2007), aggression, and self-harm (Patel and Hodes 2006). For example, a study of Tamil refugees in Canada found that, one-third of participants had directly witnessed a traumatic event such as rape or combat, and 12 % of the study group suffered from PTSD (compared with a general population prevalence rate of 1 %) (Beiser et al. 2003). A study by Rummens and Seat (2003) with refugees from Kosovo conflict found that 26.3 % of the children/youth met diagnostic criteria for PTSD as a direct result of the conflict.

Additionally, these experiences of forced migration and protracted refugee conditions also result in less than optimal physical health status including malnutrition, low birth weight, iron deficiency, high rates of infectious diseases and enteric parasites, and high rates of gastrointestinal and cardiovascular ailments (Denburg et al.

2007; Fieldman 2006; Morris et al. 2009; Oxman-Martinez and Hanley 2005; Pottie et al. 2007). Further, these experiences can also lead to family separations, fracturing or collapse of ordered relationships within families, and intensification of domestic conflicts (Boyden et al. 2002).

Forced migration conditions can also seriously limit access to employment, education and overall professional development. Thus, majority of refugees who come to western nations like Canada arrive with limited education, language fluency, and professional experience. With the enactment of the Immigration and Refugee Protection Act (IRPA) in 2002, Canada made firm commitments to sponsor refugees primarily on humanitarian grounds and removed restrictions on "admissibility" criteria based on medical, economic, educational and language proficiency that are usually applied to economic immigrants.[3] With this progressive policy measure, Canada has seen more refugees from "high risk" background from severely war-torn countries in Asia, Africa and the Middle East. Immigrant arrival data from 2000 to 2009 in Canada indicate that on average refugees 15 years and older are 4 times more likely than economic immigrants (32.3% vs. 8.43%) to have had 9 years or less of schooling and twice as likely than economic immigrants (44.4% vs. 21.1%) to have no English or French language ability upon arrival in Canada (Citizenship and Immigration Canada 2010). Since 2005, the percent of refugees 15 years and older with 9 years or less of schooling has been steadily increasing from 27.7% in 2005 to 38.3% in 2009. Current Canadian evidence indicates that people who come to Canada as refugees persistently experience high levels of unemployment, get stuck in low-paying and unstable jobs, face chronic poverty, low educational success rate, and other forms of marginalization (Access Alliance 2010; Hyman 2007). These post-migration stressors in turn have been shown to worsen the physical and mental health of refugees (Baya et al. 2008; Gifford et al. 2007; Hyman 2007; Redwood-Campbell et al. 2003; Simich et al. 2006; Wilson et al. 2010).

However, limited evidence exists about how refugee communities articulate, shape and contest these powerful transformative processes. For example, we know very little about the role that refugees play in resolving the political conflicts that resulted in their forced migration, or in negotiating repatriation, or about the political organizing they do within refugee camps to secure better humanitarian supports (e.g., increased access to education for children). Also missing is literature on how refugees contend with and transform the opportunities and challenges that resettlement brings. Our study results start to bridge this evidence gap.

---

[3] Canada receives between 25,000 to 35,000 refugees every year; this represents about 10–12% of the roughly 250,000 'permanent residents' that settle in Canada annually (CIC 2009). On average, about 11,000 refugees come as "sponsored" refugees under the Refugee and Humanitarian Resettlement stream: 7,500 as Government-Assisted Refugees (GARs) and 3,500 as Privately Sponsored Refugees (PSRs). Roughly 12,000 to 19,000 come to Canada through the "In-Canada Asylum" stream in which people apply as refugee claimants upon entering Canada and then become "permanent residents" once their claim process is approved by a quasi-judiciary body called the Immigration and Refugee Board. The remaining 5,000 settle in Canada as family dependents of people who have come as refugees (CIC 2008). From 2000 to 2009, about 280,000 refugees have settled in Canada of which 62,000 (21%) are youth between the ages of 15–24.

9.3 Study Objective and Method

In 2008, we brought together a multi-disciplinary team of academic partners, community agency partners, and eight refugee youth peer researchers in Toronto and established a community-based research project called the Refugee Youth Health Project. Peer researchers for the study included youth with lived experience of forced migration and protracted refugee experience. Peer researchers received three months of training in research. The research team then used a collaborative research design process to develop research questions for the project, with peer researchers leading as subject matter experts. Peer researchers were actively involved in all phases of the study starting from research design, to data collection, analysis, and writing (including two peer researchers in co-authoring this book chapter).

Our study focused on youth 16 to 24 years from Afghan, Karen and Sudanese communities who had come to Toronto, Canada, within the last 5 years as Government Assisted Refugees, Privately Sponsored Refugees or as refugee claimants. We intended to conduct four gender-specific and age-specific focus groups per community separating youth into 16–19 year and 20–24 year age groups. Only 10 of the 12 focus groups were conducted, however; recruitment challenges made it difficult to conduct focus groups with the younger Sudanese youth. Focus groups included 4 to 7 participants ($n = 57$) and were conducted by peer researchers of the same gender from the same community. All focus group participants completed a short demographic survey. We also conducted 13 individual follow up interviews to explore in more detail the issues that had been raised in the focus groups (total focus group and interview participants, $n = 70$). Focus groups and interviews were conducted in one of the commonly spoken native languages for each community, Sgaw for Karen participants and Dari for Afghan participants (note that the first language for some of the Afghan participants was Pashto but these participants could converse fluently in Dari). In the case of Sudanese participants, focus group and interviews were conducted in English as Sudanese peer researcher indicated that doing so would not be a barrier to participation. All were audio-taped and, where necessary, translated into English. Data were collaboratively analyzed in NVivo using inductive thematic analysis (Bryman 2001).

9.4 Community Profiles

Afghanistan, Burma (Karen refugees), and Sudan were selected for the study as these three countries have ranked within the top ten 'source countries' for sponsored Convention refugees to Canada since 2006. Also, all three communities are priority client groups for Access Alliance, the community health centre leading this research. All three groups have been facing protracted wars resulting in a large number of people being killed or displaced. UNHCR estimates that almost 2.2 million Afghan refugees remain outside of Afghanistan, despite more than five million returning to the country since 2002. Worldwide there are about 690,000 refugees from Sudan and roughly 165,000 refugees from Burma (of which 140,000 are from Karen ethnic group).

Afghanistan has been a key source country for refugees to Canada from the mid-1990s. From 2000 to 2009, Canada received about 25,500 people from Afghanistan, half of whom settled in the Toronto Census Metropolitan Area (CMA). Census 2006 data show that there are currently 18,205 people in Toronto CMA who were born in Afghanistan. Many of them came to Canada after having lived for many years in transition countries like Iran, Russia, and Pakistan (usually in urban areas). Between 2000 and 2009, roughly 10,100 people from Sudan arrived in Canada, of which 2,707 (roughly 25 %) settled in Toronto CMA. Many Sudanese refugees to Canada came via Egypt, Chad, Kenya and other neighbouring countries in Africa.

The Karen people are the largest of several minority ethnic communities who fled their Karen state (Kawthoolei) in Myanmar (Burma) following persecution by the military government from late 1980s. A large number of Karen settled in refugee camps in rural Thailand and many have lived in these camps for over 20 years. Canada has only recently begun resettling Karen refugees; since 2000, about 3,100 Karens have resettled in Canada, the majority of whom have arrived after 2006. It is estimated that there are about 500–700 Karens in the city of Toronto.

Compared to Canadian-born residents, immigrants from all three communities face disproportionately high levels of unemployment and low-income rates. For example, Census 2006 data show that, compared to national average, citizens who identify as 'Afghan ethnic origin' face double the rate of unemployment (13.3 % vs 6.4 %) and three times the rate of low-income before tax (56.8 % vs 18.4 %). Census Canada data on the Sudanese community and Karen community are not available; however, regional level data indicate that these two communities face levels of unemployment and low-income rate comparable to Afghan community.

9.5 Study Results

Table 9.1 presents key demographic information about focus group participants. The gender breakdown was proportional. Since we were not able to recruit younger Sudanese participants, we had slightly more older youth (20–24 years) compared to younger cohorts (16–19). At the time of the study, all participants had been in Canada five years or less with the majority of participants (77.7 %) less than three years. Half came to Canada as Government Assisted Refugees, 17 % came as Privately Sponsored Refugees, and 14 % came as refugee claimants. Almost half of Sudanese youth came as sponsored students through the World University Service Committee (WUSC) program. Only about 30 % indicated that they spoke English "very well;" none of the Karen youth reported that they spoke English "very well." Only 20 % of the participants were the eldest sibling in the family.

The majority of participants (88 %) was enrolled in school/college/university. Only 42 participants responded about employment status. Of these, almost half (43 %) were currently employed, with the majority of them working part-time jobs.

Table 9.1 Demographic Profile of Focus Group Participants

Variable	Percentage ($N = 57$)
Age	
16–19 years	43.9
20–24 years	56.1
Gender, Female %	49.1
Ethnicity	
Afghan	42.1
Karen	40.4
Sudanese	17.5
Length Of Stay in Canada (2009 as reference year)	
< 3 years	77.7
Arrival Immigration Status	
Government Assisted Refugees	50.0
Refugee claimant	13.8
Privately sponsored	17.2
Other (e.g. WUSC)	12.0
English Language Fluency (Spoken)	
Very well	29.3
Okay	24.1
A little	46.6

Most of the jobs were in food services, sales and factory work. A few older youth attending university were doing research assistant and office jobs.

9.5.1 Refugee Youth as "Resettlement Champions"

Study results indicate that newcomer refugee youth (as young as 16 years) are acutely aware of the resettlement challenges and needs facing their family and are playing an active role in addressing them by taking on a number of crucial roles and responsibilities. Based on our data, the resettlement responsibilities that refugee youth take on for their family can be broadly categorized into six types:

1. navigating information, services and resources;
2. serving as interpreters/translators (at home, outside and while accessing services);
3. providing economic support through paid jobs;
4. doing instrumental functions (e.g., finding housing, helping to move, getting food, taking care of family sponsorship applications and other legal matters);
5. mentoring/teaching responsibilities (to younger siblings and parents/adults)
6. and giving care and emotional support (including taking care of younger siblings and grandparents, and offering emotional support to family and friends).

While many non-refugee youth (economic immigrants or Canadian born) may also experience similar changes in their family responsibilities as they age (for e.g., helping with grocery shopping or mentoring younger siblings), the causes, the scale and implications of these changes in family responsibilities are more intense and far reaching for refugee youth groups. Unlike youth from other groups, most refugee youth do not have much choice but to take on these responsibilities; failing to do so may be detrimental to the everyday wellbeing of their family. For example, a Canadian-born youth or youth from more privileged immigrant family may willingly decide to do a part-time job to earn some pocket money. In contrast, many refugee youth take a paid job to financially support their family since their parents are not able to find jobs; they often do this at the expense of their studies and other aspirations. Similarly several refugee youth mentioned that they were primarily responsible for grocery shopping since it was difficult for their parents with low English language fluency to read the food labels and communicate with grocery store staff.

We were struck by the multitude of family responsibilities that refugee youth assume on an everyday level. We also found that younger refugee youth cohort (ages 16–19) were as likely as the older cohort (ages 19–24) to be doing all six types of responsibilities including wage labor, taking care of legal matters, and offering caregiving responsibilities to their family members.

The first two types of responsibilities (navigating information and services, and serving as interpreters/translators) were the most prominent for refugee youth from all three communities and across gender as well as the two age groups. Youth from all three communities, particularly Afghan and Karen communities, were acutely aware of the limited English language fluency and low education among their parents/guardians and the service barriers and other negative impacts that result from this. While none of the Karen youth indicated that they understood English "very well," many of them nevertheless mentioned that they were doing interpretation and service navigation roles for their family. The narratives presented at the beginning of this chapter capture the service navigation and interpreter/translator role that refugee youth do for their families. Youth also spoke about helping their neighbors and members of their community with navigating and accessing services on a regular basis.

Many youth shared about having to provide economic support to their family. Youth were particularly aware of the labor market barriers facing their parents/adult family members and about the resulting financial hardships. Quite a few youth spoke about stepping in to find jobs to contribute to household income. More than a third of the study participants were doing paid jobs and others mentioned that they were actively looking for jobs. Some youth spoke about feeling responsible to take on paid work because they see that it is easier for youth to find jobs compared to their parents in the Canadian labour market:

> In my case because we are still young, finding a job is easier for me, for us as kids. For my parents they can't find jobs. In this way I feel responsible. They rely on us (Participant from Sudanese Female Focus Group, age 20–24).

Others mentioned that severe financial difficulties facing the family presses them to start doing paid jobs and making tough decisions including dropping out of school:

> My parents can't find jobs in Canada. It affects me financial way. School wise, you can't buy certain books because you are thinking of okay, if I spend this amount of money. Because

OSAP [Ontario Student Assistance Program] doesn't give enough money to buy books and laptop, and here you are working limited job and don't have enough money and trying to differentiate which one come first: shelter, food or school. You buy certain books and the rest, library, photocopy .... So it is really a lot of pressure. Sometimes you just tend to drop out and take a semester off thinking, "okay, if I work I might be able to help". (Participant from Sudanese Female Focus Group, age 20–24)

The sense of responsibility to financially support the family by doing paid jobs was not limited to older youth. In the words of one younger Afghan youth:

Yes, before, when we used to be in Afghanistan, we didn't have to go work outside because of any financial or economical problem. Over there my father worked. But here, we all have to work and we have to support our family financially. I think this is a kind of change. (Participant from Afghan Female Focus group, age 16–19).

Several youth from all three communities (particularly older Sudanese youth) mentioned that they were sending money to their family and community back home. One Sudanese youth talked about a mixed sense of responsibility and "pressure" to provide economic support to community and villages back home to help rebuild schools, healthcare and other crucial infrastructures:

And these are my responsibilities now in Canada, they more than ever. Because, people back home looking towards you because here they think you have a lot of things to help them with. Here you go to work to help your family members but still you have to send money back home to help people back home. I also contribute to the community by sending money to rebuild the villages that I worked on... A lot of villages need to be rebuilt, schools, health care, it tends to be more pressure on us than ever. (Participant from Sudanese Female Focus Group, age 20–24).

Almost all youth highlighted that they were providing instrumental support to their family, such as buying food, food preparation, securing housing, securing utilities and materials (water, cooking/heating materials etc.), cleaning and maintenance, taking care of legal matters and so forth. Most refugee youth spoke about actively providing instrumental support even before coming to Canada. Interestingly, there are striking contrasts in the contexts and nature of instrumental functions for these youth before and after coming to Canada, particularly for refugee families who have come to Canada from rural refugee camps. Take for example, these telling narratives from Karen youth comparing their instrumental responsibilities (like getting food and securing/building housing) in refugee camps to those in Canada:

In Mae La U refugee camp we have to work harder, but in Canada the working is lighter and easier. When people move to new apartment, we need to help only loading and unloading. But there when we moved to new place, we need to help carrying things through long distance. To search for food in the jungle was also very difficult. Some time we need to sleep. In the jungle to help pull out trucks that were sink in the muddy road. The mountains are very high. In Canada we don't need to do heavy work like that. (Participant from Karen Male Focus Group, age 16–19)

When I was in the camp, I was very poor. My daily works in the house were raising animals (pig and poultry) and gardening. I got seeds from [an NGO] and grew vegetables. For the community – when I was asked to help loading and unloading food supply I helped them. Sometimes I had to go and pull timber pole and bamboo for community building and helped built also. After I came to Canada – as my parents are uneducated and all sales jobs use computers, they are at a loss to go shopping, so I had to do the shopping duty. (Participant from Karen Male Focus Group, age 20–24).

As captured above, youth in refugee camps had to help with growing food, doing difficult tasks like collecting food or building materials from the forests, and carrying, loading and unloading food supplies and other materials. In Canada, youth continue these functions of getting food for their family by helping with grocery shopping. Along the same lines, youth in refugee camps helped with finding timber and bamboo for construction and were involved in building houses. The Karen peer researchers highlighted that Karen refugee families had to move multiple times while in refugee camps due to flooding and forced displacement; in such cases, as noted above, they had to carry heavy loads and rebuild entire houses from scratch. The comparable function of securing accommodation in Canada involves helping family and friends find housing and helping them move. In fact, helping family and friends move was a recurring and important task that many youth talked about. This resonates with the fact that finding accommodation is a pressing priority for newcomers; also, newcomers may have had to move multiple times during the first few years. In other words, youth continue to perform instrumental functions for their family in Canada, but the nature and weight of these responsibilities are strikingly different.

The study documented some gender differences in the types of household functions youth take on before and after coming to Canada. For example, unlike for male participants, most female participants listed "inside the house" chores like cooking and cleaning as the most significant instrumental functions they did before coming to Canada. Male participants were more likely than female participants to highlight instrumental functions "outside" of the house such as building or repairing the house, help with moving, building roads, or getting materials. These gendered differences appear to decrease and change after coming to Canada. According to one female participant:

> Because boys and girls both go to school and study, as well as working. In Afghanistan girls were mostly at home and did house chores, and boys work outside of house. But here, everything is the same for boys and girls and there is no difference between them, girls work both in and out of the house, because they want to have something in hand in the future, I mean to be independent. (Participant from Afghan Female Focus group, age 16–19).

Many youth talked about mentoring and teaching responsibilities for younger siblings. Youth were aware that their parents often did not have the capacity or time to help children with school work. In the words of one Karen youth:

> Among young children, like the Karen newcomer kids because their parents work whole days and they come back and they are exhausted, they have no time to spend with their children to do their homework and also even if they have time they don't have the language skill, they don't know how to help them, so children lack support in terms of completing their homework (Participant from Karen Male Focus Group, age 16–19).

Older youth appear to draw on their educational experience in Canada to take an active role in mentoring younger siblings in terms of academic planning. Specifically, older youth sought to help younger siblings avoid the shortcomings and disappointments they themselves had experienced in schools. The mentoring involved reminding younger siblings that they need to decide for themselves and not necessarily depend on guidance from school:

> Now my sister is in grade 11, and she is thinking like me, she is waiting for her school to help or guide her to choose her field. I told her "No, this is not the case, now in grade 11 you can decide what you want to study, and where to go." (Participant from Afghan Female Focus Group, age 20–24).

Youth spoke about having to teach English and about the Canadian system and culture to their parents and older relatives.

Many youth were providing caregiving responsibilities as well as emotional support to family members. Several youth talked about having to look after children in the family and their aging grandparents/relatives. Some youth spoke about having to console and emotionally support their parents when their parents were feeling down because of economic and other difficulties. Similar to instrumental functions, caregiving responsibilities were not necessarily new for many youth. Particularly older youth and youth from single parent households mentioned that they did caregiving responsibilities before coming to Canada and continue to do so after coming to Canada.

In summary, study results highlight that newcomer refugee youth are deeply aware of the systemic barriers that their families face in Canada and thus take on numerous responsibilities to help their family members deal with resettlement process and challenges. These resettlement responsibilities appear to be crucial for their families' day to day wellbeing in Canada; for many refugee families, youth may be the only source of support and hope. To this extent, we argue that newcomer refugee youth are playing a vital role as "resettlement champions" for their families in Canada.

9.5.2 Making Sense of Change: Political Agency and Mental Wellbeing

Refugee youth narratives reveal that these shifts in roles and responsibilities are not smooth, clear cut transitions but rather complex and tenuous. The political agency embodied within these shifts is complicated and fragile and yet carries salient implications for their wellbeing. Most refugee youth expressed mixed perspectives about whether these resettlement responsibilities are self-initiated or imposed or a combination. Along the same lines, refugee youth talked about being simultaneously empowered, vulnerable and overwhelmed in their resettlement responsibilities. We noticed that these resettlement responsibilities had important implications for the youths' sense of self, their self-esteem, capacity for self-care (including time to relax and spend quality time with friends) and their help seeking behavior.

When we asked about the level of change in family responsibilities after coming to Canada, almost half of the youth (46 %) reported that the responsibilities had "changed a lot." Interestingly, we noticed several distinct variations. Youth who came alone clearly experienced a "big change" in responsibilities. They were also more likely to say that they have very little support. In the words of one Afghan youth:

> Here (in Canada) I am alone. There is no one to help me or be with me. In Afghanistan I was dependent on my family, because I was not working, they helped me with money. I just went to school and did nothing else. But I see a big change here, my family is not with me, I have to depend on me. I have to go to school, work, clean the house, and do everything by myself. (Participant from Afghan Male Focus Group, age 16–19).

Our survey data indicate that 60 % of Afghan youth and 55 % of Sudanese youth perceived that their responsibilities have "changed a lot" after coming to Canada compared to 22 % for Karen youth. On the other hand, when asked about how well they are adjusting to their responsibilities in Canada, half of the Afghan youth indicated "very well" while only 17 % of Karen youth answered "very well." In other words, it appears that many Afghan youth perceive that their responsibilities have changed a lot after coming to Canada but feel that they are adjusting well to these changes. In contrast, most Karen youth view that their responsibilities have not changed much after coming to Canada; some mentioned that tasks are "lighter" in Canada. Nonetheless, most Karen youth feel that they are not adjusting very well to these changes. In the case of Sudanese youth, one third of the participants indicated they are adjusting "very well" to their responsibilities. Focus group discussions show these varied perspectives across groups are closely linked to divergent experiences with forced migration.

Unlike most Karen youth, who came from rural refugee camps, many Afghan and Sudanese youth came from urban settings and mentioned that they had fewer responsibilities before coming to Canada. Thus, many Afghan and Sudanese youth perceived a marked increase in responsibilities after coming to Canada including performing instrumental functions, service navigation, providing interpretation, earning income, mentoring and caretaking responsibilities. Focus group discussions show that many Afghan youth viewed these changes in family responsibilities as opportunities. Also, study results indicate that, compared to other groups, Afghan youth appear to be more aware of settlement and community services and more likely to use services to address resettlement challenges they are facing.

In contrast, Karen youth were already carrying many instrumental and other family responsibilities before coming to Canada and thus did not perceive that the scale or burden of their multiple responsibilities had changed. Most Karen youth had low English language fluency, were poorly connected to formal services, and relied mostly on other Karen youth for help (who already had their own family responsibilities). These are potential factors why many Karen youth felt that they are not adjusting well to these post-migration changes in spite of their responsibilities becoming lighter.

Similar to Karen youth, Sudanese youth were not well connected to settlement and community services and spoke frequently about social isolation. Several mentioned that they knew very few people from Sudanese background in Canada and were expressively thrilled to meet other Sudanese youth during the focus groups for this study. At the same time, many of Sudanese youth participants had high English language fluency and were in university or college. Thus, compared to other two groups, their narratives embodied a stronger sense of individual capacity to face resettlement challenges. Unlike Afghan youth, they did not necessarily perceive these new family responsibilities as opportunities. Several, in fact, were very critical of these added responsibilities taking time away from their other priorities like studying. However, most Sudanese youth did not really perceive that they were having serious difficulties adjusting to these resettlement responsibilities.

While understanding variations across community groups is useful in developing community-geared solutions, it is important to caution against falling into cultural deterministic perspectives. In other words, these variations are not reflective of inherent cultural features of each community but rather are socially produced by macro-structural factors linked to the divergent forced migration and resettlement trajectories for the three communities.

How do then refugee youth perspectives and responses to resettlement responsibilities affect their mental wellbeing, particularly their self-esteem and capacity for self-care? Our study findings suggest this relationship is complex and tenuous. For some youth, being able to help their family made them feel good and important:

> Well now I feel I am more important to my family and everything and my brother and sister, because I really help them with their homework and everything. So I feel that I'm more important for it. After doing my homework I'm going to help my little brother and sister with their homework because they also need help with the new language and new things. So I feel really good to help them. (Interview Participant, Afghan Male, age 16–19).

For other youth, the added family responsibilities were forced obligations and often went unappreciated by their family members in ways that was emotionally upsetting for youth:

> Sometime my parents ask me to go somewhere to help them but I cannot help them, so then they told me that you have been here for a long time, why, you can speak English and you cannot help me and go there?... Sometimes my parents tell me that I'm lazy. I feel upset, I feel upset (Interview Participant, Karen Male, age 16–19)

While some youth mentioned that it was easier for youth to find jobs than adult family members, other youth (particularly those with low English and low education levels) discussed how they feel hopeless because they themselves also cannot find jobs in order to support their family:

> Whenever you apply for a job you are asked to submit your qualification high school certificate, which we unfortunately do not have. So we cannot get a job. It is not easy. We become Kyaw Thu Taw [in Sgaw language this means *'a person who is unfortunate in anything he tries to do'*] (Participant from Karen Male Focus Group, age 20–24).

Some youth mentioned that they felt emotionally disturbed for not being able to solve the core problems that their family and community face, but had aspirations for pursuing higher education in order to be able to help in the future:

> It's morally and emotionally disturbing because I see my family, my people, living in problems, having problems. I can't do anything. Well I have long-term plans. I will go to university because I need to give something to my country, to my people, because they need help and we are the ones who need to help them. (Interview Participant, Afghan Male, age 20–24).

In another paper (Shakya et al. 2010), we have discussed how refugee youth develop very strong aspirations for higher education after coming to Canada but that these aspirations are undercut by the multiple systemic barriers they face.

Many youth spoke about negative consequences for themselves from being burdened with numerous resettlement responsibilities. A number of youth mentioned that they had limited time for themselves or for self-care because of all the added responsibilities. In the words of one Sudanese youth comparing his current situation to how things were prior to migration,

> Just like *[another participant in the focus group]* said before, the school gets overshadowed. So here I can relate it to the fact that the care for myself gets overshadowed, that I tend to think of doing more things. Like when I was there [back home], because I'm obviously smiling and tend to, I mean take care of myself so much. But here there is no smile (Participant from Sudanese Male Focus Group, age 20–24).

Many youth expressed major concern about having less time to relax or do things they like. As one Karen youth put it:

> If I compare there and here, I have less time here. Because here I have to go to school at 3 o'clock come back and do my homework. Plus I go to work at part-time job. And I don't have free time. (Interview Participant, Karen Male, age 16–19).

Youth were also concerned about spending less time with family "just chilling" and how this was weakening family relationships. In the words of one Sudanese youth:

> Also I think family ties. Family ties is not as strong because there is so many stuff, so many responsibilities that you have in this country you tend to forget the old stuff. Like you know just chilling with your family and going out and all that (Participant from Sudanese Female Focus Group, age 20–24).

Other youth mentioned how they felt bad about not being able to spend time with friends, including on weekends:

> Sometimes on Saturday we like to spend time with friends, a friend calls but then my work is not done, so then I feel bad for refusing to go with my friends. And I feel like it's time for me to enjoy, for example, on Saturdays, a time for me to enjoy, to be happy, but then I have to complete all the unfinished work. And so it makes me feel sad, and sometimes upset about it. But then on the other hand when I think about it these works are not more than people work, it's my role so then I have to complete it and, and I go ahead and do complete that. (Interview participant, Karen Female, age 16–19)

On the one hand, refugee youth are doing many chores for their family and friends. At the same time, they feel that they do not have quality time to spend with their family and friends. The irony of this situation is troubling.

Overall, 83 % of study participants indicated that they need more support to fulfill their resettlement responsibilities. When we asked about where they go for help, we noticed some variations across the three communities. As noted earlier, compared to Karen and Sudanese youth, Afghan youth were more familiar with settlement and community services and used them more frequently. Unlike the other two groups, the Afghan community is fairly large and has a well established history of settlement in Canada. Several Afghan community leaders have founded exemplary ethno-specific and settlement agencies to provide services to the Afghan community. Afghan youth and their families appear to be well linked to these services and supports. Though there are ethno-specific and settlement agencies serving the Sudanese community in Toronto, only some spoke about using these services. Most Sudanese youth mentioned that they rely more on themselves. The Sudanese community is quite dispersed in their settlement patterns in Toronto and is not necessarily closely connected geographically and socially as compared to the Afghan and Karen communities. The political tensions between northern and southern Sudanese communities also result in some division. In contrast, Karen youth mentioned that their key source of help was other Karen youth who had come a few years earlier or those with strong education and English language fluency. In the words of one Karen youth:

> I would like to say a very difficult situation like this is really hard to cross through. But just as the wise Karen saying goes "bushes depend on island and island depends on bushes". Likewise, the only fortunate thing for us here is we have some educated Karens who help us in finding jobs, or going to get health care and so on. So it makes us easier to cross. While we come here, if those people are not with us it will be really difficult for us. We are glad of our Karen who help us and settle here earlier. They show us ways to cross difficulties, so we are able to cross it one by one smoothly (Participant from Karen Male Focus Group, age 20–24)

Since the Karen community is fairly new in Canada, there are no Karen-specific community agencies. A number of settlement agencies in Toronto have collaborated with Karen leaders to establish the Karen Partnership Group to better coordinate services for the Karen community. Nonetheless, as captured in the above narrative, for most Karen families in Toronto the vital source of support is this group of educated Karen youth leaders (participants provided names of half a dozen of them) who go out of their way to help. Some settlement and community agencies have begun to hire these youth leaders as outreach workers specifically to connect other Karen youth and their families to formal services. While this has helped to improve employment prospects for these Karen youth leaders, many of them appear overwhelmed since the need greatly exceed what this small group of youth outreach workers can provide within work hours. Also, like many newcomers working in settlement and community agency sector, they face barriers in progressing to decision-making and management positions to be able to influence broader level programmatic changes within these agencies.

At the same time, some Karen youth spoke sadly about not having anybody or any place to go for help:

> I don't go anywhere... I simply don't find anybody or anyplace who I think would be able to help me or support me (Interview Participant, Karen Female, age 16–19).

In terms of mental health support, none of the youth spoke of seeking professional mental health services. Many said that they either "pray," "sleep it off" or "cry" when they are feeling down. Most youth across all groups did mention that their friends were the most important source of emotional support and inspiration for them. The following quote by an Afghan youth resonates with what many youth had to say about the important role that friends play:

The only thing, in Canada I have is my friends because do we do need to like talk to them. Because I don't have relatives in Canada and the only thing that makes me happy, which keeps me energetic and happy and is my friends. They encourage me. Because you know I wasn't expecting this much problems in Canada. Like employment problems, financial problems, and being isolated from family. But they encourage me and they inspire me, and whenever I felt sick they came to me, they visited me. (Interview Participant, Afghan Male, age 20–24).

9.6 Discussion: Implications for Critical Theory and Refugee Resettlement Policy

Refugee youth in our study shared with us the significant reconfiguration and intensification of their responsibilities to their family and community after coming to Canada. Responsibilities refugee youth mentioned include navigating services, doing interpretation, earning income, doing instrumental functions, mentoring/teaching, as well as caretaking responsibilities and giving emotional support. To some extent these are common changes that youth in general go through as they age. However, the scale and intensity of these changes are more pronounced for youth with refugee experience. These resettlement responsibilities that refugee youth adopt are vital for their families' everyday wellbeing in Canada. To this extent, refugee youth are serving as "resettlement champions" in Canada for their families.

At the same time, our findings highlight that refugee youth tread a thin line between empowerment and vulnerability in their role as resettlement champions for their families. Most refugee youth expressed mixed perspectives about whether resettlement responsibilities were self-initiated or imposed or whether they felt empowered, burdened or overwhelmed by these changes. Some variations across the three communities were observed closely linked to the different patterns of forced migration and resettlement for each community.

Study findings suggest that the multiple resettlement responsibilities that youth take on had negative consequences on their capacity for self-care, leisure time to spend with family and friends (which they highly value), and other aspirations (including educational) that, if met, could improve their settlement experiences. While these are risks for mental health, most youth mentioned that they do not seek mental health services and instead just "cry" and "pray" when they are in distress or rely on their immediate circle of friends (who also face multiple difficulties of their own). Some refugee youth appear to be experiencing acute social isolation. Some youth did view these changes as opportunities and sources of empowerment. However, the fact that 83 % of study participants indicated that they need more support to deal with these changes in family responsibilities highlights a clear gap in formal services. Of particular concern are newly resettled refugee communities who came from rural refugee camps, such as the Karens.

These findings have important implications for policy and for critical theory. Can we build on the leadership role that refugee youth play in helping their families resettle in Canada without exacerbating their vulnerabilities and compounding their burden? Under what conditions are these roles empowering versus overwhelming? Youth taking on leadership role in their family and community is a common and often a positive process. For refugee youth, however, the multitude and the enormous weight of resettlement responsibilities they have to assume in the face of minimal professional support appear overwhelming with damaging risks to their mental wellbeing. What is the root cause of this and can it be rectified?

A closer examination of Canadian refugee resettlement policy reveals that current policy framework (or lack of equity focused policies) is the key cause of the negative intensification of resettlement responsibilities on refugee youth. In other words, refugee youth appear to be taking on a multitude of family and community responsibilities because of lack of supportive policies and formal services. For example, gaps in professional interpretation services and ineffective language training programs means that the burden of providing interpretation (including in medical visits) is being downloaded on youth members of the family, who themselves may not have strong official language fluency. Similarly, the acute difficulties that adult refugees are facing in the labour market is pressuring youth to step in and enter the labour market, often at the expense of other priorities such as education. Foregoing higher education for immediate "survival jobs" can stream marginalized youth into protracted cycles of low-wage and insecure employment trajectory.

Canadian policy makers boast about having a "non-discriminatory" resettlement process for refugees particularly after the enactment of IRPA. As noted earlier, Canada has seen a rise in the number of refugees that may not necessarily have a strong educational background, work qualification, or good health. However, apart from an initial year of financial and settlement service support, other equity-focused policy complements to build educational, professional and political capacities among refugees are largely lacking. Such policy gaps can result in refugees being "assimilated into poverty" (see Portes and Zhou, 1993 for discussion of "segmented assimilation"). The hopes that refugees have for safety, security, rights, citizenship, and improved socio-economic conditions and improved health in resettlement nations are often undercut by exclusionary and punitive government policies that seek to control, contain or exclude refugees.

The following Canadian policies exemplify how governments often apply punitive and exclusionary treatments towards refugees that contradict international humanitarian commitments:

1. Government Assisted Refugees are required to repay their transportation loan to travel to Canada. For a family of 5, this debt can easily total $10,000 which they are required to repay from the minimal income they get from resettlement assistance program or earned income.
2. Government Assisted Refugees cannot choose where in Canada they want to settle. Instead, they are 'destined' to various parts of Canada, including to remote areas, to fill quota needs.
3. Refugee claimants are not eligible to apply for financial assistance when pursuing post-secondary education.

4. Since September 2012, refugee claimants are no longer eligible for federal health insurance coverage.
5. Refugee determination process and family reunification process are excessively stringent, lengthy and stressful.

There is an urgent need to eliminate these damaging policies. Sadly, however, the conservative Harper government in Canada is doing just the reverse by recently passing Bill C-31 that give more control to government to selectively exclude, detain, and persecute refugee groups. Under Bill C-31, the Harper government promises to speed up refugee determination process. However, they plan to do this by barring certain types of refugees (particularly "mass arrival refugees" or refugees deemed to have come through "irregular arrivals") from having fair review process and subjecting them to detention and hasty deportation.

More broadly, the systemic marginalization that refugees experience in Canada is reflective of a lack of proactive equity focused and refugee-sensitive policies to match the humanitarian commitment. Most refugee communities, including the three communities in this study, continue to face unemployment and poverty rates that are three or more times higher than those of average Canadians. However, policy measures to improve employment services or welfare provisions have not been forthcoming. Current employment services run by government and community agencies make little attempts to understand and overcome the root causes of labour market barriers facing refugee groups. In fact, they have been criticized for inadvertently or intentionally streaming refugees (and other marginalized groups) into precarious, low-skill, and low-paying types of jobs rather than enabling them to pursue more stable employment/career pathways.

Education rights advocacy organizations in Canada like People for Education (2011) and Coalition for Equal Access to Education (2002) have documented extensive provincial and national level evidence about declining professional support for English/French language learners in schools at a time when the number of students that require this support is increasing. According to People for Education (2011), 29 % of schools in Greater Toronto Area that report having English/French language learners do not have teachers who specialize in teaching English/French to newcomers. This is largely due to policy implementation gap. Funding formula to schools for English/French language training is based on number of English/French language learners. However, this government grant is open and not legislated to be used specifically for English/French language training programs (in policy language, this grant is 'unsweatered'). School administrators suffering from overall funding cuts to education end up using this grant to cover infrastructure and other expenses (Coalition for Equal Access to Education 2002; Community Social Planning Council of Toronto 2005; People for Education 2011). Refugee youth with pre-migration disruptions in education are acutely impacted by this practice with adverse consequences on their educational trajectory. Moreover, English/French language training programs and schools in Canada are not sensitive to learning difficulties caused by long gaps in education and/or by trauma, thus are failing to provide necessary pedagogical supports to enable refugees to develop language fluency and succeed academically (Coalition for Equal Access to Education 2002). These examples highlight lack of equity focus in current policies.

These policy limitations are indicative of a broader problem of the division between politics and ethics within humanitarianism. Post-colonial scholars based in Canada including Himani Bannerji, Rinaldo Walcott, Vijay Agnew, and Ilan Kapoor, (building on writings by Edward Said, Franz Fanon, Gayatri Spivak, Homi Babha, and Stuart Hall) and scholars of "bio-politics" such Peter Nyers, Liisa Malkki, and Diedre Fassin (influenced by writing of Michel Foucault and Giorgio Agamben) have exposed the flaws within mainstream humanitarian policies. Their insights reveal how current refugee resettlement policies result in "compassionate repression" of refugees such that they remain in a "state of exception" as "speechless emissaries." Worse, dominant policy and public discourse in resettlement nations like Canada often portray refugees as non-productive "dependents" and "burdens" who unnecessarily drain taxpayer money or are risk to national security and health. Negative perceptions about refugees by policy makers and general public become particularly pronounced during recessions. At present in Canada, any equity focused policies for refugees are being labeled as being "unfair" towards average taxpaying citizens and are being categorically eliminated one by one by the conservative Harper government.

The lack of refugee sensitive policies and the claw backs of existing equity focused policies is the root cause of the adverse trends and consequences within shifts in family responsibilities for refugee youth in resettlement context. Punitive and exclusionary policies make these shifts in family responsibilities obligatory for refugee youth and thus exacerbate their vulnerabilities and mental health risks. In other words, refugee youth are serving as resettlement champions for their families with harmful consequences on their wellbeing and aspirations.

The first and the most important step to rectify this is recognize the crucial role that refugee youth are playing as resettlement champions and to involve them in leadership capacity (as paid employment opportunities wherever possible) within research, policy making and service planning for refugee youth and their families. This can result not just in better refugee sensitive policies but also improved career and economic pathways for these youth and their families who are facing acute labor market barriers. Our study findings highlight that refugees have an intimate understanding of the systemic conditions that produce the challenges they face and are constantly confronting them to improve conditions for their families. They also have rich insights on policy and programmatic solutions. For example, one youth rightfully gave a concrete policy recommendation to hire people without Canadian experience:

> There are some services but there are not enough. I had those kind of services like resume, it is important to make resume but it is not the thing that will get you the job. I feel like, I don't know if this is possible but making sure that every organization or every company has hired those people who are, like, have some job postings for people who do not have Canadian experience. Make sure it is in the *policy* of the company to stress this thing. (Participant from Sudanese Female Focus Group, age 20–24)

Many youth provided detailed recommendations about how to make policies and services more youth-friendly and empowering. Among other things, they emphasized the need for more youth staff, youth-friendly spaces, and opportunities for networking and learning from peers (about what not to do and how to access helpful professional services). Many emphasized the need to reach newcomer youth with youth-friendly programs from the very first day of arrival in order to prevent social isolation. One participant was articulate about the need for their community to get more involved in governmental politics to find broader solutions:

> I mean Afghans in Ontario. We have 70,000 people but we don't have a Member of Parliament, we don't have anyone to represent us in parliament, in Provincial parliament, in City Councils. I mean we should do something. We should stick together, we should work in cooperation with each other, we should raise the problems, we should try to find the solutions. (Interview Participant, Afghan Male, age 20–24).

These and other youth narratives presented in this chapter are counterpoints to mainstream perceptions of refugees as passive and helpless victims. We refer to these everyday strategies of marginalized people to understand, respond to, and contest systemic inequalities and injustices as transformative resilience. There is an urgent need to tap into this capacity for transformative resilience among refugee youth. Our experience of working with refugee youth as co-researchers clearly indicates that refugee youth can do professional quality research. In order to develop real solutions, we call on researchers, policy makers, and service sector leaders working on refugee issues to involve refugees as empowered (and meaningfully employed) partners in research, policy-making, and service planning.

References

Access Alliance Multicultural Health and Community Services. (2010). *Literature review: Health issues of government assisted refugees*. Toronto: Access Alliance.

Anstiss, H., Ziaian, T., Procter, N., & Warland, J. (2009). Help-seeking for mental health problems in young refugees: A review of the literature with implications for policy, practice, and research. *Transcultural Psychiatry, 46,* 584–607.

Babha, H. (2003). Culture's in between. In S. Hall & P. D. Guy (Eds.), *Questions of cultural identity*. London: Sage Publication. Pg 57.

Baya, K., Simich, L., & Bukhari, S. (2008). A Study of Sudanese women's resettlement experiences. In S. Guruge & E. Collins (Eds.), *Working with immigrant women: Issues and strategies for mental health professionals* (pp. 157–176). Toronto: Centre for Addiction and Mental Health.

Beiser, M. (2005). The health of immigrants and refugees in Canada. *Canadian Journal of Public Health, 96*(Suppl.2), S30–S44.

Beiser, M., Simich, L., & Pandalangat, N. (2003). Community in distress: Mental health needs and help-seeking in the Tamil community in Toronto. *International Migration, 41*(5), 233–245.

Bottrell, D. (2009). Understanding 'marginal' perspectives. Towards a social theory of resilience. *Qualitative Social Work, 8,* 321–339.

Boyden, J., de Berry, J., Feeny, T., & Hart, J. (2002). Children affected by armed conflict in South Asia: A review of trends and issues identified through secondary research. Refugee Studies Centre Working Paper No. 7. Oxford, University of Oxford, Refugee Studies Centre.

Brough, M., Gorman, D., Ramirez, E., & Westoby, P. (2003). Young refugees talk about well-being: A qualitative analysis of refugee youth mental health from three states. *Australian Journal of Social Issues, 38*(2), 193–209.

Bryman, A. (2001). *Social research methods*. Oxford: Oxford University Press.

Cooperrider, D., & Srivastva, S. (1987). Appreciative inquiry in organizational life. In W. Pasmore & R. Woodman (Eds.), *Research in organizational change and development* (Vol. 1). Greenwich: JAI Press.

Coalition for Equal Access to Education. (2002). *English as a second language education: Context, current responses and recommendations for new directions*. Calgary: Coalition for Equal Access to Education.

Community Social Planning Council of Toronto. (2005). *Renewing Toronto's ESL programs: Charting a course towards more effective ESL program delivery*. Toronto: Community Social Planning Council of Toronto

Denburg, A., Rashid, M., Brophy, J., Curtis, T., Malloy, P., Audley, J., Pegg, W., Hoffman, S., & Banerji, A. (2007). Initial health screening results for Karen refugees: A retrospective review. *Canadian Communicable Disease Report, 33*(13), 16–22.

Dlamini, S. N., Wolfe, B., Anucha, U., & Chung Yan, M. (2009). Engaging the Canadian diaspora: Youth social identities in a Canadian border city. *McGill Journal of Education, 44*(3), 405–433.

Fassin, D. (2005). Compassion and repression: The moral economy of immigration policies in France. *Cultural Anthropology, 20*(3), 362–387.

Fazel, M., & Stein, A. (2002). The mental health of refugee children. *Archives of Disease in Childhood, 87*, 366–370.

Fergus, S., & Zimmerman, M. A. (2005). Adolescent resilience: A framework for understanding healthy development in the face of risk. *Annual Review of Public Health, 26*, 399–419.

Geltman, P. L., Grant-Knight, W., Mehta, S. D., Lloyd-Travaglini, C., Lustig, S., Landgraf, J. M., & Wise, P. H. (2005). The "lost boys of Sudan": Functional and behavioral health of unaccompanied refugee minors re-settled in the United States. *Archives of Pediatrics & Adolescent Medicine, 159*, 585–591.

Gifford, S. M., Bakopanos, C., Kaplan, I., & Correa-Velez, I. (2007). Meaning or measurement? Researching the social contexts of health and settlement among newly-arrived refugee youth in Melbourne, Australia. *Journal of Refugee Studies, 20*(3), 414–440.

Goodman, J. H. (2004). Coping with trauma and hardship among unaccompanied refugee youths from Sudan. *Qualitative Health Research, 14*(9), 1177–1196.

Heptinstall, E., Sethna, V., & Taylor, E. (2004). PTSD and depression in refugee children: Association with pre-migration trauma and post-migration stress. *European Child and Adolescent Psychiatry, 13*, 373–380.

Hyman, I. (2007). Immigration and health: Reviewing evidence of the healthy immigrant effect in Canada. CERIS Working Paper No.55. Joint Centre of Excellence for Research in Immigration and Settlement, Toronto.

Hyman, I., Vu, N., & Beiser, M. (2000). Post-migration stresses among Southeast Asian refugee youth in Canada: A research note. *Journal of Comparative Family Studies, 31*, 281–293.

Kretzmann, J. P., & McKnight, J. L. (1993). *Building communities from the inside out: A path towards finding and mobilising a communit's assets*. Chicago: ACTA Publications.

Kumsa, K. K. (2006). 'No, I'am not a refugee!' The poetics of be-longing among young Oromos in Toronto. *Journal of Refugee Studies, 19*(2), 230–255.

Lustig, S. L., Kia-Keating, M., Knight, W. G., Geltman, P., Ellis, H., Kinzie, J. D., & Saxe, G. N. (2004). Review of child and adolescent refugee mental health. *Journal of the American Academy of Child and Adolescent Psychiatry, 43*, 24–36.

Magro, K. (2007). Overcoming the trauma of war: Literacy challenges of adult learners. *Education Canada, 47*(1), 70–74.

Magro, K. (2009). Expanding conceptions of intelligence: lessons learned from refugees and newcomers to Canada. *Gifted and Talented International, 24*(1), 79–92.

Malkki, L. (2007). Commentary: The politics of trauma and asylum: Universal and their effects. *Ethos, 35*(3), 336–343.

Montgomery, E., & Foldspang, A. (2007). Discrimination, mental problems and social adaptation in young refugees. *Journal of Public Health, 18,* 156–161.

Morris, M. D., Popper, S. T., Rodwell, T. C., Brodine, S. K., & Brouwer, K. C. (2009). Health care barriers of refugees post-resettlement. *Journal of Community Health, 34,* 529–538.

Ni Raghallaigh, M., & Gilligan, R. (2010). Active survival in the lives of unaccompanied minors: Coping strategies, resilience, and the relevance of religion. *Child and Family Social Work, 15,* 226–237.

Nyers, P. (1999). Emergency or emerging identities? Refugees and transformations in world order. *Millennium: Journal of International Studies, 28*(1), 1–26.

Oxman-Martinez, J., & Hanley, J. (2005). *Health and social services for Canada's multicultural population: Challenges for equity.* Ottawa: Heritage Canada.

Patel, N., & Hodes, M. (2006). Violent deliberate self-harm amongst adolescent refugees. *European Child and Adolescent Psychiatry, 15,* 367–370.

People for Education. (2011). *Support for newcomer students. In, 2011 people for education annual report.* Toronto: People for Education.

Portes, A., & Zhou, M. (1993). The new second generation: Segmented assimilation and its variant. *The Annals of the American Academy of Political and Social Science, 530*(1), 74–96.

Portes, A., & Rumbaut, R. G. (2001). *Legacies: The story of the immigrant second generation.* Berkeley: University of California Press.

Pottie, K., Janakiram, P., Topp, P., & McCarthy, A. (2007). Prevalence of selected preventable and treatable diseases among government- assisted refugees: Implications for primary care providers. *Canadian Family Physician, 53*(11), 1928–1934.

Pumariega, A. J., Rothe, E., & Pumariega, J. B. (2005). Mental health of immigrants and refugees. *Community Mental Health Journal, 41,* 581–597.

Redwood-Campbell, L., Fowler, N., Kaczorowski, J., Molinaro, E., Robinson, S., & Howard, M. (2003). How are new refugees doing in Canada? *Canadian Journal of Public Health, 94*(5), 381–385.

Rousseau, C., Drapeau, A., & Platt, R. (2004). Family environment and emotional and behavioural symptoms in adolescent Cambodian refugees: Influence of time, gender, and acculturation. *Medicine, Conflict and Survival, 20,* 151–165.

Rummens, J. A., & Seat, R. (2003). Assessing the impact of the Kosovo conflict on the mental health and well-being of newcomer Serbian children and youth in the greater Toronto area. CERIS Working Paper No. 25. Toronto: Joint Centre of Excellence for Research on Immigration and Settlement.

Shakya, Y. B., Guruge, S., Hynie, M., Akbari, A., Malik, M., & Alley, S. (2010) Aspirations for higher education among newcomer refugee youth in Toronto: Expectations, challenges, and strategies. *Refuge, 27*(2), 65–78.

Simich, L., Hamilton, H., & Baya, B. K. (2006). Mental Distress, Economic Hardship and Expectations of Life in Canada among Sudanese Newcomers. *Transcultural Psychiatry, 43*(3), 419–445.

Simich, L., Wu, F., & Nerad, S. (2007). Status and health security: An exploratory study of irregular immigrants in Toronto. *Canadian Journal of Public Health, 98*(5), 369–373.

Soroor, W., & Popal, Z. (2005). *Bridging the gap: Understanding the mental health needs of Afghan youth.* Report commissioned by the Ministry of Children and Youth Services.

Vanderbilt, A. E., & Shaw, S. D. (2008). Conceptualizing and re-evaluating resilience across levels of risk, time and domains of competence. *Clinical Child and Family Psychology Review, 11,* 30–58.

Wenzel, T., Kastrup, M., & Eisenman, D. (2007). Survivors of torture: A hidden population. In P. Walker & E. Barnett (Eds.), *Immigrant medicine* (pp. 653–663). Philadelphia: Saunders.

Wilson, R. M., Murtaza, R., & Shakya, Y. B. (2010). Pre-migration and post-migration determinants of mental health for newly arrived refugees in Toronto. *Canadian Issues. Immigrant Mental Health, Summer, 2010,* 45–50.

Zembylas, M. (2010). Agamben's theory of biopower and immigrants/refugees/asylum seekers: Discourses of citzenship and the implications for cirriculum theorizing. *Journal of Curriculum Theorizing, 26*(2), 31–45.

Chapter 10
A Social Entrepreneurship Framework for Mental Health Equity: The Program Model of the Canadian Centre for Victims of Torture

Sean A. Kidd, Kwame J. McKenzie and Mulugeta Abai

Abstract Social entrepreneurs, generating unique and highly leveraged responses to major social problems, forming strong connections within communities and creating social capital, are increasingly sources of solutions to complex problems in under-resourced settings. This chapter uses a social entrepreneurship lens to examine the work of an internationally recognized organization serving victims of torture and political oppression. Key components of social entrepreneurism promote an effective response in fragmented and under-resourced health service contexts characterized by narrow, individualistic conceptualizations of mental illness and treatment. The social entrepreneurship framework can be useful in guiding individuals and services early in their development and in providing decision makers with criteria against which they can identify services to have the greatest impact on immigrant and refugee health.

Keywords Refugee · Torture · Service · Intervention · PTSD · Social entrepreneur

10.1 Mental Health Services for Immigrants and Refugees—Questions of Access and Adequacy

In contrast with the increasing recognition of the importance of addressing mental health as a public health concern there remain numerous fundamental shortcomings in the solutions generated. Specifically, while we have a better understanding of the social and economic costs of mental illness and have developed a range of effective interventions, access to adequate treatment and services remains a major problem.

S. A. Kidd (✉) · K. J. McKenzie
Department of Psychiatry and Centre for Addiction and Mental Health,
University of Toronto, Toronto, Canada
e-mail: sean.kidd@camh.net

M. Abai
Canadian Centre for Victims of Torture, Toronto, Canada

In high-income countries, fewer than half of individuals with mental illness receive adequate treatment- 41 % in the United States (Wang et al. 2005) and in many low-income countries a ratio of one psychiatrist to 1 million people is common (Saxena et al. 2007).

This problem of providing effective and accessible services to individuals struggling with mental health concerns is further compounded for newcomers. It is not a problem of heightened rates of illness, as there is every indication that immigrants do not on average suffer from poorer mental health than non-immigrants (Tiwari and Wang 2008). This is a consistent finding across many developed countries though there are some exceptions, such as indications of higher rates of psychosis among individuals of African-Caribbean descent in the UK (Cantor-Graae and Selton 2005). Where the challenge lies, in terms of the provision of adequate care to immigrant populations, is in service access. Most immigrants, particularly racialized immigrants, are not accessing mental health care when it is needed (Alegria et al. 2008; Tiwari and Wang 2008). In this area, immigrants have much in common with other marginalized groups that do not have adequate access to care (e.g., sexual and gender minorities or homeless persons). While the overall rates of mental illness for many immigrant groups is on average lower, when illness is experienced they are far less likely to receive care. It is around this issue of access that the disparities in mental health emerge, and in which the impacts of mental illness are exacerbated.

The question of the origin of this disparity in service access and the associated worsened course of illness would seem to lie both in barriers to accessing care (such as a lack of awareness of the available services; lengthy waitlists for available services; lack of health insurance; language barriers) and the lack of appropriate models of care (Wu et al. 2005). It is this latter problem in the delivery of services to immigrants that is the focus of this chapter. Specifically, we will be focusing on services for newcomers who have fled countries in which they have suffered from political oppression, violence and torture.

Fundamentally, the difficulty in developing effective mental health services and service networks for immigrants and refugees lies both in difficulty defining the problem and the associated conceptualization of solutions. The shortcoming of problem definition that is present in most western contexts is one of service systems not employing a social determinants framework (WHO 2008). Mental illness is understood as a circumscribed problem of an individual that is framed in the form of the decontextualized presence or absence of a certain number of symptoms (e.g., criteria of the Diagnostic and Statistical Manual of Mental Disorders; DSM-IV). Flowing from this definition of mental illness are treatments that are illness-focused and typically applied as individual-level interventions. Ideally, these interventions are "evidence-based", with evidence defined as demonstrated effectiveness in randomized trials which are optimized when interventions are circumscribed and amenable to being manualized. This approach is reified by siloed and poorly integrated funding streams that provide little encouragement, if not active discouragement, of the development of services or integrated systems that address the social determinants of health. From a cultural perspective, the problem of having such narrow definitions of illness and treatment is compounded by the fact that many persons immigrating to western contexts do not understand mental illness within such a framework.

A second difficulty that impedes effective efforts to address mental health disparities for immigrant and refugee groups is what appears to be a poorly coordinated approach to generating solutions. Looking to the research, it is immediately evident that there is a preponderance of research documenting risk factors and rates of illness that is greatly out of proportion with the study of the effectiveness of culturally appropriate interventions. Outcome studies are scarce and even more rare are randomized trials examining culturally grounded interventions (Aisenberg 2008; La Roche and Christopher 2009). In most Western service settings, the most common effort to address mental health equity has been the provision of "cultural competence" trainings. In these trainings providers are given general instruction regarding ways of adapting their practice to be more appropriate to the range of communities accessing their services. The problem with this strategy is that such trainings are highly variable in content and quality and there is no definitive indication that they actually impact the services received (Bhui et al. 2007).

10.2 Survivors of Torture and Political Oppression

While there is a general agreement that it is difficult to generate accurate estimates as to the number of refugees who have experienced torture, due to both variability in context and questions about rates of disclosure, it is agreed that the numbers are substantial. It is estimated that between 5 and 35 % of refugees have been tortured (Campbell 2007), with the numbers of those having experienced prolonged periods of political oppression likely much higher. It is suspected that these numbers are increasing given that the number of nations engaging in systematic torture increased from 93 in 1992 to 132 in 2004 (Amnesty International 2004). The generally agreed upon definition of torture is that of the United Nations (1987; pp. 197–198), which views torture as "... any act by which severe pain or suffering, whether physical or mental, is intentionally inflicted on a person for such purposes as obtaining from him or a third person information or a confession, punishing him for an act he committed, or intimidating or coercing him or a third person, or for any reason based on discrimination of any kind, when such pain or suffering is inflicted by or at the instigation of or with the consent or acquiescence of a public official or other person acting in an official capacity."

The long term impacts of torture are, for many, profound in physical and mental health domains with the harm carried forward from individuals, to family, community, and cultural levels of impact (Abai 2011). The most common psychological problem identified is posttraumatic stress disorder, with rates of PTSD ranging from 25–65 % of those tortured (Kinzie 2011). Rates of PTSD are predicted by the cumulative exposure to traumatizing events, the time since the traumatic circumstances took place, and the level of political terror experienced (Steel et al. 2009). While PTSD is the predominant focus of much of the torture research, many other impacts are equally if not more prevalent. Somatic problems typically emerge first, with other difficulties emerging over time including high rates of anxiety and depressive disorders and psychosis, and a range of other long term impacts such as irritability, suspiciousness, guilt, insomnia, and memory impairments (Abai and Sawicki 1997; Campbell 2007; Kinzie 2009, 2011). Furthermore, the effects of torture on an individual have been found to differ as a function of cultural background with, for example, East Asian persons more often experiencing depression (Campbell 2007). Other effects of torture, beyond the individual level, include higher rates of divorce (Gordon 2001) and higher rates of psychosomatic problems and depression among the children of torture survivors (Kira 2002). Overall, poorer outcomes are associated with prolonged displacement and better outcomes linked to permanent placement (Steel et al. 2009).

Generally speaking, torture victims and their families struggle with a broad constellation of physical and mental health concerns (Domovich et al. 1984). They face contexts of tremendous adversity escaping the countries and contexts in which torture took place and face numerous financial and legal challenges in developing safe and stable living circumstances (Gray 1998). All of these challenges are occurring, at least in Canadian and U.S. contexts, in social and legal environments that increasingly see refugees as frauds and in which there is an increasing risk of categorization as illegal, with the associated break up of families, confinement, and deportation (Macklin 2005).

10.3 Models of Care and Support for Victims of Torture: The Evidence

The challenges in developing effective service models for torture survivors are significant and complex. Treatments and services need to address more frequent and severe physical and mental illness symptoms (Domovich et al. 1984), fewer available social resources (Mollica et al. 1998), and more severe consequences associated with deportation. Just as there is little guidance in treatment literatures for all marginalized populations, literature on effective treatments for torture victims is likewise very sparse (Campbell 2007). There have been some case studies, with several completed by Basoglu and colleagues, indicating that cognitive behavioural therapy for PTSD is promising (Basoglu and Aker 1996; Basoglu 1998; Basoglu et al. 2004). There is an emphasis on multidisciplinary models of care which include attention to psychological and physical health (Campbell 2007; Fabri 2011) along with attention to legal (Germain and Velez 2011) and spiritual needs (McKinney 2011), family-level intervention (Weine et al. 2008) and involvement in political advocacy (Gray 1998).

Case studies of services for torture survivors describe services that are grounded in community participation (see McKinney 2007; Ramaliu and Thurston 2003). This includes support for micro-enterprises, self-help groups, and the use of volunteers as "culture brokers" who help refugees negotiate dominant cultures in their new environment. These elements are present in services that provide some components of traditional case management and access to medical services along with support for political advocacy activities. It has been cautioned, however, that a drift towards services in which political advocacy is the predominant or sole emphasis are less effective (Basoglu 2006).

General themes running across the torture survivor service literature involve the need to rebuild the identity of persons affected by torture, with one of the most damaging impacts of torture involving its impact upon individual and community identities (Abai 2011; Ramaliu and Thurston 2003). Interventions, grounded in attention to the social determinants of health, must help individuals and communities rebuild a sense of control and agency, rebuild the capacity for having trusting relationships, and help people move past crippling levels of fear (Basoglu 2006; Gray 1998; McKinney 2011; Winter 2011). Furthermore, there is a general agreement that to have a meaningful impact such services need to provide support for a substantial amount of time given the extent and chronicity of the problems faced (Abai and Sawicki 1997; Campbell 2007).

There are two challenges to the comprehensiveness and depth of the intervention literature as described above. First, is the much-referenced lack of randomized trials (e.g., Campbell 2007; Fabri 2011; Kinzie 2011). There is a risk, however, in this criticism in that it can tend to conflate interventions with services. These authors are correct in noting a need to extend the extensive number of controlled trials of psychotherapeutic and pharmacotherapy interventions to torture survivor populations. It is indeed not clear that existing literature generalizes to this group. The conflation problem arises, however, in that the holistic service approaches that are generally understood to be effective are not amenable to randomized trial designs. This problem is further compounded by the tremendous diversity of the clients of such organizations. What is needed, and what is the second challenge, is a framework or model that can be used to help understand how effective services for torture survivors operate. Some components of these services might be evaluated through randomized trials but many, and certainly the impacts of the services as a whole, cannot.

10.4 Social Entrepreneurship: A Promising Framework

One way of considering the attributes of non-profit organizations that have succeeded in delivering services to marginalized groups such as survivors of torture and political oppression, despite limited resources, is to use the lens of social entrepreneurship. The concept of social entrepreneurship (SE) emerged in the 1980s, growing largely out of Bill Drayton's work in identifying and supporting individuals who were effectively addressing major social problems in developing countries (Bornstein 2007). He and others sought to identify persons who had developed innovative and effective ways of unraveling highly complex systems of oppression, apathy, and dependency to mobilize communities and effect change. These were persons and services which employed highly leveraged approaches—having identified targets for intervention that might yield large systemic change.

While there is some contention as to the meaning of the SE construct, it is generally taken to be defined as individuals and groups who (i) identify and develop a solution that address unmet needs, (ii) are "relentless" in their effort to create social value, (iii) are continuously engaged in innovation and act despite adversity and resource limitations, (iv) are highly embedded in the communities and networks related to their work, (v) generate social capital and, (v) have developed sustainable and transferable solutions (Paredo and McLean 2006; Myers and Nelson 2011; Shaw and Carter 2007).

There have been several recent calls for the use of the social entrepreneur framework to address health equity (e.g., Drayton et al. 2006; Germak and Singh 2010; Savaya et al. 2008; Wei-Skillern 2010), in large part driven by its applicability to the problems underlying health inequity. Social entrepreneurs are highly effective in connecting multiple sectors and bridging siloed systems (Drayton et al. 2006; Harting et al. 2010). Such an approach is directly relevant to mental health equity which is a function of many health determinants and suffers in most contexts due to fragmented and poorly coordinated service systems. Social entrepreneurs also generate community-based solutions to problems, an approach that is relevant if not necessary to effectively addressing mental illness in many ethnocultural contexts.

10.5 The Example of the Canadian Centre for Victims of Torture

The Canadian Centre for Victims of Torture (CCVT) is an example of a service whose development and operations can be readily understood within a social entrepreneurship model. CCVT, located in Toronto, Ontario, has identified as its mission to provide comprehensive mental health, legal, medical and psychosocial support to survivors of torture and political oppression. CCVT is the second largest organization in the world that works with survivors of torture and war. CCVT has assisted approximately over 14,000 survivors from 136 countries living in Canada. For the past 34 years, CCVT has supported an average of 1,500 clients annually with their clientele including equal proportions of adult men and women and nearly one half of their clients being youth, children, and seniors.

Building from a conceptualization of the impacts of torture and political violence as being systemic, with the primarily impact being that of dissolution of bonds within family and community networks and identities, CCVT conceptualizes intervention as being one of "reconstitution." This process of reconstitution, of systems, families, networks and communities, is framed as being only possible when driven by the survivors themselves. The role of staff is to create a conducive environment where recovery can take place. It is a process within which survivors are assisted in moving from victims to active community members.

One of the central concepts of the Canadian Centre for Victims of Torture is to see itself as a community. CCVT has a paid core staff of less than fifteen, approximately fifty professionals (lawyers and medical professionals) working voluntarily, and 250 volunteers who assist in every aspect of the organization and acting as a bridge to the community at large. The conceptualization is one of this group regarding itself as a community which can provide a bridge for an individual to move from isolation to contact with others, a place in which network relationships can develop and in which families can find support in re-establishing themselves. It is also a community which is connected with other communities, both exile communities and the host community.

The care provided includes examination and treatment of abused bodies and inquiry about the experiences of torture that had been suffered. Care also extends through practical help in obtaining accommodation, social assistance payments and, at a later stage, career counselling and assistance in obtaining employment. Psychiatric assessment and treatment, counselling, psychotherapy on individual, family and group basis, child psychotherapy and art therapy are all available. Although clients nominally attend the CCVT on an appointment basis it is not uncommon for them simply to turn up or telephone to talk to whoever is available.

A deliberate attempt is made to create an atmosphere of informality so that clients can regard the CCVT less as a medical facility and more as a safe place, a place in which they can feel a sense of belonging. Some clients have contributed to CCVT by decorating, repairing furniture, providing refreshments at meetings and contributing their own personal and professional expertise to seminars and to publicizing the Centre's work through the media.

In this way, an effort is made to create a setting where survivors can experience themselves as participants making a contribution rather than as victims passively receiving services.

CCVT tries to establish opportunities for clients to establish a common ground with others in which they can experience a common personhood and humanity, and recover and build upon their sense of history and continuity. In this way the traumatic experience is not only approached slowly, but is also set within a larger story of an individual in a family, a network, and a community. The violence and torture are then events within a story, terrible events to be sure, and events which threaten to fracture the story completely, but they are not the whole story or the only story.

> We responded with ... a burning concern with social justice, political action, and the impatience and frustration against a confused world of passive bystanders. (Federico Allodi, CCVT Founder)

CCVT is fundamentally a social entrepreneurial organization. It has a clear social justice framework that assists in (i) bringing focus to their work, (ii) providing a compelling case for support for partners and stakeholders and, (iii) feeding into the a coherent narrative of meaning and agency that is much needed by people who have been tortured (Ramaliu and Thurston 2003). The organization is able to hold this approach of political involvement and activism alongside evidence based interventions such as pharmacotherapy and psychotherapy. In this manner they avoid falling into the problem of some organizations where political advocacy becomes the predominant or sole focus and lessening their overall effectiveness (Basoglu 2006).

CCVT is fundamentally embedded in the communities that it serves. It is not a model of service delivery by "providers" but, rather, facilitates networks of mutual support, volunteerism, and integration. This characteristic likewise has numerous benefits to the organization that are very salient to both the needs of its clients and the current socioeconomic context. With its contingent of volunteers serving roles ranging from culture brokers to lawyers and physicians, CCVT does not require a large operating budget relative to the services it provides. Furthermore, CCVT is closely in tune with the needs of the communities it services. This leads to a well-grounded and current understanding of the types of interventions which have a maximum degree of leverage. Finally, through its many social forums, the organization engages people in rebuilding the meaning, interpersonal bonds, and trust that are so profoundly damaged for many in contexts of torture (Basoglu 2006; Gray 1998; McKinney 2011; Winter 2011). This emphasis upon social connectedness also extends beyond the organization. CCVT has cultivated a range of partnerships with policy makers, other service organizations, and academic institutions. Through an adept strategy of building social capital around the organization, its ability to have an impact through advocacy, raise funds, and improve the access to social capital for its clients is greatly enhanced.

The final core characteristic of CCVT that aligns with those of social entrepreneurs is its focus on reflexivity and rapid implementation of programs. As a function of the degree of inclusion that CCVT facilitates for its participants, it has developed into an organization that is very sensitive to the needs of the communities it serves and responds to those needs. This has extended to their taking some risks in programming—providing services that communities ask for that radically depart from what might be considered traditional western models of care. When a community was concerned about their children struggling in school, they set up a homework program for teenagers. When Somali women were concerned for their personal safety as single mothers, they arranged self-defense classes. When Muslim clients would not come to group meetings in a Church basement which was at the time serving as the CCVT offices, they approached a local Imam who agreed to attend a meeting at the church to reassure their clients that attending the group would not compromise their commitment to their faith. In this manner CCVT has nimbly and effectively met the needs of a wide range of cultures. Furthermore, their responsiveness to their clients' needs and requests represents a striking and compelling difference from the contexts they have faced of degradation and powerlessness enacted through threats, violence, and myriad legal and bureaucratic barriers.

10.6 Conclusion

While equitable access to effective mental health services is a problem for all marginalized individuals and communities, the problem is exacerbated for survivors of torture. Along with facing the numerous stressors that form challenges and barriers for most immigrants, torture survivors, as individuals, families, and communities, struggle with many more significant and complex health concerns. These individuals, in western contexts, are then faced with systems of care that regularly confound native residents for whom English is a first language. These systems are based upon models that offer little attention to the social determinants of health that are pivotal for refugee well-being and, even when the interventions offered are evidence-based, the research upon which they are founded is questionably applicable. In turn, the literature on interventions and models of care for torture survivors is largely fragmented.

In this context, there is a need for a coherent framework into which one might place services that include evidence-based psychotherapy for PTSD, lobbying members of parliament, and homework clubs for teenagers. Social entrepreneurship is a model of understanding those addressing a broad range of major and complex social problems that is readily applicable to organizations such as CCVT. While not articulating specific interventions, it identifies core characteristics such as values grounded in social justice, innovation in generating solutions, community embeddedness and reflexivity. It can provide a tool for policy makers and service providers to better recognize and understand how effective interventions for marginalized groups develop and operate. Furthermore, as western governments increasingly align with a neo-liberal agenda of offloading social responsibility to communities, we are increasingly faced with contexts in which models for understanding community-driven solutions are desperately needed. It would be beneficial if future inquiry was undertaken to refine our understanding of how organizations such as CCVT attain their impacts. This will likely involve integrating rigorous case studies with much called for and arguably over-emphasized randomized trials of the intervention components of service organizations.

References

Abai, M., & Sawicki, L. (1997). Toward a community based approach to healing: A case study of the Canadian Centre for Victims of Torture. *Refuge, 15,* 32–33.
Aisenberg, E. (2008). Evidence-based practice in mental health care to ethnic minority communities: Has its practice fallen short of its evidence? *Social Work, 53,* 297–306.
Alegria, M., Chatterji, P., Wells, K., Cao, Z., Chen, C., Takeuchi, D., et al. (2008). Disparity in depression treatment among racial and ethnic minority populations in the United States. *Psychiatric Services, 11*(1), 264–1272.
Amnesty International. (2004) Amnesty International report, London.
Basoglu, M. (1998). Behavioral and cognitive treatment of survivors of torture. In J. Jaranson & M. Popkin (Eds.), *Caring for victims of torture* (pp. 131–148). Washington, DC: American Psychiatric Press.
Basoglu, M. (2006). Rehabilitation of traumatized refugees and survivors of torture. *British Medical Journal, 333,* 1230–1231.
Basoglu, M., & Aker, T. (1996). Cognitive-behavioral treatment of torture survivors: A case study. *Torture, 6,* 61–65.
Basoglu, M., Ekblad, S., Baarnheilm, S., & Livanou, M. (2004). Cognitive-behavioral treatment of tortured asylum seekers: A case study. *Journal of Anxiety Disorders, 18,* 357–369.
Bhui, K., Warfa, N., Edonya, P., McKenzie, K., & Bhugra, D. (2007). Cultural competence in mental health care: A review of model evaluations. *BMC Health Services Research, 7,* 15.
Bornstein, D. (2007). *How to change the world: Social entrepreneurs and the power of new ideas.* New York City: Oxford University Press.
Campbell, T. (2007). Psychological assessment, diagnosis, and treatment of torture survivors: A review. *Clinical Psychology Review, 27,* 628–641.
Cantor-Graae, E., & Selton, J. (2005). Schizophrenia and migration: A meta-analysis and review. *American Journal of Psychiatry, 162,* 12–24.

Domovich, E., Berger, P., Wawer, M., Etlin, D., & Marshall, J. (1984). Human torture: Description and sequelae of 104 cases. *Canadian Family Physician, 30,* 827–830.

Drayton, B., Brown, C., & Hillhouse, K. (2006). Integrating social entrepreneurs into the "Health for All" framework. *Bulletin of the World Health Organization, 84,* 591.

Fabri, M. (2011). Best, promising, and emerging practices in the treatment of trauma: What can we apply to our work with torture survivors? *Torture, 21,* 27–38.

Germak, A., & Singh, K. (2010). Social entrepreneurship: Changing the way social workers do business. *Administration in Social Work, 34,* 79–95

Germain, R., & Velez, L. (2011). Legal services: Best, promising, and emerging practices. *Torture, 21,* 56–60.

Gordon, M. (2001). Domestic violence in families. In E. Garrity, T. Keane, & F. Tuma (Eds.), *The mental health consequences of torture* (pp. 227–245). New York: Plenum Publishers.

Gray, G. (1998). Treatment of survivors of political torture: Administrative and clinical issues. *Journal of Ambulatory Care and Management, 21,* 39–55.

Harting, J., Kunst, A., Kwan, A., & Stronks, K. (2010). A 'health broker' role as a catalyst of change to promote health: An experiment in deprived Dutch neighbourhoods. *Health Promotion International.* Advance Access.

Kinzie J. (2009). The effects of war: A comparison of Somali and Bosnian refugee psychiatric patients. *World Association of Cultural Psychiatry's 2nd World Congress,* Norcia, Italy, 2009.

Kinzie, J. (2011). Guidelines for psychiatric care of torture survivors. *Torture, 21,* 18–26.

Kira, I. (2002). Torture assessment and treatment: The wraparound approach. *Traumatology, 8*(1), 23–51.

LaRoche, M., & Christopher, M. (2009). Changing paradigms from empirically supported treatment to evidence based practice: A cultural perspective. *Professional Psychology: Research and Practice, 40,* 396–402.

Macklin, A. (2005). Disappearing refugees: Reflections on the Canada-US safe third country agreement. *Human Rights Law Review, 36,* 365–426.

McKinney, K. (2007). Culture, power, and practice in a psychosocial program for survivors of torture and refugee trauma. *Transcultural Psychiatry, 44,* 482–503.

Mollica, R., McInnes, K., Pham, T., Smith-Fawzi, M., Murphy, E., & Lin, L. (1998). The dose–effect relationship between torture and psychiatric symptoms in Vietnamese ex-political detainees and a comparison group. *Journal of Nervous and Mental Disease, 186*(9), 543–553.

Myers, P., & Nelson, T. (2011). Considering social capital in context of social entrepreneurship. In A. Fayolle & H. Matley (Eds.) *Handbook of research on social entrepreneurship.* Cheltenham: Edward Elgar.

Paredo, A., & McLean, M. (2006). Social entrepreneurship: A critical review of the concept. *Journal of World Business, 41,* 56–65.

Ramaliu, A., & Thurston, W. (2003). Identifying best practices of community participation in providing services to refugee survivors of torture: A case description. *Journal of Immigrant Health, 5,* 165–172.

Savaya, R., Packer, P., Stange, D., & Namir, O. (2008). Social entrepreneurship: Capacity building among workers in public human service agencies. *Administration in Social Work, 32,* 65–86.

Saxena, S., Thornicroft, G., Knapp, M., & Whiteford, H. (2007). Resources for mental health: Scarcity, inequity, and inefficiency. *Lancet, 370,* 878–889.

Shaw, E., & Carter, S. (2007). Social entrepreneurship: Theoretical antecedents and empirical analysis of entrepreneurial processes and outcomes. *Journal of Small Business and Enterprise Development, 14,* 418–434.

Steel, Z., Chey, T., Silove, D., Marnane, C., Bryant, R., & Ommeren, M. (2009). Association of torture and other potentially traumatic events with mental health outcomes among populations exposed to mass conflict and displacement. *Journal of the American Medical Association, 302,* 537–549.

Tiwari, S., & Wang, J. (2008). Ethnic differences in mental health service use among White, Chinese, South Asian and South East Asian populations living in Canada. *Social Psychiatry and Psychiatric Epidemiology, 43*(2008), 866–871.

United Nations Convention Against Torture and Other Cruel, Inhuman or Degrading Treatment or Punishment. (1987). GA Res. 39/46, 39 GAOR Supplement (No. 51) at 197, U.N. Document A/39/51, opened for signature 4 February 1985, entered into force 26 June, 1987. New York: Author.

Wang, P., Lane, M., Olfson, M., Pincus, H., Wells, K., & Kessler, R. (2005). 12-Month use of mental health services in the United States. *Archives of General Psychiatry, 62,* 629–640.

Wei-Skillern, J. (2010). Networks as a type of social entrepreneurship to advance public health. *Preventing Chronic Disease, 7,* 1–5.

Weine, S., Kulauzovic, Y., Klebic, A., Besic, S., Mujagic, A., Muzurovic, J. & Rolland, J. (2008). Evaluating a multiple-family group access intervention for refugees with PTSD. *Journal of Marital and Family Therapy, 34,* 149–164.

Winter, A. (2011). Social services: Effective practices in serving survivors of torture. *Torture, 21,* 48–55.

World Health Organization. (2008). *Closing the gap in a generation: Health equity through action on the social determinants of health.* Geneva: WHO Press.

World Health Organization. (2009). *Improving health systems and services for mental health.* Geneva: WHO Press.

Wu, Z., Penning, M., & Schimmele, C. (2005). Immigrant status and unmet health care needs. *Canadian Journal of Public Health, 96,* 369–373.

Chapter 11
The Role of Settlement Agencies in Promoting Refugee Resilience

Biljana Vasilevska

> *To focus exclusively on services is to misunderstand the nature of settlement and the full influence of settlement agencies. In fact, the name—service provider organizations—is misleading and makes the mistake of assuming that what governments pay for is what agencies are.*
>
> —Burstein 2010, p. 6

Abstract How do settlement service providers promote resilience amongst refugee clients? Connections are made with people, not organizations. However, the personality of individual workers is not the primary predictor of a client's success and resilience. Settlement workers exercise varying levels of flexibility in order to meet a client's unique needs, and the degree of flexibility is a product of the agency's culture, its policies and programming options, and the professional support available to its staff. This chapter examines how individual settlement workers can support the settlement and resilience of both individual refugees and the communities that they are a part of, and how individual staff are supported by the broader settlement service provision community, including within the workplace.

Keywords Settlement · Refugee · Resilience

What are settlement agencies, which are called Service Providing Organizations (SPOs) by government funders, and Immigrant Serving Organizations (ISOs), by agencies themselves? Burstein reminds us that what an agency is contracted to do is not the totality of what an agency does. Just as the acronym differs according to perspective, there is no uniform model of what a settlement agency does or ought to do.

In Canada, settlement agencies are generally non-profit enterprises that were created in response to local needs to serve immigrants, and very few have a presence outside of the area where they were founded. The exceptions are large "multi-service" agencies, such as YM/YWCAs or Family Service Associations, whose settlement

---

B. Vasilevska (✉)
Department of Health, Aging and Society, McMaster University, Hamilton, Canada
e-mail: vasileb@mcmaster.ca

services are but one unit within a larger structure. In some cases, a large multi-service agency offers coordination or support to smaller settlement agencies, but little direct settlement programming. Settlement agencies are located in big cities, in suburbs and in rural regions; some "ethno-specific" agencies offer a wide range of services to clients who are from one region of the world, while others serve a multi-ethnic clientele. Regardless of location or client profile, their common features are a deep concern for the wellbeing and successful integration of newcomers to Canada, and a set of shared practices to help accomplish this mandate. These practices may include helping newcomers find housing, offering language classes, assisting with completing forms, orienting clients to the transit system in their new city, finding doctors and perhaps interpreting during medical visits. However, these processes are rarely as straightforward as they seem.

"Settlement worker" is a description and not necessarily a formal job title. Job titles include settlement worker, settlement counsellor, language aid, cultural broker, multi-cultural broker, settlement social service worker, and others.[1] Job descriptions vary by agency, with some workers officially only providing interpretation and translation, but generally settlement work involves providing material and emotional support to clients, and sometimes exercising critical judgement about significant life choices, such as where the client should live and how problems within the family should be handled. While settlement workers typically strive to have the client make the ultimate decision, refugees, who have had no opportunity to prepare for migration, often rely heavily on the settlement worker. One psychologist provides this (informal) job description of the settlement worker: "they have to deal with absolutely everything, from enrolling children in school to dealing with someone who is schizophrenic and decompressing in their office."

This chapter explores how settlement agencies support the resilience of recent refugees. At a fundamental level, it is the individual worker, not the agency, who works with a client, and that person must possess the necessary skills, aptitude, and local knowledge to support their clients. However, the role of the worker is always mediated by the context in which she works.

11.1 Theoretical Grounding

The focus of this chapter is on the settlement worker and the settlement agency, rather than the refugee. The role of the settlement worker is to support the first stages of building a new life, and it is assumed that refugees arrive with strengths, or personal and social resources which allowed them to survive their difficult pre-migration experiences. Any refugee who has come to Canada has already demonstrated resilience, or "the ability to forge adaptive trajectories" (Theron et al. 2011) and has shown to some degree "positive adaptation in the face of significant adversity" (Luthar et al. 2002).

---

[1] Credentialed professions, such as social workers and psychologists, can also engage in settlement work, but are usually referred to by their professional designation, leaving the "nuts and bolts" of starting a life in Canada to settlement workers within their agency.

As Pickren (this volume) explains, the concept of resilience has evolved from a focus on children and their personal attributes to a more socially contextualized understanding which examines process and change. To make sense of refugee resilience, a theory is needed that is both cross-culturally valid, and admits continued development into adulthood. Ungar (2011) suggests that there are many ambiguities in the construct of resilience, and that researchers have been challenged "to account simultaneously for the individual and the environment in the same explanatory model." Ungar argues that greater emphasis needs to be paid to ecological factors, and has articulated four principles to help do so: decentrality, complexity, atypicality and cultural relativity. He maintains that these principles are a direction that theory can move towards, and that they can be used to plan and evaluate programs and interventions. Importantly, Ungar's contribution addresses some critiques of resilience theory (see Mohaupt 2008), in particular the limits to operationalization. The study findings presented in this chapter are organized around these four principles, which are helpful for interpreting the role of the settlement worker in the settlement agency context, and in understanding how the two support refugee resilience.

Decentrality conceptually changes the focus of analysis from the individual to what the environment provides, and particularly what the environment makes available to those who face greater adversity (for example, those who are low income or unfamiliar with "the system").

Complexity involves recognizing the interconnectedness of refugees' needs and non-linearity in the process of settlement and adaptation. For example, without stable housing, stable employment is difficult to find. And of course, a newcomer who lacks knowledge of an official language of the resettlement country will have difficulty addressing housing or employment problems.

Atypicality. Atypicality addresses an over-reliance on a common dichotomous view of factors that affect resilience—whereby something is either defined as a *risk* or as a *protective* factor. For example, associating with one's ethnic community is commonly considered to be protective, and failing to do so is a risk. Atypicality re-focuses the discussion on the adaptive process and examines how environmental factors can be adaptive in some situations and maladaptive in others. Ungar writes:

… researching resilience as a process requires less focus on predetermined outcomes to judge the success of growth trajectories and more emphasis on understanding the functionality of behavior when alternative pathways to development are blocked. (Ungar 2011, p. 8)

Cultural relativity describes the belief that values and behaviour are culturally determined and that to understand what has motivated a particular behaviour, one must understand what value is ascribed to it in a person's culture. When refugees resettle in a new country, there is almost necessarily a clash of cultures—this is almost a cliché. Yet we sometimes fail to understand why some newcomers struggle in adapting to new norms, and this is because the cultural practices of the resettlement country are taken as normative. Cultural relativity in this case is not about assigning value to behaviors, but rather about recognizing that different values exist.

11.2 Two Studies about Refugee Resilience

The findings presented in this chapter come from two studies that investigated factors that promote refugee resilience during settlement in Canada, the first focusing on perspectives of settlement agencies, and the second on perspectives of refugees. As part of a Canada-wide environmental scan on support services available to refugees, data collection consisted of semi-structured interviews with 182 respondents and a review of documents produced by settlement agencies. Respondents included settlement workers, program coordinators, managers, social workers, psychologists, psychiatrists and civil servants from 40 different agencies. An additional 100 respondents participated in-depth individual and group interviews during five site visits: four sites were individual settlement agencies, and one, a five-agency consortium. In a related study with recent refugees, 32 refugees from Afghanistan, Burma, Ethiopia, and Colombia participated in in-depth interviews conducted in their first language by trained peer interviewers. Transcripts were produced for each interview, and translated in to English, when necessary, by the peer interviewers. Funding for the two studies was provided by Citizenship and Immigration Canada and by Human Resources and Skills Development Canada, respectively, and the research was conducted under the auspices of the Centre for Addiction and Mental Health and Ryerson University, Toronto

11.3 Methods

Documents, field notes and interview transcripts were analyzed to answer the question, "How do settlement agencies support refugee resilience?" where resilience is defined as "the ability to forge adaptive trajectories" (Theron et al. 2011). By using qualitative methods of constant comparison and iterative thematic analysis three primary categories of support emerged: abilities (knowledge and skills), processes, and goal-oriented movements ("adaptive trajectories"). During analysis, it became apparent that settlement workers, not agencies, serve clients, and that workers are embedded within a particular social and political context. Based on the importance that respondents attached to agency context in the interviews, further analysis focused in greater depth on the qualities of the agency environment, rather than the qualities of the individual settlement worker.

11.4 Findings

For many refugees, personal interaction with a settlement worker takes primacy over the agency or institution that employs the worker. Settlement workers, however, always view their work in relation to their agency, their profession and a government policy context. While individual-level factors such as the strength of the client-worker relationship and the worker's experience are important to both refugees and settlement workers, the discussion here highlights four contextual factors that affect how settlement workers support refugee resilience: working conditions, policies, community support, and professional support.

11.4.1 Workers, Not Agencies, Serve Clients

> When we make a referral [for a client], we make a referral to a person, not to an agency. We need to know what is going to happen. It is not written policy; it is the way everybody prefers to do business. It is, 'I know you. We have met. I have this person.' We are basically entrusting somebody's life to somebody, not to something. (Settlement program manager in Ontario)

The Personal Connection Matters

When a client approaches any support system for help—whether alone, on the advice of a friend, or via a professional referral—nothing matters as much as having another person actively engage with them, someone whom they can trust. Safe surroundings and warm decor in the waiting room; innovative and accessible programs; sound fiscal management and multiple certified staff: none of these hallmarks of "a good agency" matter as much as a welcoming interaction with a person who is genuinely interested in helping.

Many refugees either come from traditional societies where they have had little experience with formal service agencies or they have had very good reason to distrust organizations and governments in the past. Thus, the first cultural barrier to serving recent refugees needs to be overcome by making connections both personal and trustworthy. Settlement workers embody an agency's programming and give life to the rooms and corridors. The connection with the individual settlement worker determines the ultimate success of the service relationship. As two recent refugees relate:

> My story is all about taking a risk and I did not have advice from anyone except G-.[2] She was my only role model and she opened doors for me. If there were such people like her in our community, it would be great. Because when you come here if someone believes in you, keeps telling you it is possible to do things, encourages you to go ahead, regardless of all the challenges, and shows you the path to take, then eventually you will start challenging yourself.... finding a mentor was my biggest challenge. (Ethiopian Male)
> The social worker that received me was very kind. She soon discovered that I was a psychologist, and she was... my main guide, because she was the one that told me 'no, with your profession... you have a lot to offer to this country. Try to find a volunteer job in your profession... there are more possibilities in Toronto because it's a big city.' So she was the one that most opened my eyes. (Colombian Female)

---

[2] All proper names have been anonymized in this chapter.

The Worker's Experience Matters

Not only must a service provider be caring, but she needs to be experienced enough to provide personalized service. A community liaison in Vancouver explains:

> What happens with the newcomers is that everybody SHOWERS them with information. I don't. I give them specific information, and then they can come back for more information. Because I know what happens. They come in with a bunch of papers and say 'I don't know what to do, where to go!'

One reason many settlement workers can provide personalized service is because they have also been immigrants to Canada, if not necessarily refugees. The comment above, "I know what happens" expresses the worker's personal experience of settlement. Settlement agencies often hire newcomers to increase the capacity of the agency to serve its clients. Professionally trained foreign-born staff add value based on their insights and cultural knowledge. As the manager of as settlement agency in Windsor, Ontario explains, "I was a government-assisted refugee myself, so I knew what I was looking for." This agency designed an innovative program which had emotional well-being as a core element, and the program design was strongly informed by the experiences of the refugee-turned-settlement manager. As well, "ethnic matching" in settlement agencies increases service use (Wayland 2010), as the foreign-born worker is able to draw in clients and speak their language.

Being an immigrant is not a requirement for providing excellent services. Native-born settlement workers also have much to offer recent refugees, as they can serve as invaluable mentors and guides, and can provide indigenous wisdom about labour markets and other opportunities. At a minimum, they must have insights into different cultures and be open and flexible when encountering them. A program manager gives this example:

> My husband used to be a lawyer, and we were helping a Salvadorean family. I was the translator, and I warned him, 'they are going to offer us coffee and cake, and we will have to accept.' He said, 'I can't do that.' He did of course! For him that was a real, professional code that he was going to have to break.

11.4.2 Workers Operate Within a Context

While relationships develop with individual workers, the personality or skill of a worker is not the sole factor that determines how well a settlement worker can support a client's positive adaptation. The most skilled and resourceful workers operate in an agency environment that offers possibilities and constraints. Irrespective of the agency's size, its location (whether urban, suburban, or more rural), and the clients it serves (whether ethno-specific or multi-ethnic), contextual factors affect the workers ability to promote resilience. The first two factors, working conditions and policy context, were frequently discussed by study participants as constraints or hurdles; the third, community support, was seen as an opportunity, while the final factor, professional support, was discussed as both a constraint and an opportunity.

Working Conditions

The employment conditions that significantly affect settlement workers are low pay, precarious contract work, heavy case loads, and emotionally demanding work, which contribute to burnout and high turnover in some organizations.[3] The difficult working conditions were a concern voiced by almost every social worker, psychologist, coordinator and manager of settlement services who participated in the study. For example, one agency employs "multi-cultural brokers" as translators, liaisons, and general systems navigators. Two senior staff expressed great concern for their colleagues:

> **Social Worker**: It's the pressure on these brokers, ... because they are really the people that walk that middle line. They get pressure from us [at the agency] to help them get into the [ethnic] communities and help those communities.... They're always in the middle, and those brokers pay a high price for the work that they do. They don't get the funding for it, they don't get the time that they need, and we [at the agency] don't get money to build up those other leaders.
>
> **Community Development worker:** Just at a personal level, even their mental health, we forget about it. It's like this person in the middle being bombarded from all directions and there's not really enough support, ... so it can weigh down on people.
>
> **Social Worker:** That's where I find the systems clash because mainstream culture will look at that and say, "The community should take care of itself." Well, they don't understand the depth and breadth of what it takes to get the community to do that.

Settlement workers are necessary to achieve the goal of strengthening ethnic communities where the less-empowered members (usually women and youth) are actively engaged, but at a "high price" to their wellbeing. A psychologist in Vancouver reflects on the material conditions of the job and the lack of training or support in handling emotionally complicated interactions with clients:

> Settlement counsellors themselves have often come from similar circumstances as the group that they are working with. So they really need self-care skills to work with this population.... They really need to have some skills around boundaries, how to manage a population of people who have learned to be helpless, because of the situation they are in. They are not helpless people necessarily, but they have LEARNED to be helpless, EXPERIENCE themselves to be helpless, and then become reliant on the settlement worker to be the source of help. There's a big payoff professionally for being the person who can help, but there's also a huge amount of damage that can happen from being that only source of help, because they are the often only person who can speak for [the client] in that language.... They are underpaid, they are always on contract, they never know when their job is going to be cut, and they never know if ... they will have a job next year.

Additionally, many settlement workers work part-time and most professional development opportunities are available only to full-time staff.

These working conditions are often a reflection of the service agreements which settlement agencies have with their program funders. In recent years, service contracts have been shortened to as little as one year so that agencies cannot be certain of their continued receipt of funding.

---

[3] Over 80 % of the participants in the Refugee Mental Health Practices study who were agency staff were female, a proportion that the most recent complete Census data on the job category "Community and social service workers," where 78 % are female (Statistics Canada 2006).

Policy Context

> The fact that settlement organizations depend so heavily on governments for support and programming means that they are correspondingly impacted by changes in government capacity and orientation. (Burstein 2010, p. 11)

The types of settlement programs and their admission criteria affect workers' ability to support their clients, and these program constraints are often not under the direct control of the agency, but are a function of the larger economic and policy context. The settlement sector in Canada has undergone structural change within the last two decades. The current relationship between settlement agencies and their government funders is characterized by a lack of autonomy in designing and delivering programming, and heightened restraint and scrutiny in funding (Richmond and Shields 2004), resulting in funding disparities and gaps in where they are located with respect to where newcomers settle (Sadiq 2004).

The most common services are settlement assistance, job search, and English as a Second Language instruction. Going under different names in different jurisdictions, these are generally government funded and designed with different eligibility requirements resulting in variations in services offered to clients. For example, federally-funded language instruction programs are often restricted to those who have immigrant status, denying refugee claimants (asylum seekers) access to this resource. Meanwhile, provincial and municipal governments implement other restrictions. Waiting lists are another barrier to properly supporting clients. At the time of this study there was a six month waiting list for language instruction in the city of Calgary, and a home support program for mothers of pre-schoolers in Toronto had approximately 200 families on its waiting list. Popularity of programs or greater numbers of newcomers are not the only factors behind these waiting lists; in the case of Calgary, the oil boom had driven up the cost of living, and wages for ESL instructors had not kept pace, resulting in a diminished supply of qualified instructors. This is an example of how of larger economic realities and policy decisions have effects over which settlement worker and agencies have no control.

Furthermore, clients are often frustrated by the confusing system, and may feel angry when they realize that they are ineligible for some programs. Some clients ascribe this experience to a generic "Canadian way of doing business." A recent refugee from Colombia describes his encounter with bureaucracy:

> In Colombia... they are very personalized and the people that attend to you take the time to explain practically everything that you have to do, one single person; you don't need to pass by five, only one. Here in Canada, they attend to you for five seconds... and then they pass you on to the next person. So,... you are going in circles for half an hour around the whole building, ending up at another person to ask them a question that could've been answered by the first person.

Many settlement agencies would prefer to offer the seamless, personalized services described, but they face pragmatic hurdles, as explained by a program manager from Hamilton, Ontario:

> It is always better for the client when it is more of a one-stop shop, but there is always the issue of space. That is one of the issues. The other issue is English. I'd say eighty percent of all our interactions with our clients are in their first language.... you need to be able to refer to a place that has got a bank of languages and that can do this stuff.... it is a tricky business because those [refugee] groups, they change. The high-needs group of the 1980s is not the high-needs group of the 1990s or of this millennium.

Refugee clients cannot be expected to be aware of the range of available services nor how to access them. Adding further complications, their needs change over time, particularly as a consequence of political events and changes to immigration and refugee policies. Moreover, sector-wide issues, economic instability and lower government funding have resulted in many settlement agencies closing, particularly in Ontario, the largest immigrant receiving province in Canada. Agencies across Canada have been working to diversify their funding stream to be less reliant on government funding, and therefore, less susceptible to policy changes.

Community Support

No settlement service provider can be expected to provide all of the social support that a refugee needs. The goal of settlement services is to assist newcomers in integrating into the broader community, and not to create dependence. Thus, an agency's connection with outside resources also affects settlement workers' abilities. An example from a settlement provider in Windsor, Ontario provides lessons on long-term community engagement and support: Settlement workers in the agency felt overwhelmed with the number of refugee clients who required ongoing emotional support. The closest hospital-based psychiatric services were in another town, requiring a two-hour bus ride and a months-long waiting list, and very few clients required specialized hospital treatment. Feeling that local solutions were required, the agency wrote to every practicing psychologist and psychiatrist in the city, stating that their clients required therapeutic services. At first this bold request resulted in a number of clients receiving free counselling; however, long term *pro bono* services were not sustainable and it became apparent that not all clients were receiving culturally appropriate care. Ultimately, two lasting community partnerships emerged. In one case, a psychologist recognized that isolation itself was a common risk factor for refugees. She initiated a weekend expressive arts and ESL program open to all ages and ethnicities and run entirely by volunteers. The drumming, painting, drawing and sculpture activities were immensely popular with the adult and child clients, as was the fact that people of various backgrounds came together. Volunteers also benefitted, stating that they came to know people in their city that they never would have met, and that they appreciated the warm recognition from program participants when they saw one another on the streets or in a supermarket. An older man from Somalia explains how participating in the arts program helped him, and led him to befriend the Karen family (from Burma) seated near him in the program:

> ... if you stay like this [i.e. seated quietly] you become CRAZY. You have to think a lot about this and this and this and this. But when we are together with A [the organizer], we

> are very busy, laughing... After half an hour drumming, then we feel the whole day we are happy.... But you have to tell them so they learn... to make a friendship. Like this family, they are Burmese. I'm a Somali. We [live] nearby. We like each other.... I get a taxi, they come with me.... This is how people help each other.

Similarly, a community liaison worker in Vancouver explains the value of connecting refugees to services outside of the settlement agency:

> It's important to realize that a lot of people don't trust institutions. I think it's more important, for me, for newcomers to be more integrated with community and to be involved with community activities AND institutions, not just institutions, because they're not treated the same way.... Really, in everyday life.... [refugees] are just like anybody else, and I think that is helpful for them in community events.

Professional Support for Workers

Professional support is linked closely with working conditions. Challenges that settlement workers face lead to burnout and high turnover. Workers tend to rely on informal social support from their peers and occasional debriefing with social workers, psychologists and psychiatrist, for example, when they have been asked to act as an interpreter during particularly difficult interactions. In the agencies studies, informal, collegial supports were typically available, but formal professional support, such as systematic use of debriefing or training in communication skills, was not evident at any of the agencies. Where such support existed, it tended to be as part of induction into a regulated profession. Thus, social workers, psychologists and medical professionals often benefitted from mandatory case reviews and debriefings with peers and supervisors, whereas the settlement counsellors, language aids, and others with lower-paid, less secure positions often had little such formal support. A psychologist who works with survivors of torture provides her own life as an example:

> Have you heard of the expression "compassion fatigue"? That is my EVERY DAY PROBLEM. If I didn't have an almost perfect personal life—having been happily married for 37 years, having good support from my husband, I wouldn't last long here.

Professional support benefits service providers in terms of increasing their own capacity for working with refugees. In some areas, professional support systems have evolved through a Communities of Practice (CoP) model (see works of Etienne Wenger for more on this model). Those who participate in formal CoP activities, often via phone and in-person meetings, find them invaluable for bridging services across agencies and for strengthening goodwill and trust amongst colleagues. However, our research suggests that these formal CoP structures have not been implemented for front-line settlement workers. A psychologist in Vancouver explains the link with the local coordinating group in which she participates, and its benefits to clients, "I don't think you can do this work in isolation, and I think it's an incredible disservice to NOT be connected. I use [various community services] in a cooperative fashion. Any service that I can use, I use. I can't do the work without linking them."

11.5 Discussion

11.5.1 *Operationalizing Resilience in Settlement Agencies*

Resilience is understood as a process rather than a fixed quality. The individual settlement worker supports her client's changing needs over time, and she herself must constantly negotiate the conditions, constraints and opportunities within her own place of employment. Ungar's four principles help to explicate how an agency as a whole can support its workers and by extension, refugee resilience, and what policy makers should consider.

Decentrality

Considering the settlement agency as the sole point of intervention contradicts the decentrality principle. If, for example, the settlement worker's goal is to help a refugee find employment and quality housing, then both labour policies and affordable housing stocks would need to be aligned. A Community Liaison Worker in Vancouver explains,

> The waiting list for housing is two or three years. I spend most of my time writing letters of advocacy—one, two, three, four, five, you know. Especially when they are homeless... It is very difficult to have individual contact with someone in [the housing authority].

The newcomer and settlement worker are expected to negotiate problematic systems in order to solve a problem of being homeless or under-housed, yet an immigrant serving agency usually has no control over housing stocks and housing policies unless it provides housing itself. One large agency in the study owns an apartment building and provides supportive housing, defined as non-permanent, safe housing while a client tries to resolve other issues. This agency has been able to provide the "one stop shop" by having housing, therapy, language instruction, community development, and many other programs and supports under one "administrative roof." But few cities have such a comprehensive settlement agency that can take a systems approach to meeting refugees' needs.

Complexity

Workers in the settlement sector are well-versed in complexity when meeting clients' interconnected needs. One agency described its service model as "holistic, integrated practice," (HIP):

> Sometimes the psychologist will be working with a client who has some housing needs, or children's services [needs]. And if you don't address these problems, things will just spiral down, so you really have to have this holistic integrated approach in helping the whole person.

Narrowly formulated settlement goals and interventions are a violation of the complexity principle. Programming premised on discrete, unvarying program units (e.g. 10 counselling sessions, three meetings with an employment counsellor, or 500 h of ESL instruction) or uniform outcomes defined by standardized protocols do not address complex realities. Settlement agencies are loath to set such limits and often stretch services beyond what they are contracted to offer, with overload and burnout being common consequences. In short, settlement workers and agencies embrace complexity in service provision, but face challenges to doing so.

Atypicality

Atypically requires taking a radical client-centred perspective on positive adaptation. For example, instead of dropping out of school being unambiguously considered a risk factor for a refugee youth, that teenager may take pride in now being able to contribute to the household finances; he is as a result considered in a much more positive light in his community, and given responsibilities and prestige reserved for adults. Another example is a refugee who avoids associating with his cultural community; while perhaps being considered a risk factor (for isolation and loss of cultural identity), this refugee may want to learn English more quickly, or may have been marginalized within that community pre-migration (say, as a sexual or religious minority) and feels little allegiance to it. Thus, avoiding contact with people from the same ethnic community may be a positive adaptation, rather than a risk factor.

One counsellor explained how she embraced atypically and changed her practice:

> In most conventional psychotherapy you would never see a client in their home, so that's one way of going outside of the box. You'd never advocate for them; you probably won't even make them a cup of coffee. You might not see other members of the family.... Something I've learned is that... you're not just working with family, you're working with the whole community. In some conventional therapy, the focus is very much on the individual. But you realize that sometimes the best possible thing is keeping the whole family together but in a way that is supportive of everybody. So you really respect the holding structure, which is the family.... You don't try to get this person healthy at the expense of all these other people who are devastated.

One should note, however, that simply because a behaviour is adaptive in the short term, it may not continue to be positive. Perhaps one of the biggest challenges to atypicality is time: Time is required to build trust between settlement workers and their clients. This is where the experience and knowledge of the individual worker becomes an asset in meeting clients' specific needs.

Cultural Relativity

In the above example, a counsellor changed her conventional practice, acting partly on the principle of cultural relativity. An internationally trained medical professional, now employed as a cultural aid and medical translator in a refugee health clinic in Calgary, gives another example of practice informed by acknowledging different cultural values. He explains how he worked with one client from his own culture who was initially diagnosed with depression and anxiety:

If you always follow the protocol for depression or for anxiety for what questions you should ask, it doesn't work all the time, if I ask the question "what is your mood?" or "do you still enjoy some activities?" We should go for risk factors. I know my culture, in which there are risk factors that precipitate anxiety or depression. One factor is domestic violence. Through that we explored the problem of this patient's relationship [and] violence.

11.6 Conclusion

What does it mean to be a service provider? Is it just providing an apartment?... When we have, let's say, a family support worker assigned to a teenager... what they DO is they spend a couple of hours every week with the youngster. Take the youngster places. Go out to lunches. That's part of the job. So there is an interesting fine line, because that's what people need most–somebody who CARES about them that they can share those joys and sorrows with. We ALL need that.... many [refugees] became our translators. They were also trained as counsellors, so the lines very often got blurred. To me, it's very important that people DO care about the refugees. (Service Manager in British Columbia)

The fostering of refugee resilience happens at multiple levels, including for the individual client, the family, and the community, as well as for the settlement worker who may need ongoing support in working with clients who have complex needs. Settlement workers are well-situated to provide individual support and to support refugee communities in becoming resilient. However it is important not to focus only on the individual worker and how her personality or unique skills support resilience. The context of her workplace and the professional and community resources which she can access are fundamental to her own wellbeing and to her ability to support her clients.

References

Burstein, M. (2010). *Reconfiguring settlement and integration: A service provider strategy for innovation and results.* Canadian Immigrant Settlement Sector Alliance—l'Alliance canadienne du secteur de l'établissement des immigrant. Retrieved from integration-net.ca:81/infocentre/2010/007_2.pdf.
Luthar, S. S., Cicchetti, D., & Becker, B. (2002). The construct of resilience: A critical evaluation and guidelines for future for. *Child Development, 71*(3), 543–562.
Mohaupt, S. (2008). Review article: Resilience and social exclusion. *Social Policy & Society, 8*(1), 63–71.
Richmond, T., & Shields, J. (2004). NGO Restructuring: Constraints and consequences. *Canadian Review of Social Policy, 53,* 53–67.
Sadiq, K. D. (2004). The two-tier settlement system: A review of current newcomer settlement services in Canada. *CERIS Working Paper No. 34*.
Statistics Canada. (2006). Census of population, statistics Canada catalogue no. 97-559-XCB2006011 (Canada, Code01).
Theron, L., Cameron, C. A., Didkowsky, N., Lau, C., Liebenberg, L., and Ungar, M. (2011). A "Day in the Lives" of Four Resilient Youths: Cultural Roots of Resilience. *Youth & Society, 43* (3) 799–818. doi: 10.1177/0044118X11402853

Ungar, M. (2011). The social ecology of resilience: Addressing contextual and cultural ambiguity of a nascent construct. *American Journal of Orthopsychiatry, 81*(1), 1–17.
Ungar, M., Brown, M., Liebenberg, L, Othman, R., Kwong, W. M., Armstrong., et al. (2007). Unique pathways to resilience across cultures. *Adolescnce, 42,* 287–310.
Wayland, S. (2010). Integration of immigrants through local public services. *Region of Peel Immigration Discussion Paper.* Peel Human Services: Peel Region, Ontario.

Chapter 12
Mental Healthcare Policy for Refugees in Canada

Kwame J. McKenzie, Andrew Tuck and Branka Agic

Abstract Existing services do not meet the needs of refugees with physical or psychological difficulties. To promote health and to prevent the development of mental and physical illness in the refugee population there is a need for three areas of policy action: (1) Public policy that minimizes the impact of social risk factors for physical and mental illness; (2) Equitable access to a full range of health, social care and legal services that are capable of delivering appropriate and high quality care; and (3) Public bodies that organize to fulfill their duties under national and international law.

Keywords Mental health · Mental illness · Canada · Refugees · Policy development · Health equity · Social policy · Health promotion · Post-migration determinants · Barriers to care

Worldwide there are about 10 million refugees. The vast majority live in low-income countries, some in refugee camps and only a minority travel to high-income countries (Office of the United Nations High Commissioner for Refugees 2006a).

Though there has been a downward trend in the total number of refugees, the mental health impacts of migration have not decreased as there is an upward trend in the numbers of people displaced within their own countries.

Only 25,000 refugees each year come to Canada. This is about 10 % of the 250,000 immigrants that arrive annually but it makes Canada one of the top ranking destinations among high income countries for refugees (Citizenship and Immigration Canada 2011; Office of the United Nations High Commissioner for Refugees 2007).

Canada's national mental health strategy, launched in May 2012, tackles a wide range of issues and presents recommendations for change (Mental Health Commission of Canada 2012). But while the strategy recognizes the need to improve the

---

K. J. McKenzie (✉) · A. Tuck
Department of Psychiatry and Centre for Addiction and Mental Health,
University of Toronto, Toronto, Canada
e-mail: kwame.mckenzie@camh.ca

B. Agic
Health Equity Unit, Centre for Addiction and Mental Health,
Toronto, Canada

service response for immigrant and refugee populations, there is no specific guidance for refugee mental health services despite the fact that there may be differences between the needs of refugee and other immigrant groups.

Effective policy is based on evidence; a clear conceptualization of the needs of the population to be targeted and a sound logical model of how these needs can be met. So before outlining possible policy directions it is best to define the problem.

12.1 Mental Illness and Mental Health in Refugees

The mental health of refugees is rarely discussed. Using the WHO framework, mental health is a state of well-being in which an individual realizes his or her own abilities, can cope with the normal stresses of life, can work productively and is able to make a contribution to his or her community. Mental health is more than the absence of mental illness it is the foundation for individual well-being and the effective functioning of a community.

A mental illness is different. It is a pattern of thinking or behaviour which is generally associated with subjective distress or disability that occurs in an individual, and which is not a part of normal development of culture.

Mental health is about how people live and thrive in a society. It is about positive health in the widest sense. It is not about clinical encounters or diagnoses. Using the analogy of diabetes to consider the difference between mental health and illness policies and services: mental health would be analogous to having policies that make sure people are able to look after their diets and exercise to ensure they can do the things that they can do, live to a ripe old age and decrease the risk of a number of health problems including diabetes. Mental illness would be similar to policies that identify diabetes, work out the severity and use a combination of therapies to try to treat it.

Policy to promote mental health and policy to prevent mental illness are different things, though clear evidence-based strategies have been reported for both. Strategies to promote mental health may, on a population basis, decrease the rates of mental illness and may decrease individual risk, but the purpose of the strategy is to promote mental health.

Good studies which measure well-being and mental health are difficult to identify though there is work on physical and mental illness needs.

Refugees can present with complex medical needs, including infectious diseases, psychiatric disorders and complications from injuries due to trauma, including torture and violence. This complexity is in part because of the rates of illness in their countries of origin but is significantly influenced by the exposure to the social determinants of health and access to care in their new host nation.

With regards to mental illness, there is also a potential problem as health professionals may have difficulty discriminating between normal reactions to pre- and post-migration stressors and mental illness. The majority of asylum-seekers and refugees have no mental illness (Watters 2001; Summerfield 2003). They use their own resources and coping strategies to deal with the difficulties encountered in their country of origin, during migration, in their new host country and in the asylum process. They are resilient people.

The confusion comes because studies in high-income countries show that levels of psychopathology and mental illness, in particular anxiety and depression, are higher in refugee groups than in the general population (Burnett and Peel 2001). Refugees resettled in Western countries may be up to 10 times more likely to have post-traumatic stress disorder (PTSD) than age-matched general populations in those countries (Fazel et al. 2005). Other studies suggest that there may be more somatic presentation of psychological problems among asylum-seekers and refugees (Tribe 2002; Van Ommeren et al. 2002). A recent review of the rates of mental health problems in immigrant and refugee populations in Canada has reported that one of the few consistent findings is of higher rates of common mental disorders in refugee groups (Hansson et al. 2012).

Though there are higher rates of psychological problems in refugee groups it does not mean that all those presenting with what may seem to be psychological problems have a mental illness rather than a reasonable and transient reaction to the life circumstances.

There are issues of validity in transcultural epidemiology. Describing the extent of psychopathology in refugees can be problematic (Van Ommeren 2003). Many assume that PTSD will be prevalent in these groups because of the factors in their countries of origin that caused them to migrate and seek asylum elsewhere. But the diagnosis of PTSD may cause professionals to focus on pre-migration problems, potentially neglecting the effect of continuing adversities caused by asylum policies and social context. PTSD and PTSD treatments have been criticized as Western concepts that are inappropriate for refugee groups (Bracken et al. 1995; Summerfield 1999).

There is considerable evidence that post-migration problems have a significant impact on mental illness rates. A Norwegian study compared the admission diagnoses of refugee applicants with those whose applications had been accepted and were given status within the country (Iverson and Morken 2004). It found that those waiting for their hearing had much higher rates of PTSD than those who had been accepted (45 % v. 11 %). This was interpreted as reflecting the high level of stress arising from the refugee process. Further support for the importance of current social factors comes from a study of 84 male Iraqi refugees in the UK (Gorst-Unsworth and Goldenberg 1998). Although 65 % of the group had suffered systematic torture in Iraq, only 11 % met the criteria for a diagnosis of PTSD. Depression was much more common (44 %), and current poor social support was found to be a stronger predictor than past trauma. Psychological morbidity was associated with separation from children, lack of contact with political organizations in exile, and few confidants and social activities.

A meta-analysis of studies comparing the mental health problems and illnesses of refugees with that of control groups from the host countries found that refugees (including asylum-seekers and internally displaced people) had an overall increase in psychopathology (Porter and Haslam 2005). However, this increase was not an inevitable consequence of acute wartime stress. Refugees, who were older, better educated, female, and of rural residence and higher socio-economic status pre-displacement had worse mental health outcomes. Morbidity was significantly associated with post-migration factors such as a lack of permanent accommodation and restricted opportunity to work.

12.2 Understanding Refugee Adversity

Most refugee applicants to Canada are from countries in conflict. Not surprisingly, many refugees have experienced pre-migration adversities that may affect their health. The process of migration can in itself be a risk factor. Journeys can be long and hazardous, and frequently lead to separation from families and communities. However, as previously stated most refugees are resilient and it is increasingly accepted that post-migration adversities, including aspects of the asylum system, social isolation, poverty and cultural alienation can compound the impacts of the pre-migration and migration process.

The factors that have an impact on psychological health of asylum-seekers have been termed the 'seven Ds'.

Of central importance is the fact that many of these can be modified in the host country. Sensitive social policy can minimize risk factors for illnesses in refugee groups and is vital for a preventive health strategy.

12.2.1 The seven D's

Discrimination: Refugees are often stigmatized in host countries. A recent report from Office of the United Nations High Commissioner for Refugees (2006b) condemned the attitudes of the politicians and press who have turned refugees into 'victims of intolerance' and 'faceless bogeymen'. There is growing evidence that perceived discrimination carries a psychological toll (McKenzie 2003; Karlsen et al. 2005).

Detention: There is growing evidence that detention substantially worsens the health of asylum-seekers (Silove et al. 2001; Fazel and Silove 2006). In addition to the impact of detention itself, there are concerns that detainees may not always have access to satisfactory health service provision (Cutler 2005).

Dispersal: In many countries there is enforced dispersal to relieve the perceived burden of refugee groups on particular parts of the country. In such countries there may be no choice of destination and they may be moved many times. This can destabilize development of social networks as well as disrupting the continuity of any care.

Destitution: While often not allowed to work, refugee applicants in many countries receive the lowest levels of income support. In the UK, pressure from activists made the government change the amounts that were paid (Patel and Kerrigan 2004; Save the Children 2005; Lewis 2007).

Delayed decisions: The length of the refugee application process adversely affects health (Steel et al. 2006). A Dutch study reported that when the process lasts for more than 2 years it more than doubled the risk of psychiatric disorder (Laban et al. 2004). But when governments try to speed up processes they can increase the number of errors. For instance, in the UK after attempts to speed up initial decision times the success rate of appeals was one in four. In some Somali nationals and Eritrean nationals the success rate of appeal was over 50 % demonstrating that there is a need for care and considerations of equity when attempting to speed up processes (Covey 2007).

Denial of the right to work: Refugee claimants are often denied the right to work. Lack of work can inhibit social integration and increase poverty. The risk of developing a mental health problem seems to be directly linked to restrictions to work.

Denial of healthcare: In many countries there are limits to access to services for refugee applicants and those whose applications fail. This leaves those at highest risk in a precarious position. Usually there is only access to free care if it is deemed immediately necessary or life-threatening.

12.3 Barriers to Healthcare

Social factors that promote ill health and denial of health care are factors that may increase the rates of mental illness in refugee groups, but even where healthcare is available problems still arise.

This is partly because of the barriers there are to getting care.

Numerous barriers to care have been cited by research. In Canada, the most often cited impediments to equitable care are language, awareness of services, socio-economic status, discrimination, and stigma.

Most people from ethnic minority groups in need of mental health care do not get it (Lai and Chau 2007). In part, this is because mainstream mental health care may be considered inconsistent with the values, expectations, and patterns of help-seeking. Those who are more educated tend to be more likely to seek services for their mental health problems and illnesses. Refugees are no different.

Language is also an issue (Sadavoy et al. 2004, Wang 2007). Although refugees may learn English or French through language courses, many continue to speak their first language at home. This may mean that they are less fluent in discussing emotions or their health needs in Canada's official languages. Because services are often promoted in official languages, and because knowledge of pathways to care is considered part of the DNA of a community and is rarely taught, refugees may not know where to go for help.

Generally, the longer someone is in Canada and the more informed they are of an official language, the more likely they are to use health services. Though interpreter services are mandated in the court system, this is rarely the case in the health system which can mean that children or non-medical staff will act as interpreters. Where translation and interpretation services are available, clinicians are rarely taught how to use them (Hansson et al. 2010).

If people do not know where to get help, they may wait until their symptoms are more severe before they receive care. A lack of knowledge or poor information about where to get care was reported as an impediment by many different groups in Canada (SAFE 2003; Li and Browne 2000; Chen and Kazanjian 2005).

Socio-economic barriers differentially affect refugee groups in Canada because they are more likely to be poor. Low income decreases access to, and utilization of, health care services. Some of the rules surrounding this such as several provinces imposing a three-month delay after arrival into Canada to receive health insurance specifically impact immigrant groups. Other, such as the proposed changes to Canada's refugee determination system and the recent cuts to the Interim Federal Health Program (IFHP) coverage affect refugees further marginalizing already vulnerable populations (Cleveland and Rousseau 2012; Department of Psychiatry University of Toronto 2012).

Other barriers such as transportation costs disproportionately impact refugee groups because they are more likely to be poor. In addition to preventing people traveling to appointments, a lack of funds can also prevent people from purchasing necessary medications (Dyck 2004).

Various ethno-cultural groups in Canada have reported that perceived racial discrimination is a barrier to care. Institutionalized discrimination has been a way of considering structural barriers to accessing mental health care. The argument has not been that practitioners directly and actively discriminate against particular groups but that the system of care works to offer poorer access and treatment to these groups. One-size-fits-all services ignore the differential needs, presentation of problems and desires of groups and could lead to poorer outcomes (Hansson et al. 2010).

Stigma of mental illness and of mental health services is a significant barrier to care. Stigma refers to the negative perceptions people have about mental health problems and illness. Historically, people who suffer from a mental health problem or illness have been ostracized by their communities and families. Stigma can be seen in all societies. In some communities, acknowledging a mental health problem can bring significant shame not just to the individual but to the entire family (O'Mahony and Donnelly 2007; Sadavoy et al. 2004; Whitley et al. 2006). Therefore, the decision to seek treatment for a mental health problem or illness is not only a personal choice, but can be a choice that may carry social consequences for the whole family.

The first line of help-seeking is often the existing community, lay healers and religious groups. Religion and spirituality are important sources of support and help in the management of stress and mental health problems and illnesses. The next line of treatment is the family practitioner followed by possible referral to secondary care such as psychiatrists. In order for refugees to get the right care they need to be able to traverse this complex pathway of referral. This is rarely integrated as a system and relies on the knowledge and persistence of individuals, families and their care providers. There is some evidence that family practitioners find it difficult to locate culturally appropriate mental health services, (SAFE 2003) so it is not surprising that refugee populations have similar difficulty.

12.4 Improving Care

If barriers to care were minimized and pathways to care were maximized there would still be a problem of potential differences in outcomes of the care that is offered. There is no comprehensive approach to improving the quality of mental illness services for refugee populations in any province or territory of Canada. However, there have been some national policy reports that are of interest.

After the Door Has Been Opened: The report of the mental health of immigrant populations by a national task force that was established in the mid-1980s has some useful findings for refugee populations (Canadian Task Force on Mental Health 1988). It is a thorough literature review and a summary of presentations and written submissions from respondents across Canada. The Task Force concluded that, while moving from one country and culture to another inevitably entails stress, it does not necessarily have to threaten mental health. The mental health of immigrants and refugees becomes a concern primarily when additional risk factors combine with the stress of migration. One of the main issues this report describes is the fact that immigrants and refugees do not have a voice in the mental health care system either from the point of view of people living with mental health problems or illnesses, or as service providers.

The Task Force noted three principles on which improved services could be built:

1. The mental health issues affecting immigrants and refugees include both issues of cause and issues of cure. To meet the mental health needs of Canada's migrants, risk-inducing factors must be mitigated and remedial services made universally accessible.
2. The steps required to prevent and treat emotional distress in immigrants involve the persons with whom migrants come into contact as much as they do the migrants themselves. Sensitizing Canadian-born persons—immigration officers, settlement workers, teachers, neighbours and mental health personnel—to the ways in which culture can affect encounters between themselves and newcomers to this country can help eliminate major sources of distress for migrants and facilitate effective mental health care.
3. The Task Force recommendations reflect the fact that no single governmental body or level of government is or can be responsible for the mental health of Canada's immigrants and refugees. For newcomers to adapt to and integrate with Canadian society, their strengths, needs and perspectives must be taken into account by decision-making bodies at each level of government, by planners and by service providers.

The report offered 27 recommendations for Citizenship and Immigration Canada, Health Canada, and other federal bodies to improve mental health for immigrant groups. These span pre-migration orientation, support for immigrant organizations, improved educational curricula in schools to better reflect Canada's diversity, improved access to professions, improved action to help develop resilient communities, the development of culturally competent services, and improved research and dissemination of research to name but a few. However, 20 years after the report was written, only 6 of the recommendations have been implemented in full.

The Senate report: Out of the Shadows at Last took evidence on mental health services for refugee and immigrants some 17 years after After the Door has been Opened (The Standing Senate Committee on Social Affairs, Science and Technology 2006). It underlined the fact that after admission to Canada, the expectation is that the delivery of programs and services related to mental health that fall into the public health care sphere will be a responsibility of the provinces and territories.

The report called for Canada's commitment to provide safe refuge to include assurances that individuals have access to health services to help them with any mental health problems they face. It identified a role for an external body to provide oversight and assessment of how well the federal government is meeting its commitments to immigrants and refugees. It recommended that:

> the federal government establish an entity for immigrants and refugees, similar to the Correctional Investigator, the Canadian Forces Ombudsman, or the RCMP External Review Committee; That this entity be authorized to investigate individual complaints as well as systemic areas of concern related to federal provision of programs and services that have an impact on the mental wellbeing of immigrants and refugees; That this entity provide an annual report to Parliament.

Even though this is a limited proposal because it only affects health care that is the responsibility of the federal government (such as healthcare provision to the RCMP, military, federal employees, Aboriginal populations on reserve and some classes of refugees), there has been no action on this recommendation.

The reasons for a lack of action are varied but they are in part structural. Citizenship and Immigration Canada has argued that its direct role in the provision of mental health services is through the Interim Federal Health Program which was in place to cover some essential medical services (Hansson et al. 2010). The responsibility for the rest of healthcare is provincial. Although Health Canada was named in the recommendations of After the Door has been Opened, they have difficulty enforcing or contributing to healthcare provision because they are a federal body that does not actively deal with service delivery. Provincial health departments are responsible for services for refugee populations.

But the fact that health and illness of refugees is split between different bodies does not stand in the way of the development of policy and building consensus in all jurisdictions. A group of practitioners from across Canada have grouped together to publish consensus guidelines for clinical preventive care for newly arriving immigrants and refugees which includes some information on common mental disorders (Pottie et al. 2011).

Despite similarly disparate bodies at different levels and having different responsibilities the UK was able to develop a consensus for action. The Royal College of Psychiatrists UK (2007) recognized that existing services in the UK did not meet the needs of refugees and asylum-seekers with physical or psychological difficulties. It responded by producing a position statement, built on a literature review and a consensus of specialists in the field from all sectors including national departments of health, specialists in the field, immigration workers and refugee charities.

It states that:

To promote health and to prevent the development of mental and physical illness the refugee and asylum seeker population of United Kingdom require three main areas of action:

1. Public policy that minimizes the impact of social risk factors for physical and mental illness;
2. Equitable access to a full range of health, social care and legal services that are capable of delivering appropriate and high quality care; and,
3. That public bodies organize to fulfill their duties under national and international law (Royal College of Psychiatrists 2007, p. 3).

The statement proposes a number of initiatives to form the basis of service development. They include health and race impact assessments of policies that affect refugees and asylum-seekers. Early targets for such assessments will include policies on dispersal, detention and the exclusion of some groups from rights under the Children Act 2004. Training is recommended for all health and social care staff in culturally sensitive and appropriate care for refugees and asylum-seekers.

The statement advises that improved services should be designed in conjunction with refugee communities. It envisages single points of access, in existing sites such as 'one-stop shops' and National Health Service walk-in clinics, which could facilitate access to, and signpost and coordinate the use of, existing health, legal, social and voluntary services. It highlights that the full range of health and related services should be available at all times throughout the asylum process in the UK, including for those whose claims have failed.

It also states that:

> The current discourse in the media and from Government concerning refugees and asylum seekers focuses on economic migrants and does not reflect the global ethical importance of the asylum system or the situations from which refugees and asylum seekers have fled. The discourse does not focus on the strengths and positive contribution of asylum seekers and refugees to society. This leads to a stigmatization of refugees and asylum seekers which has a negative impact on their health. Public bodies should develop external relations strategies capable of delivering their duty to promote good relations between the wider public and refugees and asylum seekers (Royal College of Psychiatrists 2007, p. 10.)

12.5 Health Equity and Refugee Mental Health

Both Canadian documents and the UK consensus take a health equity lens to the existing problems.

Health equity identifies differences in health outcomes between groups that can be modified. Such action can be through initiatives to decrease the impact of the social determinants of health or through improvements in the quality and appropriateness of care services that are offered.

Given the evidence above, if services are to meet the needs of refugee groups in Canada there need to be changes at, at least, three broad level levels: pubic health, system co-ordination and content of services.

1. The research demonstrates that post-migration social factors are responsible for much of the increased rates of illness in refugee groups. A change in focus so that there is an increased emphasis on prevention and promotion, as suggested by the Mental Health Commission of Canada (2012), could decrease the rate of illness. Such changes would need a cross-ministry focus at a federal and a provincial level as changes to factors such as access to work are outside the usual remit of health services. It entails a public health approach towards mental illness where the determinants of health are the focus of decreasing both rates of mental illness and the level of mental health.
2. The systems of care that are developed in provinces and territories are important. In a rational system, specialist care for a minority population is provided by specific parts of the system, but that part of the system is properly linked to other providers to facilitate ease of access to care and to ensure that each provider meets a basic standard of offering competent care to every group. The research demonstrates that access to care is promoted by a diversity of providers offering varied treatment options. But, if this is to be recognized, there needs to be good linkages between different types of providers. Mainstream health centers, charities and community organizations need to be linked. This may be facilitated by inclusion of diverse groups in decision-making. The general aim is for improved diversity of care and illness models rather than the one size fits all strategy that is currently used. But the democratization and inclusion of communities in making decisions about health also facilitates knowledge translation, needs assessment and helps to communicate what services are available. And such work needs to include clear plans for accountability with clear metrics for assessment. An early start by healthcare systems at provincial and territorial levels could be to require health equity plans from their provider units. They could also require linguistic competency strategies and fund interpretation (Hansson et al. 2010).
3. There is also a responsibility of providers within the system. Each provider unit should have a plan of how they are to deliver competent care for the refugee groups in their area. If health equity is a quality indicator, then providers need to take some responsibility in ensuring that this quality indicator is met. Though services often consider cultural competence training as a way to deliver improvements for diverse populations, studies have not shown that this alone leads to better outcomes (Bhui et al. 2007). In part, this may be because cultural competence needs to be considered not just at an individual practitioner level but also at an organizational level. From the development of improved relationships and the building of trust with communities that will facilitate pathways to care to the array of support that individual practitioners will require—for instance access to therapists who can treat post torture patients or can use culturally adapted modalities—healthcare organizations are key to the improvement or outcomes.

These general goals are clear. They give the architecture of policy at a variety of levels needed to deliver comprehensive change for mental illness in refugee populations in Canada.

However, developing policy and a political consensus to move towards them is tricky. This is partly because there needs to be bold policy initiatives to move the situation forward, but also because there need to be bold policy initiatives to stop the situation worsening.

There is an urgent need in Canada to change the rhetoric surrounding refugees. There is a sense that the term bogus is being increasingly used when talking about refugees whose applications have failed and that a dichotomy between deserving and non-deserving refugees is being made while the discussion of global ethical imperatives and how refugees enrich community are left behind (see The Economist 2010 comments).

But perhaps the most urgent need is for health and race impact assessment of current and future policies that affect refugees. Early targets for such impact assessment could include policies that exclude some groups from basic human rights such as the right to work and an analysis of the burden of illness and economic impacts of the recent changes in the IFHP and Bill C-31 (Department of Psychiatry University of Toronto 2012).

IFHP was originally created to provide temporary health coverage to convention refugees, refugee claimants, detainees in immigration detention centres and refugee claimants whose applications had failed but were still in Canada, were unable to pay for their health care services and were not covered by provincial or private health insurance. It covered medical services, including mental health services such as consultations with a physician, hospitalization and essential medication. However, in July 2012 the federal government implemented major changes to the IFHP that reduced or eliminated health care coverage for many refugee groups, except for refugees receiving support through the Resettlement Assistance Program. The reformed IFHP restricts health care coverage to "urgent and essential health services" or conditions deemed to "pose a risk to public health or public safety", depending on the category refugees belong to. Access to mental health counselling and preventive care has been eliminated for most refugees. Medication coverage is available only for conditions posing a threat to public health or safety (e.g. psychosis). Refugees in need of a health-care service that is no longer covered through the IFHP are now expected to pay for it (Department of Psychiatry University of Toronto 2012).

Bill C-31 will increase the ability of the Minister of Citizenship and Immigration in Canada to imprison refugees. The number of detainees is set to increase. It will also add news rules to the timing of applications and appeals which will increase the stress on refugees (Cleveland and Rousseau 2012).

The general aim if we are to have evidence-based policy that promotes health equity for refugees should be to use our knowledge from the international literature, understand the seven Ds and use whatever levers we have to diminish their impact. The current fear is that, contrary to its reputation of being a refugee friendly country, recent changes in Canadian policy may harm the mental health of refugees.

Increased rhetoric about bogus and non-deserving refugees may lead to increased discrimination. New powers may increase detention. Paying for health care may increase destitution. Denial of the right to work remains. And, added to all of this some refugees will be denied healthcare.

It could be argued that because of current changes in policy Canada is going backwards in its care for refugees whereas other countries such as the UK are going forwards. Canadian scholars and practitioners have developed evidence based strategies to improve the mental health of immigrant groups (Pottie et al. 2011; Hansson et al. 2012) issues and option paper. The question is whether their aspirations will be matched by appropriate Government action.

12.6 In Conclusion

The evidence to date is that there may be different rates of mental health problems in refugee populations. This is in part due to the action of the social determinants of health in countries of origin and in the new host country. There are specific factors within the process of claiming refugee status and in the status of refugees in Canada that may increase the rate of mental health problems. There are also barriers to care that may prevent refugees from getting mental health services they need. Lastly services are not configured to meet the needs of refugee populations.

If Canada is going to meet the needs of its refugee populations then, like the UK, it needs to consider developing public policy that: minimizes the impact of social risk factors for physical and mental illness; and, offers equitable access to a full range of health, social care and legal services that are capable of delivering appropriate and high quality care. But in order for this to occur, it needs to organize so that public bodies are called to account. The Standing Senate Committee (2006) made this point—they brought it out of the shadows. But the way it may be achieved and the powers that stop progress remain in the shadows.

In some ways clinicians have shown what is possible by drawing up a consensus on the clinical preventive strategies that are useful in considering the treatment of newcomers. This is the sort of co-ordination that needs to be found at every level. At the moment, targeted care for refugee groups with mental illness is all too often a charity gesture by community groups. Though Canada has accepted refugees in need of asylum because of their circumstances, and though we know that these circumstances affect mental health, there seems to be no one accountable. Canada will not make inroads into the health care gap between refugees and other groups unless it is someone's responsibility and once this is done Canada will need to consider how it can unlock the potential of refugees by improving their mental health rather than just appropriately treating mental illness.

References

Bracken, P., Giller, J., & Summerfield, D. (1995). Psychological responses to war and atrocity: The limitations of current concepts. *Social Science and Medicine, 40,* 1073–1082.

Bhui, K., Warfa, N., Edonya, P., et al. (2007). Cultural competence in mental health care: A review of model evaluations. *BMC Health Services Research, 7,* 15. doi:10.1186/1472-6963-7-15.

Burnett, A., & Peel, M. (2001). Health needs of asylum-seekers and refugees. *BMJ, 322,* 544–546.

Canadian Task Force on Mental Health. (1988). *After the door has been opened: Mental health issues affecting immigrants and refugees in Canada.* Ottawa: Canadian Task Force on Mental Health.

Chen, A. W., & Kazanjian, A. (2005). Rate of mental health service utilization by Chinese immigrants in British Columbia. *Canadian Journal of Public Health, 96,* 49–51

Citizenship and Immigration Canada. (2011). Canada facts and figures: Immigration Overview Permanent and Temporary Residents 2010. Ottawa, Ontario. http://www.cic.gc.ca/english/resources/statistics/menu-fact.asp. Accessed 15 July 2012.

Cleveland, J., & Rousseau, C. (2012). Mental Health Impact of Detention and Temporary Status for refugee claimants under Bill C-31 CMAJ. doi:10.1503/cmaj.120282.

Covey, D. (2007). Initial decision-making is still shockingly poor. Press release, 20 November. Refugee Council http://www.refugeecouncil.org.uk/news/press/2007/november/20071120.htm.

Cutler, S. (2005). Fit to be detained? Challenging the detention of asylum-seekers and migrants with health needs. Bail for Immigration Detainees. www.biduk.org.

Department of Psychiatry University of Toronto. (2012). Position Statement on the Interim Federal health program Cuts and Bill C-31. Department of Psychiatry University of Toronto website. http://www.utpsychiatry.ca/bill-c31-uoft-psychiatry-position-statement/. Accessed 23 July 2012.

The Economist. (2010). Comments to "A smaller welcome mat". http://www.economist.com/node/17733061/comments. Accessed 23 July 2012.

Dyck, I. (2004). Immigration, place and health: South Asian women's accounts of health, illness, and everyday life. Research on Immigration and Integration in the Metropolis, No. 04–05

Fazel, M., & Silove, D. (2006). Detention of refugees. *British Medical Journal, 332,* 251–252.

Fazel, M., Wheeler, J., & Danesh, J. (2005). Prevalence of serious mental disorder in 7000 refugees resettled in western countries: A systematic review. *Lancet, 365,* 1309–1314.

Gorst-Unsworth, C., & Goldenberg, E. (1998). Psychological sequelae of torture and organized violence suffered by refugees from Iraq. Trauma-related factors compared with social factors in exile. *British Journal of Psychiatry, 172,* 90–94.

Hansson, E., Tuck, A., Lurie, S., et al. (2010). *Issues and options for improving services for immigrants refugee, ethno-cultural and refugee groups in Canada.* Calgary: Mental Health Commission of Canada.

Hansson, E., Tuck, A., Lurie, S., et al. (2012). Rates of mental illness and suicidality in Immigrant, Refugee, Ethno-cultural and racialized groups in Canada: A review of the Literature. *The Canadian Journal of Psychiatry/La Revue canadienne de psychiatrie, 57*(2), 111–121

Iverson, V. C., & Morken, G. (2004). Differences in acute psychiatric admission between asylum-seekers and refugees. *Nordic Journal of Psychiatry, 58,* 465–470.

Karlsen, S., Nazroo, J. Y., McKenzie, K., et al. (2005). Racism, psychosis and common mental disorder among ethnic minority groups in England. *Psychological Medicine, 35,* 1795–1803.

Laban, C. J., Gernaat, H. B., Komproe, I. H., et al. (2004). Impact of a long term asylum procedure on the prevalence of psychiatric disorders in Iraqi asylum-seekers in the Netherlands. *Journal of Nervous and Mental Diseases, 192,* 843–851.

Lai, D., & Chau, S. (2007). Effects of service barriers on health status of older Chinese immigrants in Canada. *Social Work, 52*(3), 261–269.

Lewis, H. (2007). *Destitution in Leeds.* New York: Joseph Rowntree Charitable Trust.

Li, H. Z., & Browne, A. J. (2000). Defining mental illness and accessing mental health services: Perspectives of Asian Canadians. *Canadian Journal of Community Mental Health, 19,* 143–159.

Mental Health Commission of Canada. (2012). *Changing directions, changing lives: The mental health strategy for Canada*. Calgary: Author.
McKenzie, K. (2003). Racism and health. *British Medical Journal, 326*, 65–66.
O'Mahony, J. M., & Donnelly, T. T. (2007). The influence of culture on immigrant women's mental health care experiences from the perspectives of health care providers. *Issues in Mental Health Nursing, 28*, 453–471.
Office of the United Nations High Commissioner for Refugees. (2006a). *State of the refugees: Human displacement in the new millennium*. Oxford: Oxford University Press.
Office of the United Nations High Commissioner for Refugees. (2006b). Refugees: victims of intolerance. Refugees, 142, issue 1. UNHCR. http://www.unhcr.org/cgi-bin/texis/vtx/publ/opendoc.pdf?tbl=PUBL&id=44508b222.
Office of the United Nations High Commissioner for Refugees. (2007). 2006 Global Trends: Refugees, Asylum-seekers, Returnees, Internally Displaced and Stateless Persons. http://www.unhcr.org/4676a71d4.html. Accessed 15 July 2012.
Patel, B., & Kerrigan, S. (2004). *Hungry and homeless*. The Refugee Council
Porter, M., & Haslam, N. (2005). Pre-displacement and post-displacement factors associated with the mental health of refugees and internally displaced persons: A meta-analysis. *JAMA: The Journal of the American Medical Association, 294*, 602–612.
Pottie, K., Greenaway, C. Feightner, J., et al. (2011). Evidence-based clinical guidelines for immigrants and refugees. *CMAJ: Canadian Medical Association Journal, 183*(12), E824–E925. doi:10.1503/cmaj.090313
Royal College of Psychiatrists. (2007). Improving services for refugees and asylum seekers: Position Statement. Royal College of Psychiatrists. http://www.rcpsych.ac.uk/docs/Refugee%20asylum%20seeker%20consensus%20final.doc.
Sadavoy, J., Meier, R., & Ong, A. Y. (2004). Barriers to access to mental health services for ethnic seniors: The Toronto study. *Canadian Journal of Psychiatry, 49*, 192–199.
Save the Children. (2005). *No Place for a Child*. STC.
Silove, D., Steel, Z., & Mollica, R. (2001). Refugees—detention of asylum-seekers: Assault on health, human rights, and social development. *Lancet, 357*, 1436–1437.
Steel, Z., Silove, D., Brooks, R., et al. (2006). Impact of immigration detention and temporary protection on the mental health of refugees. *British Journal of Psychiatry, 188*, 58–64.
Summerfield, D. (1999). A critique of seven assumptions behind psychological trauma programmes in war-affected areas. *Social Science and Medicine, 48*, 1449–1462.
Summerfield, D. (2003). Mental health of refugees. *British Journal of Psychiatry, 183*, 459–460.
The Sabawoon Afghan Family Education (SAFE) and Counselling Centre. (2003). *Exploring the mental health needs of Afghans in Toronto*. CERIS, Spring issue.
The Standing Senate Committee on Social Affairs, Science and Technology. (2006). *Out of the shadows at last*. Ottawa: The Standing Senate Committee on Social Affairs, Science and Technology.
Tribe, R. (2002). Mental health of refugees and asylum-seekers. *Advances in Psychiatric Treatment, 8*, 240–247.
Van Ommeren, M. (2003). Validity issues in transcultural epidemiology. *British Journal of Psychiatry, 182*, 376–378.
Van Ommeren, M. S., Sharma G. K., et al. (2002). The relationship between somatic and PTSD symptoms among Bhutanese refugee torture survivors: Examination of comorbidity with anxiety and depression. *Journal of Traumatic Stress, 15*, 415–421.
Wang, L. (2007). *Ethnicity, spatial equity, and utilization of primary care physicians: A case study of Mainland Chinese immigrants in the Toronto CMA*. CERIS—Metropolis Centre.
Watters C (2001). Emerging paradigms in the mental health care of refugees. *Social Science & Medicine, 52*, 1709–1718.
Whitley, R., Kirmayer, L. J., & Groleau, D. (2006). Understanding immigrants' reluctance to use mental health services: A qualitative study from Montréal. *Canadian Journal of Psychiatry, 51*, 205–209.

Chapter 13
Supporting Human Trafficking Survivor Resiliency through Comprehensive Case Management

Lauren Pesso

Abstract Human trafficking, often referred to as modern-day slavery, entails the exploitation of a person for commercial sex or labor through methods that include force, fraud or coercion. Many of those human trafficking survivors who are identified have experienced significant physical, sexual, emotional, social or economic abuse at the hands of their traffickers. Professionals who work with those most vulnerable to trafficking—including refugees and internally displaced persons (IDPs), migrant workers, runaway and homeless youth, and survivors of intimate partner violence and child abuse—must be prepared to assist. Drawing on recent literature and case examples from a social service and advocacy organization that has served survivors of both sex and labor trafficking for over a decade, this chapter reviews common psychosocial needs of human trafficking survivors, factors that foster survivor resiliency, and policy and practice implications for working with this population.

Keywords Human trafficking · Modern-day slavery · Case management · Trauma

13.1 Introduction

A Latin American migrant worker in the United States is forced to pay off an ever-increasing debt to his employers and is threatened with physical harm, arrest and deportation if he speaks out. After the devastating earthquake in Haiti, a young Haitian woman is invited to live in the U.S. with family members, but once she arrives she is forced to perform housework and care for the family's children without compensation. A teenage U.S. citizen develops a romantic relationship with an older man who eventually persuades her to have sex with strangers for money. A South Asian woman working in the home of a diplomat is made to work 16-hour days for little to no pay. A group of women from Western Europe respond to an Internet advertisement seeking au pairs; when they arrive in the U.S., their passports are taken and they are forbidden from leaving the families they are assigned to.

L. Pesso (✉)
My Sisters' Place, New York, USA
e-mail: lpesso@mspny.org

Each of these scenarios is an example of human trafficking, often referred to as modern-day slavery. Refugees, internally displaced persons (IDPs), migrant workers and others among society's most vulnerable groups are among those at greatest risk for being trafficked. Though the specifics of each survivor's story will be different, many will experience trauma- and/or displacement-related stressors either before, during or upon exiting the trafficking situation, and most can benefit from some level of assistance in meeting their physical, psychosocial and other critical needs. As awareness of human trafficking increases, dedicated funding and programs have been established to help identify and assist survivors, and it is becoming more likely that those professionals (herein referred to as "service providers") who serve individuals at risk for human trafficking will at some point encounter a victim.[1] Yet many trafficking victims remain "hidden in plain sight"—either undetected or underserved—because service providers do not know what to look for, or because those services that are offered are not appropriately tailored to the survivor's rights and needs. Drawing on the author's experience working with trafficking survivors at My Sisters' Place, a New York-based domestic violence and human trafficking services agency, this chapter will discuss how comprehensive case management services that recognize trauma and displacement as common elements of a survivor's experience can help to enhance and support survivor resilience and wellbeing.

13.2 What is Human Trafficking?

While hardly a new phenomenon, human trafficking has garnered increasing attention in recent years due to advances in anti-trafficking legislation and advocacy efforts, and several definitions have been adopted globally. One of the most comprehensive definitions can be found in the United Nations *Protocol to Prevent, Suppress, and Punish Trafficking in Persons, Especially Women and Children* (also referred to as the "Palermo Protocol"), which defines human trafficking as:

> ...the recruitment, transportation, transfer, harbouring or receipt of persons, by means of the threat or use of force or other forms of coercion, of abduction, of fraud, of deception, of the abuse of power or of a position of vulnerability or of the giving or receiving of payments or benefits to achieve the consent of a person having control over another person, for the purpose of exploitation (UN General Assembly 2000, Article 3, paragraph (a)).

The Trafficking Victims Protection Act (TVPA), Federal legislation passed by U.S. Congress in 2000, goes further to delineate two forms of human trafficking: *sex trafficking*, "in which a commercial sex act is induced by force, fraud, or coercion, or in which the person induced to perform such an act has not attained 18 years of age," and *labor trafficking*, which involves the "recruitment, harboring, transportation, provision, or obtaining of a person for labor or services through the use of force, fraud, or coercion for the purpose of subjection to involuntary servitude, peonage, debt bondage, or slavery." At the crux of these and most other definitions

---

[1] The terms survivor and victim will be used interchangeably throughout this chapter.

of human trafficking is the confluence of three factors: (1) *the act* (i.e., the recruitment, transportation, transfer, harboring or receipt of a person); (2) *the means* (e.g., causing or threatening serious harm, physical restraint, debt bondage, abuse of the legal process, withholding documents, etc.); and, (3) *the purpose* (i.e., exploiting a person for commercial sex or labor) (UNHCR 2008).

Estimates of the prevalence of human trafficking vary widely, and accurate figures at the global, national and local levels have been difficult to obtain. This is likely due to a number of factors, including that the phenomenon remains largely underground, and that methodological and definitional problems exist for the field (for instance, some researchers and demographers focus only on those trafficked for sexual exploitation, while others focus only on those trafficked across national borders) (Yakushko 2009). Different reports have suggested figures from 2.45 million (Belser et al. 2005) to 27 million victims of trafficking worldwide (U.S. Department of State 2007), though many agree that human trafficking appears to be on the rise globally (Yakushko 2009).

Among the major forms of human trafficking seen throughout the world include forced labor of adults or children, sex trafficking of adults or children, bonded labor, debt bondage among migrant workers, involuntary domestic servitude, and child soldiers (U.S. Department of State 2011). Although the term "trafficking" suggests cross-border movement, such movement is not a requirement for human trafficking. Indeed, a number of the cases that the author has worked on involved survivors who were trafficked within their own countries, cities or neighborhoods. Though transportation or migration across national borders are often present in trafficking cases, an act constitutes human trafficking simply if someone forces, defrauds or coerces another person into commercial sex and/or labor.

13.3 Who Are the Victims of Human Trafficking?

While precise global figures have been difficult to obtain, data from known, reported cases suggest that trafficking victims represent a wide spectrum of society. Identified victims have come from all over the world, from both wealthy and poor countries. They are male, female and transgender, children and adults, representing a range of socioeconomic backgrounds. Yet while anyone *can* become a victim of human trafficking, some populations are at higher risk due to factors that make them more vulnerable to exploitation. Women, for instance, have represented the overwhelming number of reported victims of both sex and labor trafficking (Goodman 2011). Other vulnerable populations include refugees and IDPs; immigrants and migrant workers; victims of intimate partner, sexual and child abuse; runaway and homeless youth; victims of political violence; the chronically unemployed or underemployed; and those displaced or affected by conflict and disasters. Similarly, though any industry can employ trafficked persons, certain industries are more commonly associated with trafficking given their underground nature and/or propensity to attract society's most vulnerable. These include prostitution, pornography, erotic massage, exotic dancing, domestic servitude, sweatshops and factories, hospitality services (e.g., restaurants, bars, hotels), hair and nail salons, construction and landscaping, agriculture, and peddling/begging (Polaris Project 2010; Project REACH 2005).

13.4 Why Address Human Trafficking in the Context of Refugee Mental Health?

Just as socioeconomic and political factors force refugees into migration, factors including globalization, poverty, abuse, restrictive gender norms, and limited viable economic opportunities serve to "push" men, women and children to leave their homes in search of prospects elsewhere. Some of these individuals fall prey to traffickers and are subjected to relocation, violence, persecution, torture and separation from social supports in ways similar to refugees. Among those trafficking victims who are able to escape a trafficking situation, many encounter difficulties returning to their country or home of origin, due to factors such as shame, or fear of retribution by their traffickers. For this reason, the United Nations High Commissioner on Refugees (UNHCR) has acknowledged a "responsibility to ensure that individuals who have been trafficked and who have a well-founded fear of persecution if returned to their country of origin are recognized as refugees and afforded international protection" (UNHCR 2008, pp. 11–12). In the United States, for example, undocumented trafficking victims who were trafficked across international borders and who agree to cooperate with law enforcement in an investigation of the trafficking case may be eligible for the same benefits as refugees.

Moreover, just as refugees and migrants are often subjected to human rights abuses either prior to or during the migration and asylum-seeking processes (OHCHR 1993), human rights considerations are relevant to understanding trafficking survivors' experiences before, during and after they have been trafficked. Regardless of the form that human trafficking takes, global factors including race, class, gender, sexuality, nationality, disability, culture and age leave certain individuals in a society more susceptible to poverty, abuse, disadvantage and discrimination, and as such play a role in determining who may be most vulnerable to traffickers. Once in a trafficking situation, victims may be subjected to a range of human rights violations including slavery; torture; forced labor; cruel, inhuman and degrading treatment; and denial of the rights to self-determination, freedom of movement, and just and favorable work conditions. Those trafficking survivors who manage to escape a trafficking situation may also be denied human rights as a result of the treatment they receive once they leave. Consider, for example, a law enforcement official who seeks to restrict a survivor's movement in support of a criminal investigation, or a service provider who denies a survivor the right to choose whether, when or how to receive particular services. The rich body of knowledge in support of the rights of refugees can be adapted when working with human trafficking survivors.

Finally, the specific mental health and psychosocial needs of trafficking survivors often resemble those of refugees. Though there are some key differences that will be discussed later in the chapter, like many refugees, many trafficking survivors experience physical, sexual or emotional violence as a result of being trafficked, and many also experience displacement either as a result of being trafficked, or once they are "rescued" from a trafficking situation (an example of the latter includes victims who, connected to a city or country only through their trafficker, are rescued by law enforcement and sent alone to a shelter in another area). These experiences are often traumatic events in the lives of refugees and trafficking survivors alike—experiences which Herman (1997) suggests serve to "overwhelm the ordinary systems of care that give people a sense of control, connection, and meaning" (p. 33). Help regaining these elements in survivors' lives can be among the most valuable assistance that service providers can offer. As the field of psychosocial support for trafficking survivors remains in the early stages of development, service providers can learn much from the existing body of knowledge on helping refugees and migrants reestablish control, connection and meaning in their lives.

13.5 How Are Human Trafficking Survivors Identified?

Service providers may encounter a human trafficking survivor in a number of ways. In developed country settings such as the United States, survivors are often identified by local or federal law enforcement officials, who may conduct a formal raid of the worksite where labor or sex trafficking is believed to be taking place (e.g., a factory, farm, brothel or nightclub), or may encounter trafficking victims while investigating other crimes, such as domestic violence, sexual assault, narcotics, gambling, pornography, prostitution, labor or immigration-related offenses. If a law enforcement official who encounters potential victims is not sensitized and trained to identify human trafficking, these victims often become ensnared in the criminal justice system—arrested, for instance, on prostitution-related crimes, or placed in deportation proceedings. If the law enforcement official *has been* properly trained, and if appropriate services are available, that official may refer the identified survivor to a service provider to assist with social, psychological, medical, legal or other services.

Human trafficking survivors might also refer or present themselves for services directly—they may have escaped a trafficking situation on their own, or have been assisted by another service provider, friend, neighbor or "good Samaritan" who refers them to services. Once the staff at My Sisters' Place were trained on the dynamics of human trafficking, for instance, they began to identify survivors of sex and labor trafficking among the domestic violence clients with whom they worked (even if the clients themselves did not identity as such). For example, a domestic violence agency in a nearby county referred Isabel,[2] an immigrant woman in her 20s who had recently left an abusive husband, to My Sisters' Place for domestic violence

---

[2] All names and certain details have been changed throughout this chapter to protect the confidentiality of survivors.

Table 13.1 Red flags and possible indicators of human trafficking. (Adapted from Polaris Project (2009))

Few or no personal possessions	Excessive or inappropriate security features at home or workplace
No control of financial records or identification documents	Works excessively long/unusual hours
Limited knowledge about whereabouts	Unpaid, underpaid or paid only through tips
Loss of sense of time	Multiple residences within a brief period
Numerous inconsistencies in story	Signs of trauma, fatigue, physical restraint, injuries or abuse
Controlled/restricted communication	
Limited/restricted freedom to leave working or living conditions	Excessive fearfulness of law enforcement
	Non-cooperativeness
Recruited through false promises concerning the nature and conditions of work	Minor engaged in commercial sex and/or sexual situations beyond age-specific norms

services, including emergency shelter. However, knowing what to look for, during an early assessment staff identified certain red flags that suggested there was more to her story (see Table 13.1 for a list of Red Flags and Possible Indicators of Human Trafficking). Isabel's American citizen husband, whom she had married legally in her home country, had brought her to the U.S. under false pretenses. Once she arrived, he hid her passport, refused to give her keys to their apartment, forced her to perform household chores, and eventually compelled her to have sex with strangers at a club while he received gifts in return. Identifying that she was a victim of trafficking not only gave Isabel a new way of understanding what had happened to her, but also granted her access to certain financial benefits and legal remedies she would otherwise not have been eligible for.

13.6 The Trafficking Experience: Mental Health and Psychosocial Implications

Though the experience of being trafficked is different for each survivor, violence, isolation, threats, intimidation and fear are often present, and the emotional effects can be significant and persistent. Some traffickers employ overt physical or sexual abuse against their victims, including physical beatings, forced sex, or deprivation of food, sleep or medical care. Other traffickers use tactics that exert power and control through non-physical methods, including psychological, emotional or economic abuse. Examples that the author has encountered include clients who have endured extreme denigration; denial of contact with family, friends or other social supports; withholding of money, identification and financial documents; and threats of physical harm, arrest and deportation. Regardless of the tactics a trafficker uses, shame, humiliation and self-blame are common victim reactions.

The physical and emotional abuses suffered at the hands of traffickers are often accompanied or exacerbated by additional stressors either during or following escape from a trafficking situation. For instance, fear of retaliation by the trafficker against the survivor or the survivor's family members may be present and well founded, and may prevent victims from reporting the crime or seeking assistance. And in some countries, including the United States, trafficking survivors may be required to cooperate with law enforcement in an investigation of their trafficker(s) in order to receive legal protection and government services, a requirement that can be frightening, stressful and confusing. For example, Maria was a trafficking victim identified by law enforcement following a raid of a brothel that was implicated in an international trafficking ring, and was referred to My Sisters' Place for shelter and other services. Maria had a child who was being taken care of by her parents in her home country, and the traffickers knew where they lived. Federal law enforcement was pressuring Maria to cooperate in an investigation of the trafficking ring, but she was terrified for the welfare of her child and parents, and ultimately decided to return to her home country, despite the potential risk to her own life, rather than cooperate and put her family at risk.

Survivors whose trafficking involved international transit may also experience displacement-related stressors similar to those experienced by refugees, including loss of social support, limited ability to communicate in the dominant language, loss of previously valued social roles, inability to work or support themselves due to lack of employment authorization, uncertainty about their socioeconomic or immigration status, difficulty accessing educational, economic and other essential resources, and difficulty managing unfamiliar and complex social and legal systems (Miller and Rasco 2004; Project REACH 2005). For instance, a South Asian labor trafficking victim with whom the author met never discussed emotional or physical abuses suffered during his trafficking experience in the restaurant industry, but he was consistently distraught over his difficulty paying rent, maintaining steady employment, and sending remittances back home, which his family expected of him, and which he felt was his duty as a father, husband and son.

The response of any individual survivor to the experience of being trafficked, and the corresponding extent of their psychosocial needs and symptoms, will depend on their individual circumstances and experiences prior to, during and following the trafficking incident(s). This includes the survivor's particular socio-biological characteristics; existing coping mechanisms; prior history of trauma, abuse or mental illness; history of family, community or national-level violence; length of time spent in the trafficking situation and relationship to the trafficker; appraisal of violence experienced (e.g., threat to life, level of self-blame); type of work he/she was required to perform; perception of his/her rights and legal status; level of social, cultural or familial isolation; and perceived or actual response of society (be it friends, acquaintances, law enforcement officials or service providers) to the disclosure of the trafficking situation (Callender and Dartnall 2011; Clawson et al. 2008).

Despite what we know anecdotally about the experience of being trafficked, formal studies on the mental health and psychosocial needs of human trafficking survivors (and on evidence-based interventions to meet these needs) remain limited (Williamson et al. 2010). To date, much of the existing literature has focused on survivors' experiences of trauma, and specifically on levels of Post-Traumatic Stress Disorder (PTSD), a diagnostic category characterized by a host of biopsychosocial symptoms including intrusive memories, nightmares, flashbacks, anxiety, fear, insomnia, hyper-alertness, sadness, hopelessness, emotional instability and reactivity, shame, guilt, self-blame or self doubt, feeling withdrawn or isolated, difficulty trusting others, identification or attachment with one's abuser/trafficker, difficulties with boundaries, poor self-care or self-harm, and somatic symptoms such as headaches, stomach aches or muscle tension. Trafficking survivors may also be susceptible to anxiety, mood, dissociative, and substance-related disorders (Clawson et al. 2008; Project REACH 2005; Williamson et al. 2010).

Though not all survivors of human trafficking will become traumatized (and fewer still will meet the formal criteria for PTSD or other mental health disorders), many that the author has encountered have exhibited some post-traumatic symptoms, and these responses to trauma are often accompanied by other critical needs, including healthcare, housing, legal and social, among others. Service providers who encounter human trafficking survivors must therefore be prepared to recognize these needs and symptoms, and to adjust the care, assistance and/or referrals provided accordingly.

Once a trafficking survivor has been identified or referred for services, assessment is the first step in ascertaining their immediate and longer-term needs (Siniscalchi and Jacob 2010). Assessment will be an ongoing and iterative process that should engage the survivor in indentifying their own needs, recognizing that many factors, including a survivor's post-traumatic symptoms, limited familiarity with local systems and limited English language capacity may make initial engagement more difficult. In the author's experience, the immediate needs of most survivors include some level of concrete assistance, including access to emergency shelter or housing; food, clothing and toiletries; interpretation or translation services; legal assistance and advocacy (particularly if they are undocumented); medical and/or dental care to address urgent issues that may have been neglected while in the trafficking situation; and transportation assistance to get to legal, medical and other necessary appointments. Given the safety issues inherent in most trafficking situations, assistance developing and implementing a safety plan is also critical. Safety plans are used to assess a survivor's current level of risk, identify actual and potential safety concerns, and develop concrete options for avoiding or reducing the threat of harm and responding if safety is compromised (NHTRC 2011). In addition, if a survivor is involved with law enforcement (e.g., they escaped the trafficking situation through law enforcement assistance, or have chosen to report the crime to the authorities), the survivor may require immediate and ongoing advocacy to help them understand the roles of various law enforcement agencies involved, and ensure that their rights are being upheld. Some survivors will choose not to collaborate with law enforcement, for many reasons that may include fear, mistrust, or a desire to simply move on with their lives. This decision should be respected, though it may limit a survivor's options for assistance. In the U.S., for instance, undocumented trafficking survivors may be eligible for trafficking-specific visas and work authorization if and only if they cooperate in an investigation. However, many survivors that the author has encountered *have* articulated a desire for "justice"—for some, this means seeing their trafficker arrested or put away in jail, while for others it means gaining access to legal immigration status or work authorization. Another important role that service providers can play both initially and as services progress is to assist survivors in articulating what "justice" means in their particular context, and to advocate for their attaining a sense of justice when possible and appropriate.

In addition to receiving help in meeting their immediate material, safety and justice needs, many survivors that the author has encountered have benefited from some form of supportive counseling to help them process what they have experienced. Depending on the particular level of distress or symptoms, formal mental health services (such as psychotherapy, psychopharmacology, cognitive behavioral therapy or other evidence-based practices) may also be beneficial.[3] However, in the author's experience, few survivors have opted to engage consistently with formal mental health services, even when services at a trauma-focused mental healthcare program were offered. There may be a variety of reasons for this. Depending on the range of mental health services available in a given location, it may be difficult to identify appropriate professionals who can provide culturally-competent services in the survivor's own language, which may make it difficult, if not impossible, for a client to remain engaged. Even if appropriate services are available, some survivors will be uncomfortable or unfamiliar with Western mental health practices, particularly if they experience shame around issues of mental illness. And, because many identified survivors will be working with at least one service provider (e.g., a social worker, case manager, attorney, etc.) before they are referred for mental health services, they may be uncomfortable being asked to share their story with yet another professional. For this reason, recognizing that disempowerment, disconnection from others and displacement-related stressors may be at the core of many survivors' distress (Herman 1997), trauma-informed case management services, described in detail below, can be an effective tool in supporting survivors' psychosocial wellbeing when formal mental health interventions are either not available, not appropriate or not desired by the survivor.

13.7 Meeting the Psychosocial and Other Service Needs of Human Trafficking Survivors

The National Association of Case Management defines *case management* as "a professional practice in which [a] service recipient is a partner, to the greatest extent possible, in assessing needs, defining desired outcomes, obtaining services, treatments, and supports, and in preventing and managing crisis" (NACM 2012). A service provider serving in a case management role helps his or her client identify and coordinate a range of service needs, often among multiple agencies or partners. Though some trafficking survivors will be able to manage their needs on their own, many survivors that the author has encountered benefit greatly from the coordination and assistance that a case manager provides, particularly if the survivor's concrete needs are made more complex by their history of trauma, violence, discrimination

---

[3] For further discussion of mental health interventions for this population, see Williamson et al. (2010) and Yakushko (2009).

and/or displacement; lack of familiarity with local legal or social structures; mistrust of authority; and/or limited English language capacity.

A *human rights-based approach* to providing case management services for trafficking survivors recognizes the underlying structural and human rights concerns affecting a survivor's predicament, and supports the realization of their rights by promoting survivor empowerment and active participation in service delivery, addressing issues of discrimination, and holding service providers accountable (IHRN 2008). Moreover, case management services are considered *trauma-informed* when the service provider understands the role that violence and victimization has played in the life of the client/survivor, and delivers services in a way that supports survivor dignity, self-determination and resilience (Clawson et al. 2008; Finkelstein 2011; Project REACH 2005). An individual need not disclose a history of human rights abuses or trauma in order to receive rights-based, trauma-informed case management services (Finkelstein 2011). In fact, victims are generally better served by service providers who focus on addressing the victims' current needs rather than on conducting fact-finding investigations into the circumstances surrounding the trafficking, a service more appropriately left to attorneys (Siniscalchi and Jacob 2010). By recognizing the *possibility* of traumatic events that may have impacted the life of the survivor, while addressing the survivor's needs as he or she defines them, a service provider can do much to bolster or re-establish a survivor's sense of safety, autonomy, trust and control. Whereas *trauma-specific* services are typically provided by specialty mental health providers, any helping professional who is trained to understand how trauma, victimization and human rights violations may have impacted an individual's current needs can effectively provide trauma-informed, human rights-based care and services.

13.8 Trauma-Informed Case Management in Practice: Case Example

My Sisters' Place has provided trauma-informed case management and supportive counseling services to survivors of sex and labor trafficking for over a decade. The organization offers a range of services to survivors directly, including emergency shelter, immigration and family legal assistance, supportive counseling and advocacy, coordination with law enforcement (if desired by the survivor), and concrete assistance including food, clothing, transportation and translation/interpretation. For other survivor needs, such as mental health services, medical and dental care, and education and job training, My Sisters' Place works closely with a network of partner organizations, many of which participate in a local Anti-Trafficking Task Force that coordinates services in the region. The case description that follows provides an example of how trauma-informed, human rights-based case management services were deployed to assist one survivor move towards safety, stability and recovery:

Twenty-year-old Grace came from a small town in Latin America. She had no history of serious trauma or abuse, but her family was poor, with limited resources to help her. Grace managed to graduate from high school, but then found that she had few opportunities for employment or advanced education. When a wealthy, older acquaintance of her family's who lived in the United States suggested she come for a visit, Grace and her family were excited about the possible opportunities this might present. The acquaintance said that she would pay for Grace's ticket, help her get a visa, offer her a place to stay until she could find one of her own, and help her enroll in school. Grace excitedly arrived on a valid visa, but soon found that the situation was not what she had expected. Her host restricted Grace's movements, refusing to let her leave the home without permission, and compelling her to perform housework and to watch the host's child for no pay. Eventually, she forced Grace to perform similar tasks for her friends, also with no compensation. She became physically and verbally abusive, and numerous times denied Grace access to medical care when she was sick. When Grace ultimately overstayed her visa, her host threatened Grace with deportation and arrest should she leave or report the situation to the police. Fearful and ashamed, Grace told no one about what was happening to her.

Grace spent nearly a year living this way, until a member of a church that Grace had attended briefly suspected something and helped her escape. Unlike many trafficking survivors that My Sisters' Place works with who need emergency shelter upon leaving the trafficking situation, Grace's connections found her a safe place to live in a new neighborhood, helped her with her rent, and connected her to an organization that provided free legal assistance. Through this organization, Grace began meeting with an immigration attorney who was able to identify elements of labor trafficking in Grace's story. As she became comfortable with her attorney, Grace began to share many intimate and difficult details of her trafficking experience, as well as challenges she was experiencing now that she was free from the trafficker. Based on non-legal needs that Grace had shared with her attorney, she was referred to My Sisters' Place for additional case management services. However, she was initially hesitant to discuss her situation with someone new.

The principles of trauma-informed, human rights-based case management were applied to help address Grace's concerns. First, although it was standard practice at My Sisters' Place to conduct an in-person consultation with a new client, her case manager recognized that fear, shame and other factors might be at play, adapting the standard practice to allow this first meeting to be held over the phone, with Grace's attorney on the line, and Grace using a pseudonym. On the call, the case manager described the services that My Sisters' Place could offer, discussed the strict confidentiality policy upheld by the organization, and provided an opportunity for Grace to share any concerns about meeting with a new service provider. The decision about whether to pursue further contact was Grace's alone, and the case manager did not seek specific details of her case. Following this initial contact, Grace soon called back to say she felt comfortable sharing her real name with the case manager, and would like to schedule an in-person meeting. Grace later reported that being allowed to pursue assistance at her own pace, and not being pushed to share more than she was comfortable with, ultimately helped her make the decision to engage further.

Initial case management sessions with Grace focused primarily on meeting her immediate and concrete needs. As an undocumented victim of human trafficking,

Grace was eligible for trafficking-specific benefits through a federal assistance program. The case manager helped Grace understand her eligibility, and supported her in making her own informed decisions about how to spend the funds she was entitled to. For Grace, this meant purchasing food, clothing, toiletries and pre-paid telephone cards to call her family, with whom she had been denied contact while living with her trafficker. Because she had also been denied medical attention, the case manager connected Grace with a local health center where she could access subsidized medical care to treat a number of ongoing and persistent conditions.

As Grace's initial needs began to be met through this case manager-client relationship, she started to share more details about her trafficking experience and about how that experience was affecting her current wellbeing. Fear of encountering her trafficker and unfamiliarity with her new neighborhood made going out and meeting people difficult, and despite reconnecting by telephone with family and some friends, she had told no one other than her attorney, case manager and one church member about what she had been through. Grace was also ambivalent about reporting the crime to law enforcement. Although she had come to understand that she was a victim of a serious crime (though she had never heard the term "human trafficking" until her attorney first mentioned it to her), she was terrified of seeing her trafficker in court, and worried about possible repercussions for the trafficker's child, whom she had cared for and felt close to, should the trafficker be arrested and jailed. Grace reported feeling depressed about being so disconnected, and shared that she was having stomach aches and difficulty sleeping, but was unsure how to address these issues.

To help Grace address her fears and regain a sense of safety, she and her case manager developed a safety plan, outlining routes she could take so as to avoid seeing the trafficker, and identifying people she could call in the unlikely event that they did run into each other (including her landlord and a fellow church member). Although Grace's undocumented status meant she was not eligible to attend most school or work programs, the case manager connected Grace with a local self-sufficiency program that focused on health and wellbeing, helping Grace become more comfortable leaving her home and meeting people in her community. Grace also shared that she experienced pleasure from attending church, listening to music, writing in her journal, and dreaming about one day starting an organization that would help disadvantaged youth. Her case manager encouraged these pursuits as a way of bolstering Grace's existing coping mechanisms, while also suggesting that Grace might benefit from meeting with a therapist at a local trauma center to address some of the symptoms she was experiencing. Grace said she was not interested in meeting with another counselor, but she and her case manager agreed to revisit the option of mental health services down the road.

After several months of working together, Grace reported to the case manager that she had begun to tell a few select friends about what had happened to her, and she was surprised to find that her friends were supportive, non-blaming, and encouraging of her to report the crime. She said that because of this support, along with the activities in which she was engaged in her community, she was starting to feel less helpless and alone. Although she still suffered from stomach aches for which her doctor could find no physical cause, her sleep has improved, and she was now considering coming forward as a victim of trafficking to the authorities. Though taking this step scared her, particularly because she was undocumented, Grace had finally stopped blaming herself for what had happened to her, and she wanted to prevent others from falling prey to her trafficker in the future. She also understood that collaborating with law enforcement could eventually lead to legal immigration status and work authorization in the U.S.,[4] and Grace was eager to start the life she had hoped for. Once she made this decision, Grace's case manager was able to help facilitate meetings with appropriate law enforcement and provide emotional support before, during and following these encounters, working closely with her attorney who helped Grace understand her rights throughout the process.

Though the final outcome for Grace remains undetermined—as with many trafficking cases, the criminal justice and immigration processes can take years to unfold, and a survivor's psychosocial and other needs will likely transform many times along the way—comprehensive case management services tailored to Grace's individual needs are helping her regain a sense of safety, trust, control and mastery that will be necessary to move beyond the fear, shame and isolation of her trafficking experience.

13.9 Conclusions and Implications for Practice

Escape or rescue from a trafficking situation is often just the first step in a survivor's recovery process. Most survivors of human trafficking face some level of physical, psychosocial and cultural needs *after* they leave. As the case example above aims to show, comprehensive case management services can be effective not only in supporting a survivors' immediate and longer-term service needs, but can help bolster resiliency, facilitate self-determination and empowerment, and assist in accessing justice, all of which are crucial for healing. Service providers of any professional background who may encounter a trafficking survivor should be trained to understand the dynamics of human trafficking, trauma and displacement. Though not a replacement for trauma-specific mental health services, a service provider who shows that they understand a survivor's needs in the context of these factors, that they will work to uphold a survivor's rights, and are willing to help meet the survivor's needs on their own terms can do much to support a survivor's psychosocial wellbeing when formal mental health services are not available, not desired, or not sufficient to meet a survivors' varied and complex needs.

---

[4] Since the passage of the Trafficking Victims Protection Act in 2000, immigrant victims of human trafficking in the United States may legalize their immigration status through a number of channels.

References

Belser, P., de Cock, M., & Mehran, F. (2005). *ILO minimum estimate of forced labour in the world*. Geneva: International Labour Organization.

Callender, T., & Dartnall, L. (2011). Briefing paper: Mental health responses for victims of sexual violence and rape in resource-poor settings. Sexual violence research initiative. http://www.svri.org/MentalHealthResponses.pdf. Accessed 3 July 2012.

Clawson, H. J., Salomon, A., & Grace, L. G. (2008). *Treating the hidden wounds: Trauma treatment and mental health recovery for victims of human trafficking*. Washington, DC: U.S. Department of Health and Human Services, Office of the Assistant Secretary for Planning and Evaluation.

Finkelstein, N. (2011). Overview of Trauma & Trauma-Informed care. Presentation at the SAMHSA pre-conference training session, 73rd annual meeting of the college on problems of drug dependence, Hollywood, FL. http://conferences.jbsinternational.com/cpdd2011/pdf/Finkelstein_Overview_of_Trauma_and_Trauma-Informed_Care.pdf. Accessed 3 July 2012.

Goodman, J. L. (2011). What we know about human trafficking: Research and resources. In J. L. Goodman & D. A. Leidholdt (Eds.), *Lawyers manual on human trafficking: Pursuing justice for victims* (pp. 1–25). New York: Supreme Court of the State of New York, Appellate Division, First Department and New York State Judicial Committee on Women in the Courts.

Herman, J. (1997). *Trauma and recovery*. New York: Basic Books.

ibid. (2009). *Potential trafficking indicators*. Washington, DC: Polaris Project.

International Human Rights Network (IHRN). (2008). Human Rights Based Approaches and EU Development Policies. http://www.ihrnetwork.org/hr-based-approaches_180.htm. Accessed 3 July 2012.

Miller, K. E., & Rasco, L. M. (2004). An ecological framework for addressing the mental health of refugee communities. In K. E. Miller & L. M. Rasco (Eds.), *The mental health of refugees: Ecological approaches to healing and adaptation* (pp. 1–64). Mahwah: Lawrence Erlbaum Associates. Publishers.

National Association of Case Management (NACM). (2012). NACM definition of case management & service coordination. http://www.yournacm.com/membership/what_cm_sc.html. Accessed 3 July 2012.

National Human Trafficking Resource Center (NHTRC). (2011). *Safety planning and prevention*. Washington, DC: Polaris Project.

Office of the High Commissioner for Human Rights (OHCHR). (1993). Fact sheet no.20, refugees and human rights. http://www.ohchr.org/EN/PublicationsResources/Pages/FactSheets.aspx. Accessed 3 July 2012.

Polaris Project (2010). Identifying victims of human trafficking. Washington, DC: Polaris Project. https://na4.salesforce.com/sfc/p/300000006E4SU9hCMUCg57NBhRw4.OiMQE27h4I = . Accessed 3 July 2012.

Project REACH (2005). *Psychological Trauma and Human Trafficking*. Brookline: Project REACH.

Siniscalchi, A. R., & Jacob, B. (2010). An effective model of case management collaboration for victims of human trafficking. *Journal of global social work practice*, 3(1). http://www.globalsocialwork.org/vol3no1/Siniscalchi.html. Accessed 3 July 2012.

Trafficking Victims Protection Act of 2000, Div. A of Pub. L. No. 106-386, § 108, as amended.

UN General Assembly. (2000). Protocol to prevent, suppress and punish trafficking in persons, especially women and children, supplementing the United Nations convention against transnational organized crime. http://www.unhcr.org/refworld/docid/4720706c0.html. Accessed 3 July 2012.

UN High Commissioner for Refugees (UNHCR). (2008). Refugee protection and human trafficking. Selected legal reference materials. http://www.unhcr.org/refworld/docid/498705862.html. Accessed 3 July 2012.

U.S. Department of State. (2007). 2007 Trafficking in persons report. http://www.state.gov/g/tip/rls/tiprpt/2007/. Accessed 3 July 2012.

U.S. Department of State. (2011). 2011 Trafficking in persons report. http://www.state.gov/g/tip/rls/tiprpt/2011/. Accessed 3 July 2012.

Williamson, E., Dutch, N. M., & Clawson, H. J. (2010). *Evidence-based mental health treatment for victims of human trafficking*. Washington, DC: HHS, Office of the Assistant Secretary for Planning and Evaluation.

Yakushko, O. (2009). Human trafficking: A review for mental health professionals. *International Journal of Advanced Counseling, 31,* 158–167.

Chapter 14
Migrant Mental Health, Law, and Detention: Impacts and Alternatives

Chelsea Davis

Abstract Asylum is granted to about 30,000 of over 75,000 refugees that arrive in the U.S. each year, and most have experienced severe trauma and possibly torture.It is the role of the state to not only protect asylum seekers with mental disabilities but to foster mental health within this vulnerable population.Numerous legal barriers to addressing refugee mental health exist because of a lack of procedural safeguards in immigration proceedings and detention centers. Various options piloted in the immigration system or modeled on the criminal justice system could help ensure due process, increase resolution of cases and good case outcomes, and create a fairer system for immigrants with mental illness, particularly programs using social workers and psychologists who work with attorneys to promote access to services.More research is needed to create a system of health services and legal protections that cultivate refugee mental health and resilience.

Keywords Asylum seekers · Mental health/illness · Trauma · Immigration justice · Immigration court · Immigration detention · Forensic psychology · Appointed counsel · Procedural safeguards · Public health · Medical associations · Medicalization

14.1 Introduction

14.1.1 Theory and Evidence

The United States has not developed an immigration justice system that simultaneously has legally binding standards for ensuring justice for refugees, asylum seekers and other migrants with mental illness and provides access to services fostering mental health for those without mental disability. The current system lacks procedural safeguards to ensure due process and care for the mentally ill. Although there is little research regarding impacts of policy on, and the needs of, this vulnerable population, some is valuable for constructing a theoretical framework and potential models

C. Davis (✉)
Mailman School of Public Health (MPH), Columbia University, New York, USA
e-mail: ms.chelsea.davis@gmail.com

for mental health in the immigration and justice systems. However, considering the culturally specific needs of refugees and complicated make up of the U.S. legal and social services system, what Watters & Ingleby (2004) call the "distinctively historically determined contexts" in which mental health services are embedded, this dearth of U.S. based research is a considerable obstacle to fostering refugee and immigrant mental health.

An underlying theoretical assumption of this analysis is that it is the state's role to remove barriers to immigrant integration (Ager 2008). Although a more supportive legal environment cannot protect against all non-legal obstacles, the law is a necessary component of integration and therefore of mental wellbeing and resilience, particularly because of the negative effects of family separation (Da Lomba 2010; Strang and Ager 2010; Carswell et al. 2011). Insecure asylum status itself is associated with a range of psychological problems; the need for high-income countries such as the United States to implement immigration, healthcare, and social policies on an individual, family, and community level is paramount (Fazel et al. 2011). In the U.S. legal system (immigration court and detention centers) broad policy change and standards can focus on stable settlement and rapid resolution, harnessing of community resources, support for intact families, and reducing post migration exposure to violence and poor mental health. The system must allow for individual assessment, necessary because there are very few broad and definite trends in refugee mental health not only cross culturally or between different traumatic events, but within cultures as well. Additionally, the prevailing cultural ethos in the U.S. sees granting asylum as an act of charity when it is in fact a legal obligation (Grove and Zwi 2006). Another underlying concept is that of therapeutic jurisprudence, the idea that the law should be used to promote the well-being of the people it influences, and this "affords one plausible remedy, which is not to detain persons with severe mental illnesses at all (Ochoa et al. 2010)." This has further implications for the detention of all refugees and asylum seekers as well.

Evidence regarding the scope of the problem of mental illness in refugee populations is variable, but it is widely acknowledged that rates of PTSD, depressive disorders, anxiety disorders, sleep disorders, exhaustion and self harm are particularly high and expressed in ways reflecting both cultural background and personal experience (Pourgourides 2006; Strijk et al. 2010). One systematic review showed rates of 9 % PTSD and 5 % major depression. A Leitner Center Report (2010) claimed 62 % of Cambodian refugees in their sample had PTSD while 51 % had major depression while 80 % of a Somali refugee population presented psychoses. In refugee children, rates for significant psychological disturbance might be as high as 25 % (Fazel and Stein 2003). One mixed methods study revealed an average asylum seeker or refugee experienced between 7 and 15 traumatic events with torture accounting for 54 %, while another qualitative study of refugees an asylum seekers from over 25 countries found the mean number of traumatic events experienced to be over 18 while 81.6 % experienced torture (Carswell et al. 2011).

Responsibility to create legally enforceable standards is increased in light of recent findings regarding the relationship between post migration problems and the psychological well being of refugees and asylum seekers. Carswell et al. (2011)

claims increased psychopathology correlates with increased post migration stress; PTSD symptoms were significantly associated with increased adaptation difficulties. Risk and resilience factors in the post migration environment might have a stronger association to psychological morbidity than pre migration trauma. Carswell describes a quantitative analysis by Laban et al. (2005) that showed moderate significance between cumulative trauma and mental health problems and associations between post migration problems and mental health problems that broadly supported the hypothesis that post migration stress is related to poorer mental health. For instance, post migration problems accounted for additional variance in PTSD symptoms when pre migration trauma had been accounted for. Tribe (2002) also found that exile related stressors may be as powerful as what contributed to the need for migration. Bhugra (2004) found complementary results suggesting pre-migration preparation as a significant factor for fostering resilience, a mechanism unavailable to most asylum seekers. For children, direct experience of adverse events was associated with increased likelihood of psychological disturbance, with some kinds of disturbance more strongly associated with post migration threats. Children who were more likely to recover had experienced fewer adverse events after displacement (Fazel et al. 2011). Post migration stressors include detention, social isolation, loss of social and occupational roles and meaningful activity, loss of resources, boredom, isolation, family separation, and discrimination (Miller 1999; Watters and Ingleby 2004). Watters & Ingleby (2004) claim the locations of care for asylum seekers should shift to the post-flight environment with the growing evidence that these stressors add to the negative psychiatric effects of previous trauma.

This chapter will focus on the state of mental health care in immigration detention and immigration court proceedings. Approximately 1,400 non criminal asylum seekers are detained daily by U.S. Immigration and Customs Enforcement (ICE), the principle investigative arm of the Department of Homeland Security responsible for immigration enforcement and detention centers. The Executive Office of Immigration Review (EOIR), part of the Department of Justice, administers immigration courts, where the lack of appointed counsel is becoming evidently problematic when an asylum seeker is four to six times more likely to be granted asylum when represented (Schoenholtz and Jacobs 2002). Legal representation can therefore indirectly confer several benefits such as promoting family unification, entitlement to work, and eligibility for social services (Meffert et al. 2010), therefore mitigating post migration stressors. EOIR has made significant efforts to address problems in these systems regarding mental illness, but none of them are legally enforceable and they do not offer specific enough guidance. Various programs piloted in the immigration system or modeled on the criminal justice system could help ensure due process for mentally ill asylum seekers if implemented in the immigration system. A systems perspective is needed for dealing with justice-mental health interaction issues while the framework of therapeutic jurisprudence could potentially inform the necessary legal structures. This chapter takes into account what Watters and Ingleby (2004) describe as the overemphasis on mental health problems of refugees and the need to focus on resilience. Similarly, Bourassa (2009) claims an unnecessary pathologizing of refugees and asylum seekers which obfuscates the resiliency of this population.

The purpose of this chapter is to identify problematic mental health impacts of the immigration justice system in the U.S. and to advocate for legal standards of care for those with mental illness. At the same time, incorporating integrated services focused on fostering resilience and mental health may improve immigrant halth without medicalizing the migratory process.

14.2 State of Mental Health Care in the Immigration System

14.2.1 Detention Centers

In the United States immigration detention centers, which are mostly privately operated, have had no legally binding medical or mental health care standards[1] (Mukhopadhyay 2009). Ochoa et al. (2010) estimates that 13.5 % of detainee deaths were suicides between 2003 and 2008, while Priest & Goldstein (2008) claim suicide has become the most common cause of death among immigrant detainees and is on the rise, accounting for 18 % of deaths. Only 4–7 % of detainees received any mental health care in detention in 2008, but confidential memos suggest that at the very least 15 % of all detainees have a mental disability, commensurate with estimates from the criminal justice system (Ochoa et al. 2010). Evidence that immigrant detainees with mental illness experience longer detention than those without is growing alongside confirmation that asylum seekers' average detention stays are several months longer than the overall average (Ochoa et al. 2010), thus making asylum seekers with mental illness a doubly burdened population in detention.[2]

Evidence from the UK shows that holding asylum seekers in detention centers separates families, forces additional relocations, separates people from mainstream communities, and increases vulnerability to further trauma and suicide (Fazel and Stein 2002). Specifically for refugee or asylum seeking children, awareness of a parent's detention was an independent predictor of PTSD in one study, and worse psychological functioning arose when children had trouble contacting a parent, a very common occurrence in detention centers (Fazel et al. 2011).

---

[1] There is a recently settled class action law suit, *Franco et al. vs. Eric Holder, et al.* (First Amended Complaint dated Aug. 2, 2010). The lawsuit asks the judge to "[o]rder the government to provide all class members with adequate competency evaluations, to provide qualifying class members with appointed counsel, and to provide qualifying class members with adequate detention hearings, and [g]rant such other relief as the Court deems just and equitable…" The class represented is "[a]ll individuals who are or will be in DHS custody for removal proceedings in California, Arizona, or Washington who have been identified… as having a serious mental disorder or defect that may render them incompetent to represent themselves in detention or removal proceedings, and who [do not have a lawyer]." (http://www.aclu.org/immigrants-rights/franco-gonzales-et-al-v-holder-et-al-first-amended-class-action-complaint).

[2] Asylum seekers are often held longer in criminal detention as their immigration status causes them to be considered a flight risk and ineligible for bail (National Immigration Forum, 2011.

A multitude of studies have found evidence pointing to the deleterious effects of detention of existing mental illness (i.e. Bracken and Gorst-Unsworth 1991; Arnold et al. 2006; Keller et al. 2003; Robjant et al. 2009). "Detention and family separation can significantly contribute to increased mental disability in refugees… these psychological effects can persist for a prolonged period of time after detention (Steele et al. 2006)." The incarceration like[3] environment of detention centers can exacerbate mental illness and result in increased resource expenditures, increased hospitalizations, and a general increased need for services (Lamb 2009). PTSD, depression, anxiety, and self harm have all been shown to worsen the longer individuals stay in detention (Texas Appleseed 2010). There have been instances of detention precipitating mental illness as a result of prolonged idleness, constant threats of violence, isolation, helplessness, and guilt compounding trauma and increasing suicidal ideation (National Commission on Correctional Health Care 1992). A systematic review showed time in detention was positively and significantly associated with symptom severity and that the impact persisted long term despite slight improvement after release (Robjant et al. 2009). Length of detention and amount of transfers also correlates to lack of access and communication, particularly for doctors, attorneys, and personal relationships (Leitner Center 2010). Fazel et al. (2011) showed more transfers and relocations resulted in more mental ill health, and in 2008, for example, over 100,000 detainees were transferred once, 100,000 twice, and over 34,000 were transferred three or more times (Texas Appleseed 2010). For those without mental illness or disability, asylum seekers in detention still feel treated like criminals, have lost family contact, and are under tremendous stress. They reported to Strijk et al. (2010) that they did not experience a sense of peace or security, but rather imprisonment; they reported needing needed more purposeful activity, job training, and language training. Thus, detention not only has a potential worsening effect on mental illness but forms a formidable barrier to resilience.

Legal representation is necessary for ensuring aylum seekers' well being. Access to counsel can also be a necessary component of ensuring procedural safeguards, particularly safe release practices and safe repatriation for asylum seekers with mental illness. Prosecutorial discretion is vital for decisions to detain asylum seekers in the first place and for assessing their eligibility for alternative to detention programs, ensuring proper mental health screening, medical record transfer, and administration of proper medication—all which result in better mental health care and lower detention costs (Texas Appleseed 2010).

14.2.2 Immigration Court

The legal standards in place for recognizing and ensuring due process for those with mental illness in immigration proceedings are informal at best resulting in serious

---

[3] The environment is often not just *incarceration like*, as about half of immigrants detained are held in jails.

injustice. For example, Jesus-Rentas et al. 2010 showed that "asylum seekers with PTSD are systematically more likely to be rejected" asylum status. There are no real mechanisms for identifying mental illness in these proceedings and a lack of formal competency evaluations. Not only is there a lack of necessary direct representation but ethical guidelines for attorneys in this context are unclear. Even if a detainee is found to be mentally ill, there are not requirements for appointing counsel. Ethical guidelines for forensic mental health specialists are also precarious despite their increasing and complex role in asylum cases.

The 2010 Human Rights Watch report details the difficulty of identifying mental illness in the courtroom because many disabilities present with a lack of obvious symptoms. Without proper procedural safeguards and records documenting mental illness, a reliance on self-identification persists despite differing conceptions of mental illness and knowledge about court practices. There is very little training for court officers and judges, who often experience stress, burnout, and even secondary transference (Lustig et al. 2008), for identifying and working with people with mental illness. Stigma associated with mental illness appears to have legal consequences which can result in prolonged detention or a general misuse of medical knowledge.

There is no model for evaluating competency in immigration proceedings, and guidelines that exist resulting from past decisions are often conflicting. The longer it takes to raise and resolve the issue of competency, the longer an immigrant will be detained and mental health will further deteriorate (Finkle et al. 2009). Lack of appointed counsel greatly complicates this issue as well. There have recently been several immigration decisions regarding the issue of competency. For example, in Jaadan v. Gonzales in 2006, the Sixth Circuit Court of Appeals ruled that an "alien involved in deportation proceedings had a right to a competency hearing only to determine whether they required representation by an attorney or guardian" and that "mental incompetence would not preclude deportation (Harlow and LeBourgeois 2007)." However, section 240(b)(3) of the Immigration and Nationality Act prohibits an immigration judge from accepting an admission of removability from an unrepresented respondent who is incompetent. In Franco-Gonzalez v. Holder, filed in 2010, U.S. district court ruled that federal officials must provide representation for two men with severe mental disabilities while they fight their deportation cases. In 2010 in Lyttle v United States, et al a U.S. citizen with bipolar disorder filed suit seeking damages resulting from wrongful deportation alleging violations of the due process clause of the Fourth Amendment and equal protection clause of the Fifth Amendment. In 2010 the Board of Immigration Appeals (BIA), given nationwide jurisdiction to hear appeals from certain decisions rendered by immigration judges and district directors of the Department of Homeland Security in a wide variety of proceedings, granted remand following the discovery of a traumatic brain injury of a legal permanent resident, and DHS withdrew an appeal of an immigration judge's decision to terminate proceedings against a mentally disabled respondent. The government also contested an immigration judge's authority to terminate proceedings in 2010 while the BIA is considering the appeal of an unrepresented respondent with mental disabilities (legalactioncenter.org). A significant recent development is the Matter of M-A-M (Texas Appleseed 2010) in which the BIA vacated an order of removal for failure to inquire whether the respondent was competent. This was an attempt to set forth a framework for competency but it falls short of providing specific guidance. There is no direction on how a court may secure a mental health examination or appoint a guardian.

According to Tsankov (2007), precedent case law and existing regulations do not provide guidance about cases when an unrepresented immigrant asserts incompetency, claims incompetency after pleading, presents evidence of incompetency, and asserts competency but presents otherwise in the eyes of the judge. Evidently a lack of counsel is a substantial difficulty. To complicate matters further, in Indiana v. Edwards (2008) the Supreme Court claimed that disorganized thinking, deficits in concentration and attention, impaired expression, anxiety, and other symptoms of mental disability and distress can impair the expanded role required for self-representation even if the individual is competent. Without counsel, immigration judges cannot reject the removal of individuals who were adjudicated incompetent because the system cannot ensure a request for a competency hearing (Leitner Center 2010). Precedents and regulatory frameworks do not adequately provide guidance about procedural safeguards for mentally ill immigrants and asylum seekers, and a model for competency needs to be created. Relying on a judge to identify symptoms is also dubious because "a separation of roles between the medical expert and the immigration judge is not only proper but essential in the determination of asylum claims and the maintenance of a regime which ensures international protection for torture survivors who require it (Jones 2004)."

14.2.3 Forensic Mental Health Specialists

Issues surrounding forensic mental health are closely tied with competency evaluations, but in immigration court specifically, forensic evaluations can serve several additional purposes. There is a large base of research on the expanding role of mental health experts in asylum cases as cultural competence is necessary in assessing credibility, especially in cases where discrepancies in memory are present. They often need to corroborate symptoms of PTSD, anxiety, and depression potentially related to trauma or torture while noting possible reasons for inconsistencies (De Jesus-Rentas 2010). Various ethical issues in forensic psychiatry in terms of the immigration system include language barriers, countertransference, and ignorance regarding ethnicity. The misuse of ethnic knowledge is also a concern. Forensic evaluation in immigration proceedings can also pose as a challenge as testimony may be required about not only the client, but their family, community, and culture as a result of the provision concerning deportation resulting in extreme and unusual hardship for others, and thus the field is much broader than normal forensic psychology (Frumkin 1995). Required expertise of evaluators is expanded as they may have to estimate the mental health effects of repatriation.

Forensic psychiatrists thus have an increasingly vital role in ensuring due process for asylum seekers with mental disability despite the increasing complexity of their role as conceptions of PTSD are contested. Asylum officers' interviews last on average no more than one hour, and it is often the deciding factor in determining credibility in court.

There is an inherent tension for forensic mental health specialists between professionalism and advocacy, the duty to care and the duty to act within the standards of regulation. Pourgourides (2006) also describes the struggle to "refrain from perpetuating the assumption that people respond to hardship with psychopathology." However, a duty exists because "their understanding of the psychosocial context of the refugee experience puts them in a unique position to speak out for a group of people who are otherwise denied a voice" (Pourgourides 2006).

Meffert (2010) explores in great detail the necessity of mental health professionals in asylum processing. Their expertise in refugee trauma can make a vital contribution as they provide diagnostic information and evaluate how culture and mental health symptoms relate to a perceived lack of credibility, though taking care not to foster stereotypes and further stigmatization by employing cultural formulations. However, Meffert claims that "culture plays an important role in any forensic psychiatric evaluation, but it is critical in the evaluation of an asylum applicant." They can define potential treatment needs for asylum seekers and help immigration attorneys improve their ability to elicit trauma narratives safely and efficiently if there is representation.

Standards of forensic evaluation should be evidence based, but what evidence base actually exists regarding specifically PTSD, particularly relevant for asylum seekers, is controversial. There is great variability in studies researching rates of PTSD in refugee populations (Watters 2001). Some studies show PTSD at rates greater than 40 % in refugees (Miller 1999). Turner & Herlihy (2009) urge researchers to be careful with evidence of self reported studies of prevalence of PTSD but maintain that there is increasing epidemiological evidence of the disorder across cultures. A focus on PTSD could potentially be the best way to mobilize resources for treatment and services or could portray refugees as passive victims. Bourassa (2009) describes how PTSD became the main lens through which clinical workers began to see forced migrants and led to overuse and misuse of the diagnosis. Making appropriate diagnoses of PTSD is becoming increasingly vital (Zonana 2010).

Most problematic, however, is the ethical issue of performing a forensic examination of a client without counsel. This ethical quandary exists for psychiatrists, psychologists, public health workers, and to some extent social workers. It is "prohibited for a forensic psychiatrist to examine a person charged with a crime before that person has appointed or retained counsel" (Sadoff 2011). Guidelines from The American Academy of Psychiatry and the Law, a branch of the American Psychiatric Association (through which all psychiatrists are ethically bound) claims that

> absent a court order, psychiatrists should not perform forensic evaluations for the prosecution or the government on persons who have not consulted with legal counsel when such persons are known to be charged with criminal acts, under investigation for criminal or quasi-criminal conduct, held in government custody or detention, or being interrogated for criminal or quasi-criminal conduct, hostile acts against a government, or immigrant violations (AAPL 2008).

Guidelines from 1991 address the issue more explicitly. "Forensic psychologists do not provide professional forensic services to a defendant or any party in, or in contemplation of, a legal proceeding prior to that individual's representation by counsel, except for persons judicially determined, where appropriate, to be handling their representations pro se (AAPL 1991)." Because the 2008 guidelines do not anticipate levels on non-representation present in immigration court, the 1991 guidelines are relevant as well. Lack of appointed counsel creates arbitrary injustice if forensic psychologists cannot play their vital role in immigration court.

14.3 Multi Professional Court Based Interventions

Various pilot programs in the immigration system, implemented in the criminal justice system, or executed in other jurisdictions could give insight into what kinds of programs are needed to ensure due process and increase speedy resolution of asylum cases. This is necessary in order to fulfill the dual role needed in the immigration system–creating a more just system for asylum seekers with mental illness and aiding in fostering resilience for those who do not. Not all barriers to resilience and mental health reside within the legal system, but because the gateway to integration is through court and detention, and currently encapsulates so many of the problems in this context, it is a natural and effective locus of broad and systemic intervention. Through what the WHO calls "consolidation of expertise," incorporating aspects from mental health courts, mental health liaison programs, and alternatives to detention, a multi professional court based intervention should be created consisting of social workers, psychologists, and liaisons promoting access to services. These programs will not negate the need for legally binding standards in court and detention but presupposes policy changes remedying injustice and due process violation. As one government attorney stated, "The person doesn't just need an attorney; they need a plan for managing their care and also addressing any related issues (Human Rights Watch 2010, p. 57)."

The roles of mental health professionals need not be entirely distinct in order to create a holistic approach to resilience. Watter (2001) discusses integrating physical, psychological, and social services into a macro level analysis of care. Turner and Herlihy (2009) also advocate for a multiprofessional approach including social, physical, emotional, and legal frameworks. Because integration often relies so heavily upon legality in the U.S., this analysis and its solution needs to rest there. Watters advocates for this to take place at the institutional/policy level, service level, and treatment level. These multiprofessional court based interventions can address all three levels, necessary because of the complex associations between families, society, and pathways for mental illness risk and protective factors (Fazel et al. 2011). Similarly, Feldman (2006) claims a system that addresses the health needs of refugees would incorporate gateway services, core services, and ancillary services. Implicit is the idea that an effective and comprehensive public health system is needed to adequately create a targeted health movement that the law can facilitate.

In a study of asylum seekers in Montreal by Rousseau et al. (2001), it was found that bonds created with community organizations alleviated pain and stress from family separation, even though the psychological influence of family separation was more similar across refugee populations than the effects of trauma. Expanding upon this research, Steinglass (2001) uses it as evidence that asylum seeking is not only an experience of individual trauma but as a familial and community experience. This is further evidence that an ecological model of community psychology (Miller 1999) rather than a clinical model can better equip asylum seekers to deal with exile related stressors. Miller (1999) asserts that the two main factors that limit the use of mental health services for refugees are exile related stressors and refugees failing to seek the services. Thus, a multiprofessional model based in the court system within which an asylum seeker must participate can alleviate exile related stressors that also lay outside of its legal purview. In addition, the dual purpose of the programs resting in the legal system, to address mental illness without medicalizing or over-pathologizing refugees while fostering resilience, is achieved as psychiatric services are not negated but also not placed at the center of the intervention strategy.

Pourgourides (2006) advocates for the creation of multidisciplinary expert teams dedicated to working with asylum seekers but worries this will increase the risk of service fragmentation and marginalization as opposed to strengthening the mainstream mental health system. Access to the mainstream system decreases because of the confused nature of the asylum process, lack of knowledge about eligibility, and stigma toward mental health issues. However, these programs can be used to strengthen the broader system by generating evidence of efficacy and promoting social justice. Incorporating mental health professionals including forensic psychiatrists and increased access to mental health services does not only create policy emphasizing individual assessment and clinical approaches but also make community development and systemic change possible.

Mental health courts are relevant for several reasons. At the center of their development and success is the collaboration between the criminal justice system, mental health system, substance abuse system, and other related systems (BJA 2008). They incorporate the kind of systemic perspective needed to improve response to mental illness in the immigration system. Human Rights Watch (2010) recommends a separate docket for mentally disabled immigrants with a trained judge, a model more similar to juvenile courts. However, though these courts have been found to increase defendants' access to services, they have little control over the actual care because of the inadequacy of the mental health system in general (Boothroyd 2005). There is also the issue of how such immigrants will be identified and moved to a separate docket if self identification is still relied upon. A separate docket should and can be a component of a court intervention in order to remedy the injustice done to mentally disabled immigrants, but it does not holistically foster resilience within the entire vulnerable population.

The concept underlying mental health courts, however, should be employed in this context to asylum seekers general—therapeutic jurisprudence. It is the study of therapeutic and non therapeutic consequences of the law, when law is regarded as a social force that produces behaviors and consequences (Toki 2010). It forces us to ask whether the law can be applied in a more therapeutic way while preserving due process. Described as "the use of social science to study the extent to which a legal rule or practice promotes the psychological and physical well being of the people it affects (Toki 2010)[4]," it can allow the existing legal system to promote the well being of communities and individuals thus allowing refugees to receive needed care.

Programs implemented in the criminal justice system include court liaisons, court consultation programs, forensic clinical coordinators, forensic peer specialists, court clinics, and multi-family psycho education groups for clients of the community mental health service delivery approach known as Assertive Community Treatment (ACT). Again, success of these projects hinges on successful integration of the criminal justice, mental health, and social services systems and the immigration system could benefit from these connections (Grudzinskas 2005). Another component of success is a core position that directly manages the interactions of staff from these different systems (Steadman 1992). Additionally, legal representation is essential for the programs to be ethical and effective in immigration court settings. Court liaisons facilitate resolution of cases, assist community re-entry, provide internal and external case management, and increase alternatives to detention. In a court clinic model in Massachusetts, social workers provide forensic assessments of competency. Judges can make informed decisions via the reports of mental health professionals freeing them from assuming an inappropriate role in immigration court, as they are not mental health court judges, thus preserving and enhancing their role as independent fact finder (Grudzinskas 2005). Non-clinicians need psychiatric assistance in making appropriate dispositions (Lamb et al. 1996). This court clinic model could also assist in assessing competency in deportation proceedings (Ochoa et al. 2010), but forensic evaluations are key to all detention and deportation diversion programs (Sirotich 2009).

In California, a liaison based model the Mental Health Court Community Reintegration program was piloted in the immigration system, which linked people to treatment and provided programming on reintegration skills. "Lawyers agreed that having mental health services available in the community was both persuasive to immigration authorities and immigration judges in arguing for release, and meant people were able to reintegrate into their communities and receive treatment" (Human Rights Watch 2010, p. 59). This model of service was effective and incorporated services such as providing housing in response to immigration judges and officials' concerns regarding detainee release. Survivors of Torture, International, based in California as well, provides psychological counsel and services to individuals coming out of detention. Their executive director stated that "it's a huge relief for attorneys to have case management services available when people are released. There hasn't been a model to pull together the mental health and legal communities before (Human Rights Watch 2010, p. 59)."

ICE's budged for fiscal year 2010 included almost $ 70 million for alternatives to detention whereby immigrants can receive greater access to mental health care and

---

[4] From C. Slobogin, Therapeutic Jurisprudence: Five dilemmas to Ponder, Psychol., Pol and Law 193, 196 (1995).

avoid inappropriate detention or deportation (Ochoa et al. 2010). Continuous increase in this budget and support for these services for asylum seekers could generate immense benefit.

14.4 Conclusion

The dearth of research regarding mental health of asylum seekers results in a lack of data that constrains policy development (Ruiz-Casares et al. 2009). Research from Canada, the UK, Australia, and European countries must be built upon in order to integrate mental health programs and policy into the distinctive U.S. immigration and justice systems. A stronger research base is necessary for implementing large scale change to allow for individual mental health assessment of asylum seekers in the legal system. Policies and programs should serve to improve and integrate mental health services into the legal system without medicalizing the refugee process and undermining resilience. Legal standards for asylum seekers with mental illness are paramount alongside services focused on fostering mental health through recognition of post migration stressors. The immigration justice system is teeming with unnecessary post migration stressors; it is not only contributing to exacerbated mental illness but also foregoing its responsibility to foster resilience and mental health.

Care can be integrated into law and policy in a way that requires some clinical approaches but is conducive for fostering community based programs as well. For clinicians, the struggle to refrain from perpetuating the assumption that people respond to hardship with psychopathology is evident (Pourgourides 2006). There is concern over pigeonholing refugees into a value ridden PTSD diagnosis and fitting their testimony into biomedical models where the only important parts are the ones that are clinically significant as opposed to forming services that provide opportunities for refugees to identify what they need from mental health care (Watters 2001).

While it would be helpful for medical, psychology, and public health organizations to clarify their ethical guidelines in order to respond to mental health challenges in immigration court and detention and to advocate for effective reforms for mental health care in this system, the immigration and justice systems bear particular responsibility for insuring due process and human rights for the mentally ill. Their effort needs to be built upon evidence based psychology regarding forensic evaluation, specifically PTSD and the impacts of post migration stress and trauma on mental health. Professional medical organizations are accountable for not only appropriate ethical guidelines but the training and dissemination of information regarding services (Pourgourides 2006). Rousseau et al. (2008) describes how European pediatricians advocated for the application of UN convention to immigrant and refugee children while Swedish pediatricians defied state policy to exclude asylum seeking children from medical care. In Sweden, this resulted in the creation of a state sponsored health program for refugee children. The Transcultural Centre of the County of Stockholm published guidelines for the psychiatric treatment of asylum seekers specifically. Macro advocacy was undertaken in the UK and the Netherlands via the Breathing Space project and the Pharos School program and serve as examples of how the problem of providing care to asylum seekers spurred innovation as opposed to perpetuating a fractured system (Watters and Ingleby 2004).

Public health organizations and legal and mental health professionals need to advocate for multi-professional court based interventions, more individual assessment of asylum seekers and their specific needs, and social justice in a system where neglect and disconnectedness are leading to extremely negative mental health outcomes. As of now, "health professionals are therefore in the unenviable position of having to compensate for the consequences of policies that can be seriously detrimental to their patients' health and over which they have no control (Feldman 2006)." All health professionals need to assume responsibility for this public health problem and integrate the necessity for care and standards into the immigration justice system. The lack of appointed counsel for refugees, immigrants and asylum seekers is a particularly significant deterrent to the feasibility and success of mental health programs.

References

American Academy of Psychiatry and the Law. (2005). Ethics guidelines for the practice of forensic psychiatry.

Appleseed, Texas Appleseed, & Chicago Appleseed. (2011). Improving efficiency and ensuring justice in the immigration court system. Committee on the Judiciary, United States Senate.

Barr, H. (2001). Mental health courts: An advocate's perspective. Urban Justice Center. http://www.urbanjustice.org/publications/pdfs/mentalhealth/MentalHealthCourts.pdf. Accessed 27 Aug 2004.

Bhugra, D. (2004). Migration and mental health. *Acta Psychiatrica Scandinavica, 109*(4), 243–258.

Boothroyd, R. A., Mercado, C. C., Poythress, N. G., Christy, A., & Petrila, J. (2005). Clinical outcomes of defendants in mental health court. *Psychiatric Services, 56*(7), 829.

Bosworth, M., & Kaufman, E. (2011). Foreigners in a carceral age: Immigration and imprisonment in the US. Stanford Law & Policy Review, Vol. 22, no. 1, 2011, Oxford Legal Studies Research Paper no.34/2011.

Bourassa, J. (2009). Psychosocial interventions and mass populations. *International Social Work, 52*(6), 743.

Carswell, K., Blackburn, P., & Barker, C. (2011). The relationship between trauma, post-migration problems and the psychological well-being of refugees and asylum seekers. *International Journal of Social Psychiatry, 57*(2), 107.

Chow, W., Law, S., Andermann, L., Yang, J., Leszcz, M., Wong, J., & Sadavoy, J. (2010). Multi-family psycho-education group for assertive community treatment clients and families of culturally diverse background: A pilot study. *Community Mental Health Journal, 46*(4), 364–371.

Committee on Ethical Guidelines for Forensic Psychologists. (1991). Specialty guidelines for forensic psychologists. American Psychological Association, division 41.

Crock-Carsey, Sherri. (2006). Mental Health Court Liaison, Athens County Municipal Court Substance Abusing/Mentally Ill Court. Interview with Carolyn Turgeon, Center for Court Innovation.

De Jesus-Rentas, G., Boehnlein, J., & Sparr, L. (2010). Central american victims of gang violence as asylum seekers: The role of the forensic expert. *Journal of the American Academy of Psychiatry and the Law Online, 38*(4), 490.

Denckla, D., & Berman, G. (2001). *Rethinking the revolving door: A look at the mental health courts*. New York: Center for Court Innovation.

Fazel, M., & Stein, A. (2002). The mental health of refugee children. *Archives of Disease in Childhood, 87*(5), 366.

Fazel, M., & Stein, A. (2003). Mental health of refugee children: Comparative study. *BMJ, 327*(7407), 134.

Fazel, M., Reed, R. V., Panter-Brick, C., & Stein, A. (2011). Mental health of displaced and refugee children resettled in high-income countries: Risk and protective Factors. *The Lancet, 379*(9812), 266–282.

Feldman, R. (2006). Primary health care for refugees and asylum seekers: A review of the literature and a framework for services. *Public health 120*(9), 809–816.

Finkle, M. J., Kurth, R., Cadle, C., & Mullan J. (2009). Competency courts: A creative solution for restoring competency to the competency process. *Behavioral Sciences & the Law, 27*(5), 767–786.

Fisher, W. H., Packer, I. K., Grisso, T., McDermeit, M., & Brown, J. M. (2000). From case management to court clinic: Examining forensic system involvement of persons with severe mental illness. *Mental Health Services Research, 2*(1), 41–49.

Frumkin, I. B., & Friedland, J. (1995). Forensic evaluations in immigration cases: Evolving issues. *Behavioral Sciences & the Law, 13*(4), 477–489.

Georgetown Law Human Rights Institute. Sent 'Home' with nothing: The deportation of Jamaicans with mental disabilities. (2011). *Global health watch, the global health landscape, in global health watch 2* (pp. 210–223). London: Zed Books.

Grove, N. J., & Zwi, A. B. (2006). Our health and theirs: Forced migration, othering, and public health. *Social Science & Medicine, 62*(8), 1931–1942.

Grudzinskas, A. J.,Jr, Clayfield, J. C., Roy-Bujnowski, K., Fisher, W. H., & Richardson, M. H. (2005). Integrating the criminal justice system into mental health service delivery: The worcester diversion experience. *Behavioral Sciences & the Law, 23*(2), 277–293.

Hagan, J., & Phillips, S. (2008). Border blunders: The unanticipated human and economic costs of the US approach to immigration control, 1986-2007. *Criminology & Public Policy, 7*(1), 83–94.

Hagan, J., Eschbach, K., & Rodriguez, N. (2008). US deportation policy, family separation, and circular migration. *International Migration Review, 42*(1), 64-88, 1813–1820.

Hagan, J., Castro, B., & Rodriguez, N. (2010). The effects of US deportation policies on immigrant families and communities: Cross-border perspectives. *NCL REV, 88*, 1799–1823.

Hannaford-Agor, P., & Mott, N. (2003). Research on self-represented litigation: Preliminary results and methodological considerations. *Justice System Journal, 24*, 163.

Harlow, M. C., & LeBourgeois III, H. W. (2007). Competency hearings for aliens during deportation proceedings. *Journal of the American Academy of Psychiatry and the Law Online, 35*(4), 530.

Herinckx, H. A., Swart, S. C., Ama, S. M., Dolezal, C. D., & King, S. (2005). Rearrest and linkage to mental health services among clients of the clark county mental health court program. *Psychiatric Services, 56*(7), 853.

Hing, B. O. (2010). Systemic failure: Mental illness, detention, and deportation. *UC Davis Journal of Immigration Law and Policy*.

Human Rights Watch & American Civil Liberties Union. (2010). Deportation by default: Mental disability, unfair hearings, and indefinite detention in the US immigration system.

Jones, D. R., & Smith, S. V. (2004). Medical evidence in asylum and human rights appeals. *International Journal of Refugee Law, 16*, 381–410.

Judge David L. Bazelon Center for Mental Health Law. The role of mental health courts in system reform. Civil Rights and Human Dignity.

Judicial Council of California, Administrative Office of the Courts. (2011). Task force for criminal justice collaboration on mental health issues: Final report. Report to the Judicial Council.

Katzmann, R. A. (2008). Legal profession and the unmet needs of the immigrant poor. *The Georgetown Journal of Legal Ethics, 21*, 3.

Kerwin, D. (2005). Revisiting the need for appointed counsel. *Insight*.

Lamb, H. R., Weinberger, L. E., & Reston-Parham, C. (1996). Court intervention to address the mental health needs of mentally ill offenders. *Psychiatric Services*.

Legal Action Center, American Immigration Council. (2011). Immigrants with Mental Disabilities in Removal Proceedings, Latest Developments and Additional Resources. http://www.legalactioncenter.org/clearinghouse/litigation-issue-pages/immigrants-mental-disabilities-removal-proceedings.

Lustig, S. L., Delucchi, K., Tennakoon, L., & Kaul, B. (2008). Burnout and stress among united states immigration judges. *Annual Reviews, 12*, 14.

Mautino, Kathrin S. (2004). Mental competence in the context of immigration proceedings. *Journal of Immigrant Health, 6*(1), 1–3.

Meffert, S. M., Musalo, K., McNiel, D. E., & Binder, (2010). The role of mental health professionals in political asylum processing. *Journal of the American Academy of Psychiatry and the Law Online, 38*(4), 479.

Miller, K. E. (1999). Rethinking a familiar model: Psychotherapy and the mental health of refugees. *Journal of Contemporary Psychotherapy, 29*(4), 283–306.

Mukhopadhyay, R. (2009). Death in detention: Medical and mental health consequences of indefinite detention of immigrants in the united states. *Seattle Journal of Social Justice, 7*, 693–736.

National Immigration Forum. (2011). Immigrants behind bars: How, why, and how much? Washington D.C.

National Organization of Forensic Social Work. (1987). Code of Ethics. www.nofsw.org.

Pitsker, N. (2007). Due process for all: Applying eldridge to require appointed counsel for asylum seekers. *California Law Review, 95*(1), 169–198.

Post Deportation Human Rights Project. (2008–2009). Keeping families connected: Annual Report. Boston College: Center for Human Rights & International Justice.

Post Deportation Human Rights Project. (2009–2010). *Annual report*. Boston College: Center for Human Rights and International Justice.

Pourgourides, C. (2006). Dilemmas in the Treatment of Asylum Seekers. *Psychiatry, 6*(2), 56–58.

Ochoa, K. C., Pleasants, G. L., Penn, J. V., & Stone, D. C. (2010). Disparities in justice and care: Persons with severe mental illnesses in the US immigration detention system. *Journal of the American Academy of Psychiatry and the Law Online, 38*(3), 392.

Office of Inspector General. (2011). Management of mental health cases in immigration detention. Washington D.C.: Department of Homeland Security.

Packer, Travis, Esq. (2010). Non-Citizens with Mental Disabilities: The need for better care in detention and in court.

Priest, D, & Goldstein, A. (2008). Suicides point to gaps in treatment. The Washington Post. http://www.washingtonpost.com/wp-srv/nation/specials/immigration/cwc_d3p1.html Accessed May 2008.

Ramji-Nogales, J., Schoenholtz, A. I., & Schrag, P. G. (2007). Refugee roulette: Disparities in asylum adjudication. *Stanford Law Review, 60*(2), 295.

Robjant, K., Robbins, I., & Senior, V. (2009). Psychological distress amongst immigration detainees: A cross-sectional questionnaire study. *British Journal of Clinical Psychology, 48*(3), 275–286.

Robjant, K., Hassan, R., & Katona, C. (2009). Mental health implications of detaining asylum seekers: Systematic review. *The British Journal of Psychiatry, 194*(4), 306.

Rousseau, C., Mekki-Berrada, A., & Moreau, S. (2001). Trauma and extended separation from family among Latin American and African refugees in Montreal. *Psychiatry: Interpersonal & Biological Processes, 64*(1), 40–59.

Rousseau, C., Key, F., & Measham, T. (2005). The work of culture in the treatment of psychosis in migrant adolescents. *Clinical child psychology and psychiatry, 10*(3), 305.

Rousseau, C., Ter Kuile, S., Munoz, M., Nadeau, L., Ouimet, M. J., Kirmayer, L., & Crépeau, F. (2008). Health care access for refugees and immigrants with precarious status: Public health and human right challenges. *Canadian Journal of Public Health, 99*(4), 290–292.

Ruiz-Casares, M., Rousseau, C., Derluyn, I., Watters, C., & Crépeau, F. (2009). Right and access to healthcare for undocumented children: Addressing the gap between international conventions and disparate implementations in North America and Europe. *Social Science & Medicine, 70*(2), 329–336.

Sadoff, R. L. (2011). *Ethical issues in forensic psychiatry: Minimizing harm.* Wiley-Blackwell.

Sheikh, M., MacIntyre, C. R., & Perera, S. (2008). Preventive detention: The ethical ground where politics and health meet focus on asylum seekers in Australia. *Journal of Epidemiology and Community Health, 62*(6), 480.

Sirotich, F. (2009). The criminal justice outcomes of jail diversion programs for persons with mental illness: A review of the evidence. *Journal of the American Academy of Psychiatry and the Law Online, 37*(4), 461.

Sly, K. A., Sharples, J., Lewin, T. J., & Bench, C. J. (2009). Court outcomes for clients referred to a community mental health court liaison service. *International Journal of Law and Psychiatry, 32*(2), 92–100.

Steadman, H. J. (1992). Boundary spanners: A key component for the effective interactions of the justice and mental health systems. *Law and Human Behavior, 16*(1), 75–87.

Steadman, H. J., Davidson, S., & Brown, C. (2001). Law & psychiatry: Mental health courts: Their promise and unanswered questions. *Psychiatric Services, 52*(4), 457.

Steele, Z., Silove, D., Brooks, R., Momartin, S., Alzuhairi, B., & Susljik, I. (2006). Impact of immigration detention and temporary protection on the mental health of refugees. *The British Journal of Psychiatry, 188*(1), 58.

Steinglass, P. (2001). Forced relocation: A family researcher/clinician's perspective. *Psychiatry: Interpersonal & Biological Processes, 64*(1), 64–68.

Strijk, P. J. M., Van Meijel, B., & Gamel, C. (2010). J. Health and Social Needs of Traumatized Refugees and Asylum Seekers: An Exploratory Study. *Perspectives in Psychiatric Care.*

Texas Appleseed. (2010). *Justice for immigration's hidden population: Protecting the rights of persons with mental disabilities in the immigration court and detention system.* Austin, TX.

Toki, V. (2010). Therapeutic jurisprudence and mental health courts for maori. *International Journal of Law and Psychiatry.*

Tribe, R. (2002). Mental health of refugees and asylum-seekers. *Advances in psychiatric treatment, 8*(4), 240.

Tsankov M. E. (2007). Incompetent respondents in removal proceedings. Immigration Law Advisor, U.S. Department of Justice, Executive Office for Immigration Review, 3:1, 2009. http://www.justice.gov/eoir/vll/ILA-Newsleter/ILA%202009/vol3no4. pdf. Accessed 15 Feb 2010.

Turner, S. W., & Herlihy, J. (2009). Working with refugees and asylum seekers. *Psychiatry, Specific Populations, 8*(8), 322–324.

Walter Leitner International Human Rights Clinic. (2010). Removing refugees: U.S. deportation policy and the Cambodian-American community. Leitner Center for International Law and Justice, Fordham Law School, New York City.

Watters, C. (2001). Emerging paradigms in the mental health care of refugees. *Social Science & Medicine, 52*(11), 1709–1718.

Watters, C., & Ingleby, D. (2004). Locations of care: Meeting the mental health and social care needs of refugees in Europe. *International Journal of Law and Psychiatry, 27*(6), 549–570.

Weiskopf Consulting Services. (2000). Draft forensic mental health standards and guidelines. Presented to The New York State Conference of Local Mental Hygiene Directors.

World Health Organization. (2010). *How health systems can address health inequalities linked to migration and ethnicity.* Copenhagen: WHO Regional Office for Europe.

Zimerman, N., & Tyler, T. R. (2010). Between access to counsel and access to justice: A psychological perspective. *Fordham Urban Law Journal, 37*, 473–507.

Zonana, Howard MD. (2010). Commentar: The role of forensic psychiatry in the asylum process. *Journal of the American Academy of Psychiatry and the Law, 38*, 499–501.

Manufactured by Amazon.ca
Bolton, ON